ISOLATED ELDERS

Health and Social Intervention

Eloise Rathbone-McCuan
Washington University, St. Louis, Missouri

Joan Hashimi
University of Missouri—St. Louis

AN ASPEN PUBLICATION®
Aspen Systems Corporation
Rockville, Maryland
London
1982

8112960

Library of Congress Cataloging in Publication Data

Rathbone-McCuan, Eloise
Isolated elders.

Includes bibliographies and index.
1. Aged—Services for—United States.
2. Social isolation.
3. Aged—United States—Mental Health.
I. Hashimi, Joan. II. Title [DNLM: 1. Aged.
2. Social isolation—In old age. 3. Health services for
the aged. 4. Social work. WT 30 R234i]
HV146.R37   362.6′042   81-22848
ISBN: 0-89443-676-7   AACR2

Library of Congress Catalog Card Number: 81-22848
ISBN: 0-89443-676-7

Printed in the United States of America

1 2 3 4 5

To all the elders we have known and to whom we never said thank you.

Eloise Rathbone-McCuan

Joan Hashimi

To Dorothy, who loved me as a mother and a friend. To Claude, who explored a relationship with me and thus added a unique richness to my life. To Noche and Samson, who gave their unqualified devotion.

Eloise Rathbone-McCuan

To those in the three generations that are my context: Laura, Audrey, Carole, Rasool, Jamil, Suzanne, and Ali.

Joan Hashimi

Table of Contents

Foreword

Grow old along with me!
The best is yet to be,
The last of life, for which the first was made:
Our times are in His hand
Who saith, "A whole I planned,
Youth shows but half; trust God: see all nor be afraid!"

Robert Browning
from Rabbi Ben Ezra

As depicted by Browning, old age represents the culmination of one's existence, the crowning glory of life. Written 25 years before his own death, Browning encouraged approaching later years with his characteristic sanguine outlook, anticipating a time unencumbered by illness, pain, and loneliness.

Most Americans, of course, have a less idealized view of growing old. *Isolated Elders: Health and Social Intervention* is written for gerontologists, social workers and other health care practitioners realistically confronting the isolation of our nation's elderly. It is significant to note that in detailing the determinants of isolation and outlining possible preventive measures Drs. Rathbone-McCuan and Hashimi rarely, if ever, use the word "lonely." There is no defeatism in these pages. The authors portray problems afflicting nine distinct subgroups of America's elderly and illustrate potential intervention techniques to thwart the development of isolators.

The concept discussed here is isolation which becomes pathological. Caused by salient factors or "isolators" in the lives of the study group members, this state of isolation, if allowed to progress, invariably results in a condition which in itself is a barrier to seeking help.

The great merit in Drs. Rathbone-McCuan and Hashimi's work is found in the presentation of a generalized framework contributing to isolation in later life. They have then applied this model to the study subgroups, reflecting the heterogeneity of the elderly population, in order to demonstrate the variations in economic, social, psychological, and physiological factors which can predispose elderly members of these groups to isolation. Rather than presenting panaceas, the authors graphically portray the plight of the elderly through their very real "case studies" and suggest planning and service delivery methods of coping with these problems.

Drs. Rathbone-McCuan and Hashimi's work will be a valuable guidebook to health care practitioners in the trenches, working directly with the elderly, an ever-increasing percentage of America's population due to recent medical advances. *Isolated Elders* is a timely, welcome, and instructive addition to the field of health care of the elderly.

Jacob A. Brody, M.D.
Associate Director for Epidemiology, Demography, and Biometry Program
National Institute on Aging

Preface

In 1976, the authors became involved with the development of the St. Louis Council on Mental Health and Aging, under the sponsorship of the Greater St. Louis Mental Health Association. As educators and practitioners interested in mental health and gerontology, we felt that it was important for the elderly, their advocates, and the professionals who served them to have a forum for resources and planning. As we surveyed the community for resources and unmet needs, the problem of isolation kept reappearing as a major concern among practitioners and the aged. Many agencies considered that they provided services to prevent isolation but felt they often were unable to reach the elderly who were most isolated.

The planning and service delivery experiences of several members of the council provided a base for a published article titled "Counseling the Isolated Elderly." That article produced an invitation from Aspen Systems Corporation to write a book on intervention with the isolated elderly that could provide guidelines for health and social service practitioners.

We began conceptualizing the book and planning the field research with blind optimism. Initially we believed we could provide, for every elderly subgroup, concrete strategies for isolation intervention and prevention services. Little did we know that isolation as both a social problem and social phenomenon would prove to be the most complex and diversified issue for which social services to the elderly are planned and provided.

The field research in the early stages affirmed our suspicion that practitioners had many definitions of isolation and the isolated elderly. Isolation was perceived to be present in all of the various target populations of elderly served by a cross section of health, social, and mental health professionals. We have attempted to write an analysis of the major factors that contribute to the isolation of these diverse subgroups and suggest alternative approaches that may help to prevent, reduce, or eliminate isolation in its various manifestations.

We are grateful to our colleagues and the administrators of human service agencies for the amount and quality of information provided in the developmental stages of the book. The identification by title of formal service organizations or incorporated groups corresponds with titles that appear in public documents. Though based on actual interviews and clinical work, the names and personal characteristics of all individuals described in the case illustrations throughout the text were slightly modified in order to maintain confidentiality.

Eloise Rathbone-McCuan, Ph.D.
Washington University in St. Louis

Joan Hashimi, Ph.D.
University of Missouri-St. Louis
April 1982

Acknowledgments

Numerous persons have contributed their ideas, time, and energy to the preparation of this book. Without the input of practitioners, elderly persons, and their families, the depth of our understanding would have lacked the sensitivity we sought to introduce in the description and analysis. Caroline Wilner offered much of herself and her thinking throughout the two years and encouraged us to write about the interpersonal and intrapersonal experiences of women as they survive to be old. The perspective for analyzing the status of older veterans relied on Charles Nieberding, who facilitated many aspects of our data collection and service description. Betty Finch supplied much information about the rural elderly and shared, in detail, her medical social work experiences.

Literature, intervention strategies, and community expertise on the black elderly were provided by Barbara Crousby. Countless hours of assistance were provided by Louise Larrabure, who offered important content and perspective on the Hispanic elderly. Ann Travis shared most generously with us throughout her clinical field training in adult protective services. More than anyone else, Carl Bretcher gave an important perspective on the realities of individuals and families who have to live with the inevitable consequences of Alzheimer's disease.

We have worked with these people in an atmosphere of respect and affection. Our gratitude is extended to Claude Walter, Robert Smith, John Young, and Mary Randlett for their willingness to read and comment.

We are grateful for the financial assistance awarded for this project from the Gerontology Program at the University of Missouri-St. Louis. The supportive encouragement and feedback from Curtis Whitesel, our editor, has been very important in all phases of the project. He helped us sustain our effort to write a meaningful manuscript. The two years of technical assistance from Keith Morton at The George Warren Brown School of Social Work was of the highest quality. We also appreciate the additional assistance from Debbie Stotler of the University of Missouri-St. Louis. As authors, we were fortunate to have Camille Claymon, Linda Withers-Borth, and Ricky Fortune as special friends and colleagues.

Chapter 1

Introduction

The purpose of this book is to provide practitioners with a framework for thinking about isolation and the elderly. Three objectives served as guides: (1) to expand the conceptualization beyond the scope of social isolation into a more holistic framework, (2) to apply this conceptual framework in an analysis of nine subgroups within the elderly population frequently defined as isolated and receiving isolation-related interventions, and (3) to identify some areas of need for future professional training and research necessary to develop intervention and prevention approaches.

Isolation among the elderly has been described as a social problem, but practitioner understanding of it is tangled by fiction and fact. Social scientists and practitioners have provided numerous and varied definitions. On the one hand, this proliferation creates incomplete and unclear conceptual definitions. On the other hand, the conceptual definitions imply human need that legitimates isolation as a reason for intervention. An increasing amount of recent empirical research and practice information indicates that the elderly as a population group are not isolated. Therefore, unsupported generalizations about isolation may be contributing to yet another myth about the elderly—the myth of isolation.

Forty years ago a leading social theorist singled out isolation as a characteristic of the elderly in middle and upper middle class urban society (Parsons, 1942). Isolation research, loosely defined, was occurring before gerontology became a specialized social science and a professional specialty. It was undertaken by sociologists, psychiatrists, psychoanalysts, and others, but rarely in collaboration. Concepts of alienation (Seeman, 1959; Dean, 1961), anomie (Durkheim, 1897/ 1951), and normlessness (DeGrazia, 1948; Horney, 1949) were introduced as descriptions of human experience. The definitions of these other concepts often overlapped with descriptions of isolation. The research on the social and psychological aspects of aging in the late 1950s and early 1960s contributed more to the conceptual confusion about isolation among social gerontologists.

1

The social disengagement theory as an explanation for the social and psycho-logical aspects of the aging process (Cummings & Henry, 1961) rapidly permeated the thinking on the elderly and their interpersonal relationships. Clinical practice theorists were quick to make their permutations of intrapersonal factors based on the social disengagement theory. When the theory became widely discredited, the confusion over isolation among the elderly lingered. However, the importance of clarifying intrapersonal and interpersonal factors in the lives of the elderly was noted by Townsend, a pioneering research gerontologist. He encouraged others to make a consistent distinction between objective circumstances and subjective status—between isolation and loneliness (Townsend, 1957).

In developing the conceptual framework for this book, it was possible to build on others' work on social isolation. Much of the most meaningful research and conceptual material on social isolation was the work of Lowenthal and Bennett. Both of these women have made important contributions to the pursuit of under-standing about social isolation through empirical research and conceptualization. Some components of their work are summarized in this chapter.

Lowenthal (1964, 1968, 1975, 1976; Lowenthal, Berkman, & Associates, 1967; Lowenthal & Boler, 1965; Lowenthal & Haven, 1968; Lowenthal & Robinson, 1976; Lowenthal, Thurnher & Chirriboga, and Associates, 1975) began her exploration of isolation, mental illness, and old age on two groups of elderly. One group was composed of 534 persons 60 years and over from the psychiatric wards of San Francisco General Hospital; the other was a sample of 600 persons, 60 and older, drawn from 18 census tracts in San Francisco. The results indicated that extreme lifelong isolation was not necessarily conducive to mental illness in old age and that relative isolation might be more of a consequence than a cause. Analysis of the case histories for both groups provided a base to develop a preliminary typology of patterns of isolation that varied in degree and kind (1964).

A second study published a year later (1965) examined differences within the group drawn from the psychiatric wards. It focused on a comparison of four subgroups formed on the degree of isolation and the type of psychiatric disorder. Lowenthal examined psychological problems in earlier life among the four sub-groups and again concluded that isolation was a consequence rather than a cause of mental illness in old age. Her subsequent research began to focus on life course, adult life stage adaptation, and social interaction and intimacy patterns. Most recently she developed several frameworks that are very useful in looking at the social and psychological factors that may influence states of isolation/involvement from social networks among adults, without psychiatric problems, as they age (Lowenthal, 1968, 1975; Lowenthal, Berkman, et al., 1967; Lowenthal & Haven, 1968; Lowenthal, Thurnher, et al., 1975).

Lowenthal pointed to the need to refine the concept of isolation and suggested two dimensions that had been neglected:

1. The "rhythm of isolation" concept is intriguing because it suggests that personal patterns of fluctuation in social involvement may be established in earlier stages of the life course and may maintain considerable stability in later life.
2. The "relativity of isolation" concept suggests that individuals might evaluate their own status through a cognitive and comparative evaluation between their circumstances and those of their peers (Lowenthal, 1976).

She also proposed a framework for examining patterns of isolation/involvement in relation to commitment areas that involve interpersonal, moral, self-expressive, and self-protection/survival that have varying degrees of importance as men and women move through the aging process (Lowenthal & Robinson, 1976).

Bennett and her colleagues at Columbia University in a recent book (1980) report on the development of their research over 20 years. That text and other publications by Bennett describe their social isolation research (1973a, 1973b; Bennett & Nahemow, 1961, 1965a, 1965b, 1972). The studies were conducted on samples of elderly in different settings. These findings pointed to the importance of environments and social interaction in relation to social isolation.

The first measures she developed provided a tool for assessing social isolation from an interpersonal dimension. Additional measures on the subjective/intrapersonal dimensions have been produced and validated. These have been applied in clinical research studies where isolation has been identified in samples of elderly; those who were socially isolated received therapies to increase their socialization levels.

The latest phase of her work on social isolation is cross-national. The United States-United Kingdom Cross-National Geriatric Community Study was conducted by collaborating teams at the New York State Psychiatric Institute and the Maudsley Hospital in London. This survey provided the first opportunity to look at how isolation is distributed in random samples of the elderly in New York and London (Bennett, Cook, & Phil, 1980). Bennett in summarizing the status of her research on social isolation states:

> We have found that isolation has a negative impact on the aged; it desocializes them, hampers social adjustment and seems to reduce independence. At the present time, isolation in the aged does not correlate with the usual demographic factors in institutions though we have found that old women in the community are more readily rejected than men when they age. Isolation is not synonymous with mental disorder in the aged though it may result in some behavior patterns associated with mental disorder, specifically poor social adjustment and poor cognitive functioning. If not compensated for in time, the

effects of isolation may lead to serious and possible irreversible cognitive and other impairments. However, unlike senile mental disorder, the effects of isolation may be reversible through resocialization, remotivation, and friendly visiting programs (1980, p. 204).

Shanas (1962, 1979; Shanas, Townsend, Wedderburn, Friis, Milhøj, & Stenhouwer, 1968; Shanas & Sussman, 1977) conducted extensive research on the patterns of interaction between the aged and their families. The results of her national and cross-national research concluded that the aged were not alienated from their families. Other researchers such as Brody, Davis, Fulcomer, and Johnson (1979), Sussman (1965), Rosow (1965, 1967, 1973, 1974), and Streib (1958) all pointed out that the elderly did remain connected to relatives when a family group was available. These findings indicated that both alienation of the aged from the family and social role interactions with its members were more myth than fact.

An important preliminary model of multiple types of isolation among elderly with organic brain syndromes was described (Ernst, Beran, Safford, & Kleinhauz, 1978). Their clinical information identified three types of isolation: emotional, social, and physiological. These types exacerbated patients' deviant behavior. The isolations and increased deviancy assumed a circular pattern that increased the patients' isolation from their environment.

From a summary of selected literature, it was concluded that social isolation conceptualized on the bases of interaction patterns between the aged and family members was not adequate. The Lowenthal and Bennett analyses involving a broader range of social roles and interactions extending beyond the family seemed more useful. Other work suggested either that social isolation might be multidimensional or that, more complex than a single social dimension, there might be several distinct types of isolation. What is known about isolation is insufficient to describe, let alone explain, the diverse and complex range of situations and circumstances faced by those elderly.

Chapter 2 provides a framework for understanding the economic, physical, social, and psychological elements that may arise for older adults in a way that highlights their influence as predisposing factors contributing to isolation in later life. Isolation is conceived of as a multistaged, multidimensional, and cumulative process. This conceptual expansion has implications for intervention. It is necessary to develop more intervention strategies that encompass clinical approaches for individuals, groups, and families, the structures and functions of service programs and community-based organizations, and the focus of social policy. The discussion of intervention as it relates to the expanded conceptualization of isolation is based on a scheme for arranging the service resources typically available in a community. Since the proposed arrangement is complex, skills are specified that isolated elderly clients need to negotiate human services effectively.

The conceptual model in Chapter 2 applies to the general aged population. However, the heterogeneous structure of the aged population is associated with variations in the isolation the elderly encounter in various subgroups. Little information is available to practitioners that analyzes the dimensions and dynamics of isolation from an elderly subgroup perspective. There also are many conceptual and information gaps about interventions appropriate for specific subgroups. Nine subgroups of elderly to which this model has been applied are discussed. Factors that may be important as predisposing to isolation are analyzed for each subgroup. Consideration is given to how these factors (identified as isolators in the model) impact on the isolation process and the types of intervention they require.

Chapter 3 provides an overview of the isolators that impinge on older women as they age. The mental health of older women is an area of major interest to both authors. The isolators that confront these women reflect the consequences of changes in economic, social, psychological, and physiological factors. These changes become enmeshed with larger environmental influences that promote sexism and ageism. In providing intervention to older isolated women, it is of the utmost importance to give in-depth attention to the intrapersonal consequences of age and sex role stereotyping.

The discussion of intervention illustrates the undesired outcomes of counseling in the context of ageist and sexist practitioner attitudes. If counseling produces such negative experiences for older women, it may well push them further into another stage of more serious isolation. The value of self-help groups is emphasized because they offer an alternative to the stigma of seeking assistance in a psychiatric setting, are accessible to older women, and can be available because they are not burdensome financially. The clinical practitioner's potential consulting relationship with self-help groups involving older women is explored.

Chapter 4 analyzes the older male veteran population. It emphasizes the changing structure and characteristics of World War II veterans as compared to those of World War I. The isolation factors considered are not limited to the older individual veteran but are extended into a detailed assessment of the Veterans Administration service system. Nowhere else in this book is it so obvious that the lack of coordination among service systems limits the intervention potential. The practitioners in the VA system are isolated from each other and from their professional counterparts in community-based service organizations. These entities have services that may be of benefit to veterans if coordinated more fully with those of the VA. The chapter presents an integrated picture of isolated veterans in a large and complex service system and what might be done about reducing isolation for the older ones in their role as VA clients.

Chapter 5 presents an in-depth analysis of the elderly in Tolivar, Missouri. Rural isolators are described and efforts are made to capture the diversity of isolation among that small town's elderly. Of particular concern are older persons who retire to a small traditional community without familial roots or community ties. The absence of any resources to which they can connect is alarming. The intervention component considers the expanded role of a rural health clinic as a single organizational model for the delivery of integrated medical, social, and mental health services. As the doctor is the most acceptable source of professional help—sometimes the only source to which the rural elderly will turn—what can be done in the context of physician-connected service is important. Many of the aspects of community organization required to coordinate formal and informal resources also are detailed.

Chapter 6 introduces the problems and situations that produce isolation among the black urban elderly population. It describes problems the very isolated black elderly may face that may differ only in degree from those that impinge on a significant proportion of the black aged population. The suggested intervention centers on coordinated efforts between the black church and other agencies that service the elderly or are in a position to offer resources. The appropriate outreach role for the black church, given its formal organizational structure and the informal networks that characterize congregations and their capacity to help, is assessed.

Chapter 7 analyzes the isolators that confront Spanish-speaking elderly. Three major subgroups of Hispanic elderly (Cubans, Puerto Ricans, and Mexican-Americans) are discussed but the experiences of Mexican-Americans in California are emphasized. Some of the strategies suggested for dealing with isolators of language and cultural differences apply across Hispanic groups. However, the variables associated with the barrio or neighborhood and local community structure influence the design and provision of services to overcome isolators. The plan for intervention described is based on efforts in San Mateo County, California.

Chapter 8 considers the multiple and tragic isolators associated with family caregivers' violence and abuse toward the elderly. The isolators in this context are so overwhelming that at times they can impact on both aged victim and abuser. Interventions range from clinical issues in the management of stress associated with caregiving to the development of statewide reporting procedures, legislation to mandate professional reporting, and a network of crisis resources to reduce the risks to the elder and the burden to the caregiver.

Chapter 9 deals with alcoholism in late life. The isolation associated with alcoholism as a chronic disease or a chemical dependency behavior, the actions of the individual, and the losses associated with aging and alcoholism converge to create a circular pattern. The general invisibility of older alcoholics is analyzed and the rejection they encounter in seeking intervention is described. Older alcoholics who turn to the treatment system often are rebuffed because of their age. Similarly, those who seek involvement in programs for the mainstream senior citizen population are rejected because of their alcohol-related behaviors. The intervention recommendations emphasize the need for the alcoholism treatment specialist to have some knowledge of the aging process and for those who work with the elderly to have some knowledge of the disease of alcoholism and the dynamics of drinking behaviors.

Chapter 10 is an extensive analysis of isolators impacting on the chronic mentally ill grown old. It considers the cumulative impact of isolators related to extended periods of institutionalization or to hospital life styles during earlier life. It describes the isolation of community placement in late life if it occurs without the person's having the skills to manage daily living activities and/or an individual to provide case management. The intervention section offers a detailed guide for the individual's developing self-maintenance skills and how practitioners responsible for their management and advocacy can address the impact of environment isolators.

Chapter 11 looks at Alzheimer's disease (presenile and senile dementia) from the family system perspective, setting forth the isolators encountered by the affected individual and/or the family/primary caregiver. It analyzes how isolation can continue even after families seek medical and psychiatric help to combat the multiple stages of the illness. A caregiver, family unit, and educational approach for home management of the individual is proposed. Specific counseling strategies for working with the primary caregiver are offered. Techniques that may optimize the functional capacity of the individual before institutionalization is required are explored.

Chapter 12 is a brief authors' epilogue. It suggests important research and training issues that emerged from the previous discussions. The research factors emphasize the importance of studies that have direct application for intervention, but few resources may be available in the near future for conducting them. The suggestions for practitioner preparation emphasize the knowledge and skills that would be helpful in encountering clients from the various subgroups. The single most important intervention skill that cuts across all subgroups and their problems of isolation is the assessment of problems before any intervention is introduced.

REFERENCES

Bennett, R. Isolation and isolation-reducing programs. *Bulletin of the New York Academy of Medicine*, 1973a, *49*, 1143-1163.

Bennett, R. Living conditions and everyday needs of the aged with specific reference to social isolation. *Journal of Aging and Human Development*, 1973b, *4*, 179-198.

Bennett, R. (Ed.). *Aging, isolation and resocialization*. New York: Van Nostrand Reinhold Company, 1980.

Bennett, R., Cook, D., & Phil, M. Isolation of the aged in New York City. *Planning for the elderly in New York City: An assessment of depression, dementia and isolation*. New York: Community Council of Greater New York, 1980, pp. 26-42.

Bennett, R., & Nahemow, L. Preadmission isolation as a factor in adjustment to an old age home. In P. Hoch & J. Zubin (Eds.), *Psychopathology of aging*. New York: Grune & Stratton, Inc., 1961, pp. 285-302.

Bennett, R., & Nahemow, L. Institutional totality and criteria of social adjustment in residential settings for the aged. *Journal of Social Issues*, 1965a, *21*, 44-78.

Bennett, R., & Nahemow, L. The relations between social isolation, socialization and adjustment in residents of a home for aged. In M.P. Lawton & F. Lawton (Eds.), *Proceedings of the Institute on the Mentally Impaired Aged*. Philadelphia: Maurice Jacob Press, 1965b, pp. 98-108.

Bennett, R., & Nahemow, L. The relations between social isolation and adjustment in residents of a home for the aged. In D. Kent, P. Kastenbaum, & S. Sherwood (Eds.), *Planning and action for the elderly*. New York: Behavioral Publications, 1972, pp. 501-513.

Brody, E.M., Davis, L.J., Fulcomer, M., & Johnson, P. *Three generations of women: Comparisons of attitudes and preferences for service providers*. Paper presented at 32nd Annual Meeting of the Gerontological Society, Washington, D.C., 1979.

Cummings, E., & Henry, W.E. *Growing old*. New York: Basic Books, 1961.

Dean, D.G. Alienation: Its meaning and measurement. *American Sociological Review*, 1961, *26*, 753-758.

DeGrazia, S. *The political community: A study of anomie*. Chicago: University of Chicago Press, 1948.

Durkheim, E. *Suicide: A study in sociology* (J.A. Spaulding & G. Simpson, trans.). Glencoe, Ill.: The Free Press, 1951 (originally published in Paris: Alcan, 1897).

Ernst, P., Beran, B., Safford, F., & Kleinhauz, M. Isolation and the symptoms of chronic brain syndrome. *Gerontologist*, 1978, *18*, 468-474.

Horney, K. Culture and neurosis in sociological analysis. In L. Wilson & W. Kolg (Eds.), *Sociological analysis: An introductory text and case book*. New York: Harcourt, Brace & Co., 1949, pp. 248-251.

Lowenthal, M.F. Social isolation and mental illness in old age. *American Sociological Review*, 1964, *29*, 54-70.

Lowenthal, M.F. The relationship between social factors and mental health in the aged. In A. Simon & L.J. Epstein (Eds.), *Aging in modern society*, Psychiatric Research Report #23. Washington, D.C.: American Psychiatric Association, 1968.

Lowenthal, M.F. Psychosocial variations across the adult life source: Frontiers for research and policy. *Gerontologist*, 1975, *15*, 6-12.

Lowenthal, M.F. Toward a sociopsychological theory of change in adulthood and old age. In J.E. Birren & K.W. Schaie (Eds.), *Handbook of the psychology of aging*. New York: Van Nostrand Reinhold Company, 1976.

Lowenthal, M.F., Berkman, P.L., & Associates. *Aging and mental disorder in San Francisco*. San Francisco: Jossey-Bass, Inc., 1967.

Lowenthal, M.F., & Boler, D. Voluntary vs. involuntary social withdrawal. *Journal of Gerontology*, 1965, *20*, 363-371.

Lowenthal, M.F., & Haven, C. Interaction and adaptation: Intimacy as a critical variable. *American Sociological Review*, 1968, *33*, 20-30.

Lowenthal, M.F., & Robinson, B. Social networks and isolation. In R.H. Binstock & E. Shanas (Eds.), *Handbook of aging and the social sciences*. New York: Van Nostrand Reinhold Company, 1976.

Lowenthal, M.F., Thurnher, M., & Chirriboga, D., and Associates. *Four stages of life: A comparative study of women and men facing transition*. San Francisco: Jossey-Bass, Inc., 1975.

Parsons, T. Age and sex in the social structure of the United States. *American Sociological Review*, 1942, *7*, 604-616.

Rosow, I. The aged, family and friends. *Social Security Bulletin*, 1965, *28*, 18-20.

Rosow, I. *Social integration of the aged.* New York: The Free Press, 1967.

Rosow, I. The social context of the aging self. *Gerontologist,* 1973, *13,* 82-87.

Rosow, I. *Socialization to old age.* Berkeley, Calif.: University of California Press, 1974.

Seeman, M. On the meaning of alienation. *American Sociological Review,* 1959, *24,* 783-791.

Shanas, E. *The health of older people: A social survey.* Cambridge, Mass.: Harvard University Press, 1962.

Shanas, E. Social myth as hypothesis: The case of the family relations of older people. *Gerontologist,* 1979, *19,* 3-9.

Shanas, E., & Sussman, M.B. Family and bureaucracy: Comparative analysis and problematics. In E. Shanas & M.B. Sussman (Eds.), *Family, bureaucracy and the elderly.* Durham, N.C.: Duke University Press, 1977.

Shanas, E., Townsend, P., Wedderburn, D., Friis, H., Milhøj, P., & Stenhouwer, J. *Old people in three industrial societies.* New York: Atherton and Routledge Kegan Paul, 1968.

Streib, G.F. Family patterns in retirement. *Journal of Social Issues,* 1958, *14,* 46-60.

Sussman, M.B. Relationships of adult children with their parents in the United States. In E. Shanas & G. Streib (Eds.), *Social structure and the family: Generational relations.* Englewood Cliffs, N.J.: Prentice-Hall, Inc., 1965.

Townsend, P. *The family life of old people: An inquiry in East London.* Glencoe, Ill.: The Free Press, 1957.

Chapter 2

An Expanded Conceptualization of Isolation and Intervention

INTRODUCTION

Two of the major reasons for the confusion over the concept of isolation were discussed in Chapter 1 from the standpoint of historical usage in social science and clinical theory and multiple definitions that describe the condition, status, and situation of the elderly population. This confusion contributes to the limitations of assessment procedures and planning and providing comprehensive intervention. Therefore, an expanded conceptualization of isolation was developed that is useful for the identification of isolated individuals and subgroups and the assessment and intervention approaches for isolation-related problems.

This chapter is devoted to a general discussion of that conceptualization. The first section describes isolators, defining them as situations or events that seem to interfere with the ability of an elder to maintain personal integrity and social involvement. Figure 2-1 displays the isolators as they cluster in the biophysical, psychological, economic, and social realms and on the individual or environmental levels. Isolation as experienced by an individual is conceived of as a multistage, cumulative process and is described in the second section (Figure 2-2). Practitioner guidelines are given in the third section and summarized in Table 2-1. The clinician's intervention with the elderly as proposed is a skills-building activity to enhance the isolation-related problem-solving capacity of the elder. The final section sets forth a conceptual rearrangement of formal organizations and informal networks that are available in many communities. Figure 2-3 is an overall presentation of the rearrangement of services generally available to the elderly.

ISOLATORS

A general conceptualization of isolators is useful to enhance understanding of: the range and diversity of isolators prevalent among elderly populations and the impact of isolators, in various combinations, on the lives of older persons. For greater clarity, the isolators are organized along two dimensions. The first dimension dichotomizes them according to whether they originate at the individual or environmental level. The second divides the individual and environmental levels into four quadrants: the biophysical, psychological, social, and economic. These two dimensions generate eight subdivisions of isolators. Examples of isolators within each subdivision are listed in Figure 2-1. There is interaction and interdependence between and among isolators and the conditions, social statuses, and living situations of the elderly. The complexities of these interactions in daily living are described in the analysis of the elderly in the subgroups.

Physical Isolators

A major physical isolator at the individual level is biophysical decline. This is manifested by limitations in physical mobility, sensory losses, diminishing physical vigor and endurance, changes in physical appearance, and symptoms of specific diseases. These factors limit, alter, or prevent individual behavior (e.g., self-maintenance and social participation). Sensory losses influence patterns of daily communication and of information processing. Severe sight or hearing losses may reduce the individual's motivation to utilize opportunities to interact with others or obtain knowledge about resources.

For some people, even a slight sensory loss may create a self-perceived stigma, reinforced by the behavior of others, that reduces motivation for social interaction. Personal reactions to these losses or changes can precipitate a retreat from social opportunities and resource procurement. Progressive cognitive losses associated with organic brain disorders are likely to lessen interaction skills, reducing them to the point where it is impossible to have meaningful interaction with even the most intimate of friends and family.

An important physical isolator at the environmental level is the lack of medical and health care resources. Rehabilitation alternatives for individuals with chronic disorders may not exist. Health care settings may fail to identify and/or address social, emotional, and/or economic needs coexisting and interacting with health problems. The elderly need time with health practitioners to explain their fears and concerns, discuss symptoms, and have clear explanations of their conditions.

The organizational structure of many treatment settings where the elderly receive the greatest proportion of their medical care (e.g., private physician offices) may preclude there being time for gathering information from or providing additional information to the doctor about problems. The limited supply of geriatric specialists in all of the health professions as well as minimal inclusion of gerontological information in the training of generalists tend to isolate the elderly from the health care resources. Another isolator is the disproportionate number of inpatient and institutional resources available as compared to outpatient and community-based facilities. There is significantly uneven geographical distribution of expertise and settings in rural areas and inner city neighborhoods as compared to more affluent suburban communities where the elderly, especially the poor aged, are not concentrated.

Psychological Isolators

There are numerous isolators in the psychological-emotional quadrant at the individual level. The consequences of aging with chronic mental disorders produce a lack of social skills. This lack may produce special problems when an elderly person is moved from an institution to a community placement where additional social skills, beyond those needed in an institution, are required for daily living. Late onset problems such as phobias and depression can become isolators. Emotional responses such as fear, anger, or grief that accompany chronic illnesses may produce withdrawal from others. Adapting to changes in roles, in self-esteem, or in the perceptions of others about the individual, loss of control in the choice of residency, or reduction of social opportunities because priorities are given to younger people (i.e., youth culture values or age discrimination practices) are isolators. Shifts in social activities from intimate to impersonal contacts, from independence to dependence in relationships and decision making, or loss of a partner with whom sexual and sensual experiences are shared all can generate the sense of isolation.

There are fewer isolators at the environmental, as compared to the individual, level. Many of these involve the structure and/or availability of resources. As with the environmental level of biophysical isolators, the absence of ambulatory services and in-community supports are important, especially for elders with chronic mental illness or late onset disorders. For those with emotional isolators of a nonpsychiatric nature, the stigma associated with emotional needs labeled as "mental problems" makes their desire to seek help an unacceptable alternative. Treatment approaches that are not modified to meet the circumstances of elderly persons also may promote isolation.

Economic Isolators

Insufficient economic resources impact in countless ways as an isolator at the individual level. The elder may be unable to pay for social interaction opportunities (i.e., membership in clubs, participation fees, costs for travel) to obtain services, purchase basic necessities, or ensure personal safety. Limited economic means may restrict resources for coping with crises or preparing for long-range life transitions.

At the environmental level, isolators often are related to poverty that stems from many factors outside the individual. For example, limitations in Social Security

Figure 2-1 Isolators That Impact on the Elderly Across All Subgroups

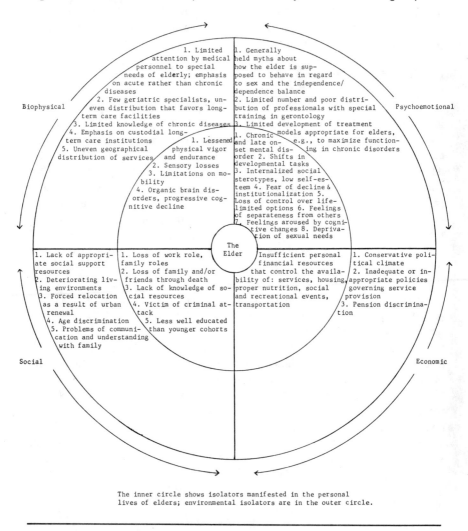

The inner circle shows isolators manifested in the personal
lives of elders; environmental isolators are in the outer circle.

benefits control the amount of some fixed income resources. Third party payments for services under major entitlements (Medicare, Medicaid, and Title XX of the Social Security Act) exert much control over what services are provided. These environmental factors can influence isolation from resources as much as, if not more than, individual level causes. The political climate of the early 1980s threatened the continuation of entitlements, employment opportunities for senior citizens, and special programs for minority and other disadvantaged elderly.

Social Isolators

Some of the factors categorized as social isolators are well documented as to their impact on the lives of the elderly. At the individual level, a major one is the change in work and family roles. The degree to which these losses are isolators depends on how they are viewed, i.e., some elders may regard retirement as an earned reward and an opportunity for new experiences while others see it as a result of diminished abilities and reduced personal worth. Other social isolators are the loss of social contacts by the death and/or disability of close family members or friends, limited knowledge about resources and how to utilize them and reduced access to them.

At an environmental level, the design of services may serve as an isolator. The attitudes and behavior of providers minimize the importance of relationships as the vehicle for providing the service. Negative stereotyping and the resultant ageism are manifest in almost every aspect of the environment. The extent to which stereotyping will affect any elderly person's life is difficult to assess. On the other hand, few elders escape some ramifications of ageism. Other environmental isolators include the hazards of deteriorating housing and/or neighborhoods or forced relocation to new and unfamiliar areas.

This conceptualization assumes that there are interactions among individual and environmental level isolators and the biophysical, psychological, economic, and social realms. These interactions are complex to the point that they encompass the totality of circumstances, events, and situations that define the daily lives of older people. It is beyond the scope of this discussion of isolators to specify all that may be involved in such interactional patterns. The examination of isolators for each population subgroup, and their assessment for possible interventions, is elaborated upon in the subgroup chapters. This discussion does provide a sample of the kinds of events and situations that place an elder at risk for becoming isolated.

THE ISOLATION PROCESS

Isolation is a process in which the elderly lose their sense of personal integrity or connection with other social resources. This process consists of four stages:

1. An isolator occurs in the life of an elder.
2. The elder evaluates the isolator in terms of its personal meaningfulness and evaluates available personal or environmental resources.
3. The individual is either (a) able to utilize resources to resolve problems or compensate for losses that result from the isolator, or (b) unable to do so.
4. The elder who needs assistance is confronted by isolation as a barrier to accessing the necessary systems.

Figure 2-2 facilitates an understanding of the isolation process. It is important to note that the presence of an isolator in the life of an elder is not a one-time happening. New isolators appear and the process begins again. However, with each new isolator the range of available resources shrinks, making resolution more and more difficult. Isolation also must be conceived of as variable, i.e., its degree can vary in terms of its extensiveness and intensiveness in the lives of elders.

The first stage of the process is relatively straightforward, a simple presence of one or a combination of isolators, such as the loss of a close friend or an incident in a social gathering that makes real the ageism that exists in the elders' environment. It is obvious that all elders are exposed to isolators, yet the occurrence of one can only be viewed as a possible precursor to isolation.

At the second stage, the elders evaluate the isolator and its potential meaning in their lives. It is at this point that they also evaluate personal and environmental resources that they may need to resolve problems or compensate for losses brought about by the isolator. The kinds of personal and social resources needed would depend much on the specific isolator. Thus the elder who loses a close friend needs the capacity and desire to establish new friendships and a close and caring family or other friend who will be supportive in a time of grief. On the other hand, the elder with Alzheimer's disease needs support from medical and psychosocial practitioners to understand how to maximize social maintenance skills and self-care capacities, help from family members, and supportive residential placement that allows for the most possible control over daily activities.

The third stage is the action phase. Individuals who have evaluated their needs and resources now attempt to use them to resolve or compensate for the isolator. If this attempt is successful, isolation will not result. The elder who has lost a close friend can develop new ones or can increase involvement with present friends, family, or social activities. However, if the deficits in personal and social resources are so extensive that the demands placed upon them are too overwhelming, then the individuals will not be able to compensate.

For example, the individual who loses a close friend and is unable to make new ones, has few meaningful solitary activities, is not used to participating in social organizations, and has a family that is distant or in a crisis period and struggling with its own needs, will become isolated as a result. Once elders are isolated, some may accept their less than satisfying lives as unavoidable and thus modify their expectations. Others may respond by neglect of self-care, withdrawal into preoccupation with self, and/or alcohol or drug misuse. These responses may further jeopardize the availability of personal and social resources. The increasing constriction of their lives and the feeling of loneliness and separation from the social whole (that lead to neglect of proper health care, states of chronic stress, and/or substance abuse) can predispose the elderly to physical and mental disorders. If such conditions are present already, isolation may cause them to become worse and vital treatment to be neglected.

Figure 2-2 The Isolation Process: Intervention Options Open to the Elderly

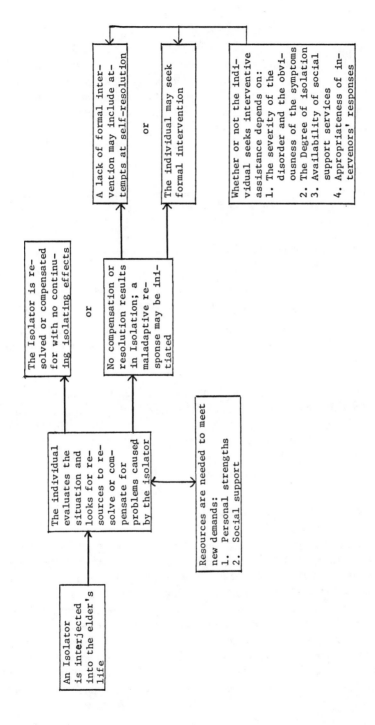

The fourth stage of the isolation process centers on help-seeking activities when significant need arises, such as emerging health problems or inadequate food. The elderly may ignore unmet needs, if possible, or attempt to restructure what few resources are present to provide for their increasingly limited existence. Thus, they direct all resources toward basic survival, with no attempt to ensure quality of survival. The isolation that first was considered a resultant condition now becomes a barrier to seeking help.

The likelihood that isolated elders will seek assistance, if at all, depends on several factors:

- The nature of the needs: physical disorder that produces painful and obvious symptoms that cannot be ignored is more likely to lead the individual to seek help.

- The degree to which the elders are isolated: the more isolated they are, the less likely they are to seek help.

- The availability of service resources: the social support resource must be available, known, and accepted by the elders.

- The degree to which the elders have had unsuccessful experiences with intervenors: those whose responses are abrupt, uncaring, or inappropriate will discourage elders from seeking future contact.

These factors all suggest that isolated elders seek assistance only under dire circumstances and even then can be discouraged easily from continuing contact with service providers. If they have a physical or mental disorder of such magnitude that they cannot seek assistance, contact could take place only through the intervention of the police, neighbors, or others to whom the situation has become known, if indeed they do become aware of it.

INTERVENTION GUIDELINES

Elderly persons caught in any stage in the isolation process need to develop more extensive social interaction skills. This section reframes clinical intervention with the elderly in a way that puts them in a position of maximum involvement in their own isolation reduction. Contact with an intervenor should prepare the elderly to better utilize all available resources, including personal strengths and the assistance of their social support network. One benefit of this approach is that it can build self-confidence for dealing with isolation; another is that it can put the elder in a state of greater preparedness to deal with future isolators.

This presentation indicates that a central problem brought about by the isolators (i.e., clients or situations) is overload on a limited social support network.

Therefore, the goal of intervention should be the development of a broader support system for the client by:

1. Providing knowledge of available social support resources. If an intervenor knows what resources are available, presents this information, then helps the elder to analyze it in relation to the isolator, the client's knowledge can be increased quickly.
2. Helping to select supports that best meet client needs. Referrals to sources that are inappropriate or not immediately available (e.g., long waiting lists or lengthy eligibility determination) can exhaust the client's energy and willingness to continue to attempt to obtain services.
3. Helping the client develop better access to supports that are available through the development of social skills. The social skills needed depend on the nature of the elder's problem and whether the desire is to expand access to informal or formal networks, or both. In general, these skills would include such diverse activities as information on how to use referral services and development of communication abilities and more assertive behaviors.
4. Legitimizing or encouraging the elderly to accept the need for and value of a broader support system in the face of the declining ability of their present social network to provide all that is needed.

To clarify how a practitioner introduces skill building into clinical intervention, the authors have developed guidelines to show how the process can begin with where the client is and go from that point to acquiring greater skills. Table 2-1 has a continuum with three positions, each representing a possible starting point for intervention. Wherever the intervention is begun, the goal is to move in the direction of Position III.

Clients at Position I can be described as having minimal functional capacity, unable to fulfill basic social support needs and unable to exist without them. Their input into the interventive effort may be little more than a brief and incomplete statement of their problem, but whatever they can contribute is valuable, both for the information needed to proceed with the process and because the elderly thus can feel a part of it. The practitioner unfamiliar with elders in this condition may interpret their lack of input as evidence of confusion related to organic brain disorder when in fact it may reflect the overwhelming situation they face with isolators.

The immediate response is to jump in and "do something" for the client. The practitioner's need to act too quickly may make clients feel pressed into taking steps they still are unsure of, urged on by a practitioner they are not comfortable in approaching and with whom they have not had the opportunity to develop trust. This approach tends to promote dependency and to rob clients of the opportunity to gain experience in problem solving and the confidence that that builds. An

Table 2-1 Continuum of Interventive Activities to Help Clients Develop Access to Social Support Networks

	Position I	Position II	Position III
What Intervention	Intervenor establishes contact with necessary resource on behalf of the client.	Joint discussion is held on problem definition and available social supports. Both practitioner and client make contacts, separately or together.	Consultation with client covers tangible needs and in some cases therapeutic intervention to resolve complex relationship problems.
What Client Situations	This is for a client who has minimal skills, no supportive contacts, and emergency need.	This is for the client with limited information and social skills who therefore feels unable to seek out and use social resources.	This is for the client with adequate basic skills but uncertain about perceptions and hesitant to implement a course of action.
Practitioner Role	The practitioner helps define need and suggests contact options, makes the contacts, later discusses them and perhaps simulates imaginary situations for the client to practice the process.	The practitioner works with the client to help crystallize needs and hoped-for solutions.	The practitioner mainly furnishes support and reassurance in making social contacts and in other therapies to resolve more complex relationship problems.
Client Role	The client's input involves defining the desired level of social need and social resource preferences.	The client completes some contacts, feeds into the decision-making process, and practices behavioral responses.	The client is responsible for the social contacts necessary to fulfill needs.
Cautions	The practitioner must be patient with and supportive of even the weakest attempts by the client to make input into the process.	The practitioner should make sure not to make any contacts or decisions that the client is capable of doing individually.	The practitioner should continue to offer support, interest, and caring concern to the client as the person attempts to resolve problems related to isolators by use of the social resource system.

Source: Hashimi, J.K. Environmental modification: Teaching social coping skills. *Social Work*, 1981, 26, 323-326.

intervention that does not foster independence and development skills at every step may risk the promotion of isolation.

Short of a crisis situation needing immediate intervention, it may be better to proceed at a slower pace, allowing the clients to gain more self-confidence. In a crisis situation where the intervenor must take immediate steps, clients still can be given the opportunity for maximizing their input but it must be facilitated by the practitioner and not thwarted by the expert's need for action.

Position II represents clients who lack the necessary information and social skills to better utilize the available social support system. They are not as disabled as those described in Position I. They could take some actions on their own behalf with proper support, guidance, and practice. However, they can be overwhelmed in fledgling attempts to seek resources either by being pressed into activities that are too difficult or by having the practitioner provide service when they could do so for themselves if reassurance and support were offered.

In Position III, the clients seem to have adequate social skills to resolve their problems but do not do so. The elderly may express uncertainty about what steps to take. In these circumstances, the practitioner assumes the role of a consultant and encourages the elderly to discuss their concerns and uncertainties.

The intervention may end at the point of resolving tangible needs emanating from the interaction between the individual and the environment isolators. Some of the elderly will move on to more complex issues. If so, the problem solving of tangible needs becomes a bridge that crosses over to a more demanding and extensive therapeutic relationship. In this type of intervention, the practitioner works with the clients to resolve isolators of a more complex nature such as a rupture in relationships with family or depression related to the death of a spouse.

The interventive guidelines emphasize the clients' need to be encouraged to assume maximal control and responsibility in decisions and to expand or better utilize their social support network. The question of how much control and responsibility the clients are capable of assuming should be determined through assessment. However, assessment frequently is hampered by problems in client-practitioner interaction. Problems in assessment cluster around:

- failures in communication and mutual understanding (e.g., the non-English-speaking elder taken to a health clinic where no staff members speak the person's own language)

- the lack of assessment to evaluate functional skills (e.g., an Alzheimer's disease patient's being considered for membership in a day care center or an elder abuse victim's ability to live alone)

- a lack of interdisciplinary assessment teams (e.g., the elderly alcoholic who may need acute hospitalization rather than placement in a state mental institution)

Clients who are misunderstood through an inadequate assessment are less likely to experience a reduction or elimination of isolation-related problems; rather, they may experience greater isolation when there is an inappropriate match between needs and prescribed interventions. In some helping episodes, the elderly may terminate intervention because they feel rejected, frustrated, or hopeless. These feelings are likely to increase isolation in that they reduce the motivation for self-initiated pursuit of intervention or create apathy and/or mistrust of the help that is made available.

A critical aspect of intervention with isolated elders is the context of that move. If the various components of the elders' possible social support resources are disconnected, it is difficult if not impossible for them to derive the fullest benefit from the help that is available. This is an important goal of many case management and linkage-building efforts. These are valuable for setting up service systems for an administrative perspective; however, their impact on the isolated elders rarely is considered in the implementation process. Direct attention to how these large-scale coordination approaches impact on the isolated elderly and their social supports is an important element of planning and evaluation.

REARRANGEMENT OF RESOURCES

The conceptualization of a formal service and informal support network arrangement, in a community context, is important in providing assistance to the isolated elderly. The conceptualization is based on some assumptions about what exists in the community:

- Both formal and informal resources are available.

- Formal resources are available from two types of service organizations: age-specific ones that provide diverse services to persons of 60 and older and problem-specific ones that offer help to adults of any age facing needs related to specific conditions, special statuses, or particular problems.

- Both types of organizations employ staff with the expertise to provide clinical interventions for individuals, families, and small groups as well as program development interventions directed toward building structures applicable to persons within the community.

The arrangement of formal and informal resources conceptualized in Figure 2-3 can become a major concern among individuals in a position to initiate and influence a communitywide rearrangement. The rearrangement as proposed here is intended to increase the accessibility, comprehensiveness, coordination, and continuity of service.

Figure 2-3 Service Resource Structure for the Isolated Elderly

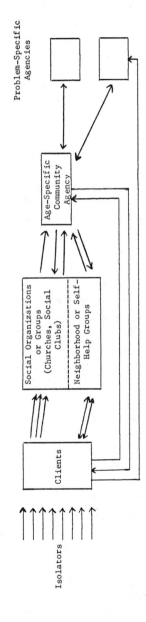
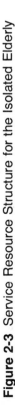

Clients are impacted upon by isolators. The ability to solve resultant problems depends on the clients' resources, general abilities, current level of functioning, nature of the stressor, and their prior experience with similar stressors.

When individuals cannot solve problems, peer groups can be helpful. With peer support and resource information made available within these groups, clients may be able to resolve their problems and need no further assistance. This would be particularly true of situations where information, friendship, and support are the principal needs. In neighborhood groups, active members are encouraged to be in contact with ill or isolated nonactive members. In cases where referral is made to formal agencies, backup social contact and support could be continued from these groups.

With a problem that does not lend itself to self or peer group solution, or with individuals who cannot make use of the group structure, referral can be made by a social group organization or by an outreach worker (perhaps an indigenous peer worker) to an age-specific service agency. This referral would be facilitated if the agency were the sponsor of the neighborhood group or had sent workers into other social organizations to provide resource information.

Situations that are not age specific (alcoholism, chronic mental disorder) would be referred to problem-specific agencies. Aftercare could be arranged with the age-specific agency.

This conceptualization has one major advantage over some others in that it assumes that needs of the isolated elderly cannot be met by organizations that are only age specific. Intervention resources usually are concentrated in problem-specific organizations. However, those entities may lack clinical and program development expertise in gerontology and have few linkages with the age-specific organizations. The potential benefits of arranging linkages between the age-specific and problem-specific organizations might include: (1) a better exchange of information between the two types of organizations, (2) more individualized and comprehensive intervention, and (3) more diversified expertise and clinical case consultation.

The arrangement also facilitates the linkage between formal and informal resources in the community. The majority of resources available to the isolated elderly are provided through informal channels. These are important because they offer acceptable and unstigmatized social support that costs nothing and is given in a personalized, caring context. Introducing the informal resources as part of the initial planning can benefit clinical and program development personnel in both types of agencies. They can perceive new ways of facilitating the informal resources without altering natural structures.

Both age-specific and problem-specific organizations in communities throughout the nation are plagued with fewer dollars to fulfill greater needs; there are serious problems with all of the third party reimbursement mechanisms and their continuation is in question; competing demands among the "truly needy" are becoming intensified; and the numbers of isolated elderly and their problems are growing. A community needs a service arrangement that puts the formal resources into a structure of economically feasible coordination that is supplemented by linkage with informal resources if it is to meet needs in the reality of fiscal constraints.

Figure 2-3 indicates how elderly clients can be serviced by a structure of the sort proposed. This general arrangement is the basis upon which the structural arrangement for each subgroup is designed. It does not reflect all the possible ways of linkage to age-specific and problem-specific organizations or those with the informal resources. It does reflect some of the most important elements to be included in a community-based resource reorganization for the isolated elderly.

While outreach is an important component in meeting the needs of isolated elders, it is unwieldly and wasteful for all age-specific and problem-specific agencies to attempt to reach individuals in the community in need of specific intervention. Resources could and should be maximized by having outreach efforts organized geographically, conducted by age-specific agencies, and connected to the range of problem-specific agencies in the same area. This means that the age-specific agency could act as a liaison between the potential client and problem-specific entities.

The function to be served by the age-specific organization includes:

- locating those in need of service in a neighborhood or geographical unit
- informing potential clients of available service in both the age-specific and problem-specific agencies
- informing the service providers of potential clients
- facilitating the coming together of the elderly and the problem-specific agency

An age-specific entity with multiple or single services delivered to the elderly or an agency that has an age-specific component with continuing contact in the neighborhoods is in the best position to further develop the outreach potential into a more formalized system.

The neighborhood can be an adjunct to a central outreach location; however, those areas must be used in a role that complements the day-to-day activity and routine gathering points, such as parks or coffee shops. Some or all parts of a neighborhood can be explored for potential outreach capacity for the isolated elderly. Some neighbors may look upon professional help as an unwelcome intrusion in the life of an elder and thus discourage professional intervention and/or try to undertake functions beyond their capacity once an at-risk person has been located. Therefore, an educational process for neighborhood outreach strategies is necessary.

Self-help groups also are a source of outreach. These, like neighborhood groups, have their own boundaries that often are kept closed to formalized linkages with organizationally sponsored outreach. However, these are excellent sources for in-home visitations with fearful elderly or those whose behaviors offend others without their knowing they have problems. Self-help group outreach also can be extremely valuable for contacts with the elders' families who may provide channels for active intervention from a formal resource.

It would be the task and responsibility of the formal service network to develop an intervention approach to assist the elderly. The conceptual arrangement indicates that this could be from either an age-specific agency source and/or another problem-specific service source. The age-specific agencies make the first contact with the elder and relate exclusively to them. These agencies, with varying degrees of adequacy, have information on resources to meet the needs that often are the elders' first priority and can provide forums for these individuals to discuss issues relevant to them as a special group.

To be able to facilitate the elderly persons' access to the problem-specific source requires some type of interorganizational linkage (popularly called coordination). The connecting process requires at least two elements: interpersonal relationships between representatives of both types of agencies and formalized service agreements. Alone, neither is sufficient and, in many instances, both are not enough to meet the needs of complex cases that require extensive liaison activity. For elderly clients less entrenched in the isolation process, having liaison with the agencies is valuable. The liaison person could act as outreach for the age-specific organization and facilitate the transfer of client service responsibility to the problem-specific group. This person also could ensure that the referral was appropriate for the requirements of the latter entity.

If the problem-specific agency can convey to the elderly that its services could be helpful, an important gain will be accomplished. Many potentially beneficial services can be provided effectively and efficiently by problem-specific agencies to help meet the elderly persons' greatest needs. These services should integrate into the components of the other formal and informal resources so that the elderly do not become even further lost or disconnected.

This brief description of isolators, the isolation process, guidelines for intervention, and social support resources lays the groundwork for the discussion of the problems and needs of the population subgroups in the next nine chapters and for examination of innovative approaches for isolation-related intervention.

Chapter 3

Older and Elderly Women: Survivors into Isolation

INTRODUCTION

Who is the older woman in our society? How does she view herself? Is she a "dear old soul" or a witch to be feared and avoided? Is she "old and brown and all but dead" or a crusty survivor of a lifetime of endurance? How does she interact with the social network that influences her life and how does she experience the massive changes that are evident today for women in general?

Fortunately there is no accurate "typical" picture of the older woman. In today's society, older women are diverse beings despite a common burden of sexism and ageism. Any time a description of an older woman or group of them is predicated on sex and/or age stereotyping, distorted images emerge that are both contradictory and cruel. This can be seen in the medical clinics where the detailed physical complaints of the older woman often are ignored as meaningless chatter. To the extent that they experience therapeutic neglect and/or inadequate services they are victims of the service systems. As such, they are at risk to feelings of helplessness and confusion and respond in ways that perpetuate loneliness and isolation.

Older women are the fastest growing segment of society and, in a sense, are survivors. They face a continuous push-and-pull struggle to live amid the double bias of sexism and ageism that promotes pain, confusion, abuse, and injustice. However, despite these experiences, many remain optimistic about reaping the merits and rewards of their survival. It is to the credit of older women that so few give up altogether. Most adequately maintain themselves as tenacious beings with strong links to the past, present, and future.

As an outgrowth of both the women's movement and the increasing awareness of gender differences that are appropriate for inclusion in gerontologists' research, a growing body of empirical information is being generated on the physical and mental health, social, and economic needs of women as they age. The question remains whether or not the theoretical and research interest in older women can change the complex set of influences that keep them in passive roles as recipients of standardized and bureaucratic professional help and can ameliorate the economic deprivation that reduces self-determination.

A beginning national advocacy movement organized by the Older Women's League is designed as a mobilization effort at the local level to integrate such efforts with larger state, regional, and national legislative and social action projects. The fiscal conservatism of the early 1980s, combined with serious fragmentations within the women's movement and a national concern among senior citizen groups to prevent destruction of the Social Security system, create a dire need for effective national advocacy for older and elderly women.

This chapter analyzes some of the characteristics of this population. Data documenting older women's growing proportion of the population and their needs form a background for the subsequent discussion of an overlapping cluster of isolators. These must be viewed in relation to age and gender variables. When significant numbers of middle-aged women begin to experience some of these isolators as they reach midlife, while others encounter them much later, an age-based conceptualization diverts attention from the gender-based factors that also are important.

This analysis of isolators incorporates both age and gender in the interpretation of an alarming state of affairs for older women. A number of cases are introduced that describe the different circumstances of older women that create the need for intervention. Sadly enough, their situations reflect additional problems of isolation they encounter in the process of being ''helped.'' Where they received services and from whom varies considerably. That variation suggests that many older women may be isolated from entry points to individualized and coordinated services. The description of intervention encompasses interpersonal informal and professionally provided helping plus programmatic levels of assistance that are designed to serve groups of women. Interventions oriented to individuals, groups, and families all require the practitioner's sensitive consideration of age and gender.

The brief review of an alternative program development framework incorporates the principle of integration between and among service networks in an arrangement that strengthens self-advocacy and self-help in older women. The context offers neither an original nor a definitive direction for avoiding the pitfalls of ageism and sexism in the provision of services to older women but does describe how existing services might best be organized and used in the reality of today's resources.

CHARACTERISTICS OF WOMEN AND THE AGING PROCESS

Research on older women has increased and has been legitimized in disciplines such as psychology, gerontology, and sociology, bringing with it new data to substantiate or repudiate historical and existing images of this population. However, there is a need to be aware that what often are mistaken for new data in reality simply form a new and different method of interpreting old information (Seltzer, 1979). It is only recently that old data on current and future numbers of older women have been reexamined with interpretations that call for urgent and immediate concern about them as a rapidly expanding at-risk segment of the total population.

Random selection of statistical information to describe older women and their circumstances is risky. Such numbers may lead to generalized impressions that bury or distort differences among the various subgroups that have similar or different needs. Practitioners should be cautious in generalizing from data that do not provide clear breakdowns of the age categories of older and elderly women in the samples. To do otherwise can encourage an inappropriate if not inaccurate understanding of age-related issues that vary between middle-aged women who may be economically disadvantaged because of job market conditions and elderly women who become deprived on pension benefits when they are widowed.

Statistics can be used to describe several groups of "older" women based on chronological age; discussion of their problems based on clearly defined age categories helps clarify which ones are the focal point. For example, by focusing on those who are 75 and older, their institutional problems can be put in proper perspective since these issues arise most frequently for such women. Setting up a clearly defined age category to cover those who are too young to receive Social Security benefits and lack other pension or third party sources to cover the cost of health care and social services can highlight the financial needs of that group, which may be different from those of women 60 and older who are eligible for benefits through the Older Americans Act entitlement for benefits and services.

In 1977 there were 13.9 million women 65 years and older, as compared to 9.5 million men in the same age range (a 31.7 percent difference). By 2035 there are expected to be 33.4 million older women as compared to 22.4 million older men (a 32.9 percent edge). That ratio is projected to increase further by the year 2050 (Uhlenberg, 1979). There is considerable debate over why men typically die at a much earlier age than women. It has been argued this can be attributed to genetic differences (Waldron, 1976a, 1976b), to heavier use of tobacco among men (Retherford, 1974, 1975), and to the masculine sex roles that lead to both greater risk taking and to greater occupational stress (Johnson, 1977). The differences in life expectancy and the possible reasons for them are receiving increasing attention in policy formulation for the elderly and chronically impaired (Federal Council on Aging, 1977).

The women who in 1982 were 70 and older could be referred to appropriately as those of the Depression Era, meaning that they were at their peak childbearing years during that time. They had the lowest fertility rate of any group of American women right down to the present. Patterns of childbearing are important in that they change from one generation to another and influence the course of women's lives. Of the women who are now 65 and older, 22 percent never had a child, 23 percent had only one, and 22 percent had only two. This lower fertility rate means that one-third of this cohort have no surviving children. They also are likely to have lived many years without a husband.

Females' longer life expectancy, combined with the custom of their marrying men older than they are, increases the probability they will survive their husbands. It also may mean that while the wife may care for the ailing older husband through incapacity in the late years, there will be no spouse to care for her in a similar manner. This pattern contributes to a higher probability of institutionalization for elderly women. Today almost two-thirds of those 65 years and older are widowed. The projected rate of younger groups who will be placed in nursing homes is unknown, but 70 percent of the current nursing home population is composed of women over age 75 (National Institute on Aging and National Institute of Mental Health, 1978).

The economic situation for the 1980s cohort of elderly women is not good. Economic deprivation is a major barrier to their achieving a better quality of life in old age. A principal solution to these problems is pension reform. Women are not covered adequately either as workers or as wives. Only 37 percent of women applying for Social Security based on their own earnings had a continuous work record since 1937, which reflects their intermittent labor force participation. Only 21 percent of retired women as compared to 47 percent of retired men are covered under private pension plans.

One-third of widows and one-fourth of divorced or never married women 70 years and older receive 85 percent of their income from Social Security. In 1976, 42 percent of those 73 or older lived in poverty. The median income of unmarried women 62 to 72 was $4,000. For women 73 or older, the median income dropped to $3,000. Of all Social Security beneficiaries still poor enough to qualify for Supplementary Security Income, two out of three are women (Womanpower, 1980). When or if pension and other retirement policies are reformed to acknowledge the work patterns of women to compensate them justly for their lifetimes of work, they will not have to make choices between food and heat, between independent living and institutionalization (Womanpower, 1980).

A wide range of physical problems is more common among older women than older men. These disorders have as much impact on the quality of the women's lives as their impoverished economic status. They are more likely to experience strokes, visual impairment, hypertension, arthritis, diabetes, and perhaps senile dementia. Five times as many older women than men experience osteoporosis (a condition in which the bones become brittle and fragile, making fractures of hips and vertebrae likely). Stress incontinence and cryptogenic drop attacks (falling without becoming unconscious but unable to get up) also are more common to older women than to older men. Certain dermatological changes seem to have more impact on women than on men when the cosmetic aspect of the physical aging process is considered (Ortmeyer, 1979; Kerschner & Tiberi, 1978).

Much more information must be collected to obtain a solid empirical basis for understanding some of the illness and disability differences between older men and women and the shifting patterns of illness-related behavior of females as they grow older. The only major cause of death where women have a higher mortality rate than men is diabetes mellitus; it also is the only potentially fatal chronic condition in which women have a higher morbidity rate than males (Gove & Hughes, 1979). Yet the role of mild forms of illness appears to differentiate between the two groups in that acute ailments are much more common than chronic ones among women but, paradoxically, the leading causes of death do not tend to be the main causes of illness (Verbrugge, 1976).

To obtain a better understanding of potential differences between younger and older women, or women as they age in relation to health problems and illness behaviors, samples of individuals should be compared. Few such data are available on all female samples. Research on different age cohorts might provide much-needed clarification on how being alone during midlife without adequate income and preventive health care can influence long-range health patterns as women get older.

While there are some differences between women who are elderly now and those who will be soon, there are general trends that can be expected to persist:

- There is a likelihood that women will continue to be alone for a significant proportion of their later years.

- There will be difficulty obtaining health insurance after being widowed because of existing physical health problems and the high cost of individual policy rates since access to group health insurance generally is tied to employment (Sommers, 1980).

- There will continue to be a limited range of ambulatory health care available to older women despite the appropriateness of these outpatient services, such as the usefulness but limited availability of ambulatory gynecologic services (Pelegrina, 1977).

- There will be a continuing struggle to find alternative life styles that are valuable for their well-being but at the same time may be counter to the accepted traditional styles of women living alone and trying to make it on too few resources (Matthews, 1979).

One group of women in a broad age range from 35 to 64 has come to be known as "displaced homemakers." As a group, some never have worked outside the home (Holden, 1979a, 1979b). After spending a significant portion of their lives as homemakers, they experience an abrupt end to financial support because of divorce, separation, widowhood, disability of a spouse, or termination of Aid to Families with Dependent Children. According to Department of Labor statistics, in 1977 there were 155,000 unemployed widowed and divorced middle-aged women between the ages of 46 and 64; 122,000 of them looking for full-time and 33,000 for part-time work. Of 32,000 separated women, 26,000 were seeking full-time and 6,000 part-time jobs (Womanpower, 1980). Until recently, they had no services directed toward facilitating their entry into new social and economic roles. Their numbers are significant and far greater than can be accommodated by the number of programs scattered around the country that face the loss of federal funding. If the network of Displaced Homemaker Programs loses that financial base without state and local funding replacements, a major human service model for midlife and reentry women will cease in many communities. Other programs throughout the United States have already been impacted by cuts in federal spending for human service entitlements during fiscal years 1981 and 1982. Programs have been eliminated if they relied solely on federal funds, rather than diversifying their base of financing through community support.

These data are significant in any discussion of older women and form the bases for selecting the isolators analyzed in this chapter as common to many of them. Some of these isolators are more frequent among women of very advanced age as compared to either their male counterparts or somewhat younger females. More large-scale survey research is needed on the distribution of these isolators and what combination may be most significant for special subgroups such as minorities (Dancy, 1977), shopping bag women (Schein, 1979), those who never married, the chronically impaired, and lesbians (National Institute on Aging, 1978).

ISOLATORS AS THEY ARE MANIFEST IN OLDER WOMEN

As this discussion indicates, the isolators older women experience in their personal lives are related to issues and events in the broader society that reinforce the impact of those isolators. Several important isolators are depicted in Figure 3-1. The inner circle identifies personal isolators, the outer circle those emanating from society. The quadrants in both circles indicate societal and personal isolators in the social, physical, psychological, and economic sectors.

The sector on physical isolators notes that women experience prevalence rates for some chronic conditions that limit social involvement yet few physicians are trained in geriatric medicine. In addition, many physicians do not recognize the important gender issues in treating older women patients.

In the psychological sector, personal isolators include the internalized social stereotypes and the personal meaning of physical changes. The stereotypes limit life style alternatives. The woman who can view herself only as wife and mother

Figure 3-1 Isolators Most Important for Late Life Women

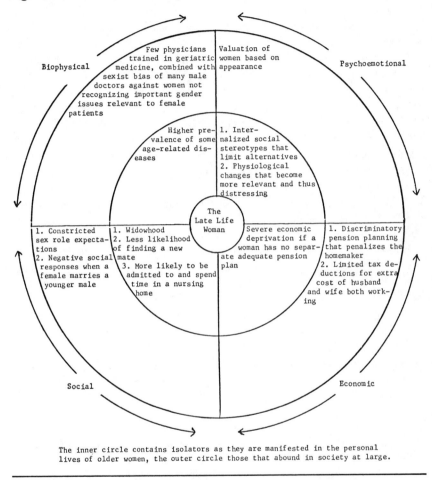

The inner circle contains isolators as they are manifested in the personal lives of older women, the outer circle those that abound in society at large.

will have particular difficulty adjusting to the older status when more important roles no longer are available. If a woman believes she is valued only to the degree that she is attractive (defined as youthfulness), age-related changes will make her feel less desirable and wanted. Both of these isolators are reflections of the societal values that elevate youthful attractiveness.

In the social sector, personal isolators include widowhood and a lesser probability of remarriage. A woman is much more likely to spend her final years in a nursing home. This is related to the greater likelihood of becoming a widow and perhaps also to the way she is viewed by others as unable to manage alone. These isolators are bolstered by the general conception of the older female as dependent.

There are more negative social responses when a woman marries a younger man, despite the logic of such a union. For unless dramatic medical discoveries are made, women will continue to outlive their spouses and spend long years in widowhood.

Less attention is paid in this chapter to economic isolators, although they are very important as constrictors in older women's lives. Whether pension income is derived through survivor benefits or her own work history, the older woman alone tends to be so limited financially that the expenses of social involvement are a luxury she cannot afford. This issue must be faced on a national level in advocacy for changes in pension and Social Security laws that recognize the years a woman spends as homemaker and the likelihood that, if she did work, it was in a lower paying job that could only result in lower pension income.

The extent to which practitioners fall short in their attempts to evaluate the influence of age and gender-related isolators among older female clients is striking. However, in all fairness to practitioners, the process of assessment is not easy. Few clinical guidelines have yet emerged from the various research approaches that have been applied to the sociological and psychological studies of older women. Methods incorporated in a life cycle perspective, historical and generational analysis, and network evaluation are not readily useful when clinical or programmatic intervention assessment is the goal.

However, practitioners should consider at least one theoretical framework for investigating social networks and isolation even though its primary purpose is to contribute to social science theory rather than to clinical intervention theory (Dono, Falber, Kail, Letwak, Sherman, & Siegel, 1979). It takes into account the usual dimensions of the amount of interaction with others and the identification of significant others, and incorporates measures of both the subjective and actual experiences of social involvement.

There are several other concepts that could be incorporated into the design of assessment tools. First is the "rhythm of isolation" that refers to an individual's pattern of social involvement and withdrawal. The second is the "relativity of isolation"—an individual's pattern of cognitive and comparative assessment of the "usual" behavior of those considered as peers. Attention should be directed to: (a) the extent to which dyadic and multiple networks may complement or substitute for each other, (b) the extent to which cognitive awareness and perceptions of the various networks change over time, (c) whether an increase in the degree of commitment in one or more networks may compensate for age-linked losses in others, and (d) whether past commitments have symbolic significance, thus compensating at least in part for the lack of current behavioral involvement (Lowenthal & Robinson, 1976).

In the dyadic relationship, many sources of isolation can occur that have significant impact on older women. The best understood of these relationships is the marital situation. For older women, the death of the spouse is considered the most isolating of crisis events associated with marriage. However, retirement also can prove to be an isolator that affects both wife and husband. Wives can be affected negatively during this transition period by what the husband anticipates and experiences before and during retirement and the degree to which these elements are shared and/or change the usual pattern of their lives.

The impact of loss of income can weigh heavily upon both husband and wife (Holden, 1979a, 1979b). Reduced income may prevent the wife from continuing her previous life style, force her to deal with more demands for financial management, and overwhelm her with dread of poverty-ridden circumstances. In addition to the economic circumstances, a major change in life style can arise from the one in which a woman is involved in meaningful social relationships beyond the dyad of husband and wife; this can lead to gradual or abrupt loss of such activities because they conflict with the increasing demands the retired husband can make. The demands increase because of his loss of social relationships with previous work roles.

Older women have reported that they enjoy the additional opportunity for companionship with retired husbands (Blood & Wolfe, 1960), but too little research has been conducted on their perspectives to know with any degree of certainty under what circumstances the retirement can produce isolating circumstances for the wife. In the future, as more two-career families move toward retirement, more consideration will have to be given to the additional impact if their jobs end at different times.

Efforts have been made to identify different categories of older women: the "pioneers," who have experienced contact with activist ideas; the "professionals," who have survived in the male-dominated professions; the "Penelopes," who live in a traditional husband-centered world; and the "Portnoy's mothers," who are child oriented and confronted with painful emptiness when their offspring leave the household (Bart, 1975). Women who center their life styles on their relationship with their spouses are the ones likely to find that experience increases once the spouse retires. To the extent that the image of high personal satisfaction after the retirement constitutes a stereotype for the older woman and her response to her husband's new role, it also is a barrier to considering some of the consequences isolating those women who give up part or all of their social world to meet the relational needs of the retired spouse (Turner, 1979).

Other less frequently considered isolators can find the older woman, when she retires, required to adapt to her husband's postretirement plans that were made either without consideration of her needs or that she later determined were less acceptable for other reasons (Blieszner & Szinovacz, 1979; Barfield & Morgan, 1978). For many women, the issue of geographical relocation to another community after the husband's retirement can be appealing when being planned but prove unsatisfactory once the couple has moved.

An older woman also may find that her spouse cannot adjust to social opportunities through participating with her friends in routines she developed before retirement and has attempted to extend to him. He may have no desire to become involved in activities she initiates and may resent the fact that she continues to be involved if he does not enjoy them. The older woman is placed in a very difficult bind if he tells her on the one hand, "I don't want you to just sit around the house because I am" and on the other hand, "You are gone so much and spend so much time with your friends that I never see you." A similar no-win situation can arise when economic circumstances lead the older woman to seek employment or when she chooses not to schedule her retirement to complement her spouse's.

Her decision to continue to work, or to go to work, can be motivated by economic or personal needs or a combination of both. When the husband directly challenges the importance of her employment, when she herself is caught in feelings of guilt about what is good for her vs. him; or when her continued work is an economic necessity while at the same time producing much loneliness for the spouse; her choices are not simple. Often there is no one with whom she can confer in making the decision so she decides in favor of what is good for her spouse, then lives with its consequences for herself. If it works out to their mutual satisfaction, she may be able to rationalize that this was the best way to preserve their marriage. However, it may not prove satisfactory and she may realize the price she has paid, but she will suffer in silence because she perceived the decision to be her duty to her husband and their marriage. To respond otherwise would be a direct violation of what she considers her appropriate role as wife.

When considering dyadic relationships as a source of isolation or as the resolution of isolation problems, it is important to consider sibling and friend relationships (Hess, 1979). Studies in the 1960s and 1970s on friendship among the elderly are inconsistent. They suggest that some older people never form new friendships and that others have more friends than when they were younger. Women, more so than men, appear to have a certain flexibility in the object of close relationships (Blau, 1961; Cantor, 1979). However, little is known about how they experience isolation when close friends die or when in late life they find themselves without geographical access to friends and/or unable to maintain relationships at a distance. A few illustrations can clarify the types of circumstances in which friendship can play important roles in the lives of older women in diverse ways.

Milly Seaver

Milly, who had never been married, lived in the same community where she had taught school. She described a long history of good and close friendships that had always sustained her and, in her words, had supplemented limited family relationships. These friendships were very meaningful and had proved to be a source of social support. She described her fears of being lonely once she had to face mandatory retirement. She decided that it made sense for her to find another retired school teacher or some other woman she thought she might be able to live with. This decision had potential advantages as well as disadvantages. She knew she would benefit economically from sharing expenses and thought she would enjoy adapting to living with someone after many years of being alone.

Milly thought at first that it would be easy to find someone with whom she could develop such an arrangement. Her first route was through her circle of a few close friends. As she approached both of the women she thought might find the arrangement acceptable it began to appear as though "too much intimacy would breed contempt." She said:

"I was inviting them to consider moving into my home and each of us had households and daily habits that we were really not willing to alter very much. I had a trial with one of my friends and it almost proved to be the end of our friendship. Thus I gave that idea up because I felt it would only ruin our friendship.

"I sat alone in my house for the first year of my retirement. I participated in every social opportunity that became available to me and I explored all that was of interest in the way of new hobbies, but I missed the routine of being connected to the school, having contact with the children and their families so I knew that I had to do something.

"At that time, the church that I have belonged to for years decided that it would make a commitment to support refugee families to relocate in our community. We had few congregation funds to do so and the minister had asked whether members of the church thought that they could open their homes to these families if the church could supplement what the families were given by the government.

"At first I thought that it was my Christian duty as a member of the church to make my home available so I volunteered. Now, two years later, I have had two families living with me. First was a Vietnamese couple with two children and they stayed only a few months. Then I had an opportunity to have a young Cuban woman move in with me who had a retarded child. The fact that I have them living with me is one of the best experiences of my life. I have been able to have a family; it is like having a daughter and a grandson that I never had before. They can stay with me as long as I'm alive if that is what they want.

"This situation really worked out far better for me than living with one of my friends because what I really wanted was another purpose to my life after I had retired and I think that I just misread what having a friend live in my house was all about. I wanted a reason for living and I might have tried to put that expectation onto friends without even knowing it.

"As to your question about friendship and isolation; I would caution other older women, especially women who have never married and had a number of friends, to recognize what friendships mean and not try to make arrangements that won't work out. I could have ended up without my friends if they or I had tried to accommodate too much to circumstances which didn't fit our wants and needs."

Shara Larsen

Shara had been widowed in midlife and married Bud shortly after her first husband had died and her two sons had graduated from college. She was in comfortable economic circumstances and her second husband had retired twice, first from the Army and then from an industrial consulting firm. She had never lived in frequent association with women she called her friends even though through the years she had many acquaintances, mothers of her children's friends, and the wives of her husband's business associates. She prided herself on being "the" woman in the lives of her two husbands, and on the close relationships she had maintained with her two sons and their families. She had always felt closest to the men in her life. Shara reflected on how she had constructed her life around these primary relationships:

"I suppose that I have always felt that the men I married were really my best friends. They and my sons took up most of my time and emotions. I never felt that it was necessary for me to develop closer relationships with women. I wasn't in need of them. When Bud retired, we considered moving to Florida to one of the retirement communities that he thought he might like, but I talked him out of that.

"We both have had good health and ample economic resources to live just about any way we saw fit so I suggested that we just use these years of good health to travel. That is just what we have been doing and enjoying it very much. We have met a lot of interesting retired couples on various tours. It has been fun meeting those people. We travel with them for a while and get to know them well enough on the trips, and then after it's over we all return to our separate lives. Bud and I don't feel the need for more close relationships with other couples."

When asked if she had thought about what she might do if her husband died, she quickly responded:

"Certainly, I'll go to live with my youngest son and his wife. I have already talked about this with them and we have made plans. I think that they'll want to relocate to a more southern climate so when the time comes I will invest some of my capital to make sure that they have an adequate house for themselves with a small attached apartment for me.

"I think that my daughter-in-law will probably go back to get an advanced degree because I'll be there to help her take care of their children and give her the assistance she needs to run her household and go to school. At that point I think I'll be ready to start participating in senior citizen activities and it's for sure that I'll then meet a number of women who I can do things with because there are so many widowed women who participate in these programs."

Belle Osborne

Belle was 64 and had been very involved with her husband's home care as an in-home renal dialysis patient who had been maintained on a kidney machine for five years. Her major supportive functions included acting as the person who supervised and monitored his dialysis three times a week. Her view of friendship and the importance of friends in her life was very different from Milly's or Shara's:

"Before Clarence had to go on dialysis we were very involved with lots of people and I enjoyed having the opportunity to spend time with several close friends, but his illness certainly did change our social life. Fortunately, I didn't lose my close friendships as these women have been friends for so many years. Sometimes when you expect the least from friends you get the very most from them.

"My very best friend actually learned how to monitor Clarence's dialysis machine in case of a need for an emergency backup person. She really did that out of love for me and has never asked anything in return. I hope the day will come when I can repay all of her kindnesses. She is really the only person who knows how hard it has been on me to try to care for him at home.

"When I can get him scheduled at the clinic in order to have some free time for myself, she and I always spend some of that time together. Sometimes I just pour my frustrations out and she listens so well. Some of the other wives I know with similar problems don't seem to have anybody to talk to, so I try to lend them some of the support she has given me. That makes me feel like I can give to others what she so generously gives to me."

These three cases illustrate the diversity of friendships in the lives of older women. Milly's case suggests that a woman with a social network of friends was able to assess how those relationships should not be used to fill personal needs and how they could be used to keep her as actively engaged as she cared to be. To the extent that older women with this type of friendship network can make such a realistic assessment of friendship potential, they probably are able to maximize the positive returns because they are aware of themselves, understand their friends, and have mutual respect.

Shara is a woman who has had a very satisfying life with few if any female friends she considers close. Her social and emotional needs for intimate relationships have been met through her two marriages and her family. She is realistic about her future need for some social life if she becomes widowed and to construct another form of involvement through participation in groups where she will meet other women. She intends that these relationships not be a replacement for family involvement but a supplement to it. She is somewhat less realistic in planning for her future role living with her son because she may not have considered all potential problems.

Belle is a woman who perceives her long-standing close friendship as one of her greatest gifts. She expresses her dependency on her friend and her gratitude. The friendship provides her with an opportunity to be replenished and supported as she attempts to sustain a difficult care-giving relationship with her spouse.

ISOLATION IN THE CONTEXT OF INTERPERSONAL RELATIONSHIPS

In recent years, some attention has been given to the role of siblings in the lives of older people (Gubrium, 1975). More information is needed to determine the extent to which the presence of supportive sibling relationships can serve functions that are similar to those of close friendships. There appears to be change in the relationship of siblings as they age; sometimes they do not grow supportive and close until late in life. There is an element of functional supportiveness between older women and their sisters and/or brothers.

These kinds of arrangements are fostered most easily when there is close geographical proximity and where there is some type of mutual dependency. Sometimes this involves joint living arrangements with a sharing of personal skills such as the trade-off in which the older women perform domestic functions in exchange for a brother's providing home repair or transportation. In other cases, it is shared social activity. However, little consideration has been given to the type of isolation that can arise when an older woman is unable, for whatever reasons, to have access to the support of a sibling relationship if she desires it. The consequences of lifelong estrangements from siblings also can have an isolating impact on some older women, especially if they have lost other important social bonds or feel the need to settle longstanding hostilities or unintentional neglect.

It was the intention in this section to avoid the topic of widowhood as an isolator because it is the one event in the lives of a large proportion of older women that many authors have addressed (Atchley, 1975; Arling, 1976; Berardo, 1970; Lopata, 1979). However, one aspect of widowhood that seems too little recognized as an isolator is the effect of persistent recall of past intimacy with a spouse to the point where it blocks the older woman from developing effective social interactions. It may come in the form of unresolved grief that does not get worked out or it can be manifested as an avoidance mechanism for women who surround themselves with memories of a husband and their past life together to avoid developing new relationships. This pattern may be a form of adaptation in cases where the woman's social skills are seriously deficient. She may lack the ability to structure opportunities to meet and interact with both men and women. While it would be inappropriate to thrust social skills training onto an older woman merely because someone evaluates her as deficient in those areas, it would be equally unacceptable for her not to have the opportunity to learn new abilities. To learn these skills requires support and encouragement, but not coercion.

The discussion of isolators, in the context of social relationships, has concentrated on dyadic relationships that seem important for older women and that can promote or reduce isolation. Multiple person networks can serve a similar function and can be vehicles for older women to avoid isolation through extended family, work, leisure time activities, voluntary associations, or helping.

Rapidly accumulating data suggest that families remain connected to older women (Brody, 1981). Women over 80 were more likely to see their children than those below that age. Socioeconomic status of families has been found to have some relation to contact between children and aged parents. Older persons with lower-class backgrounds have more children and tend to live with them more than do their middle-class counterparts. These data tend to dispel the myth that in. general the elderly are isolated from family life and raise questions about how and why this myth has been perpetuated (Cantor, 1979).

It still is shocking to see the extent to which older women in mental health and clinical settings have been viewed as clients with problems, in isolation from their families. The majority of these women were treated as though they did not have families, or that their relationships with them reflected such estrangement that there was no use in assessing their situation in a family network context. Various forms of the family (as distinct from neighborhood peer groups), friends, and other multiple group networks may provide the major protective factor against isolation. When older women lack the option of involvement with the family in a variety of physical, social, and psychological roles, isolation can become a reality.

It is necessary only to compare the range of circumstances or family forms among older women to realize that there is no single pattern of relationships that can always assure that these connections will protect them against isolation. However, in some forms or structures, it may be easier for older women to maintain a humanizing experience within their families. Family contact can be enriching when there is an opportunity for interdependency and mutual exchanges (as compared to one-dimensional dependency), equality of relationships among the generations, and effective supports for the older woman that benefit her and all other members. For some older women the nonisolating balance they can attain in relationship to their families may require that they become "liberated" in such ways as:

- learning how to make decisions without relying on family members to make them or to subvert their own well-being for the good of others

- selecting activities that broaden their social network to ensure personal growth

- arranging or maintaining a life style that allows them personal freedom even at the expense of making family members uncomfortable because the elderly are trying to be too independent.

Enmeshing an aging mother into a family may serve to isolate her from her own potential by isolating her within the family system. Simply stated, an older woman can experience isolators in the context of her family if she is not allowed to, or strives to, attain what is for her a personally appropriate balance between independence and dependence.

For increasing numbers of older women and their relatives, intrafamily relationships cannot be defined automatically or remain fixed. Given the rapid rate and profound scope in the changing status of women, there are no universally accepted roles or functions that family members will assume on behalf of the elderly or that these women will assume on their own behalf. Most older women do not have cognitive maps for being mothers, grandmothers, or great-grandmothers. Therefore, tensions become predictable when interactions lead to misinterpretations and misunderstandings about who wants and needs what from whom, across and within generations. The lack of clarity may be greatest in times of crisis. Crises occur more frequently as a result of something that happens to the older woman, such as the death of her spouse or an illness, but they also can develop in younger generations through traumatic events such as divorce, loss of job, or illness.

Older women might fare better in family relationships if they were socialized or resocialized to develop goals for themselves rather than to define only personal goals directly linked to relatives. A focus on self has been a motivating principle for a small proportion of older women as compared to the large proportion who have been affected by what is good for other people. It is not intended to promote a simplistic analysis of feminism as an alternative to the cohorts of older and elderly women. Rather, it is to say that older women should be encouraged to act and perceive themselves in their later life with a sense of self that is not totally influenced by a sense of family, within the limits of health and economic restrictions. This is the older woman's right, even though it may be lost sight of by well-meaning family.

At a more concrete level, lack of financial support for health care and social, medical, nutrition, housing, and leisure services places restrictions on the older woman that impinge on her relatives and their interactions with her. Intimacy and support certainly is not assured in the midst of economic affluence but poverty or near poverty is such a common state of affairs that many older women's relationships or interactions with their families are linked economically. Until entitlement—a universal right to available support systems—becomes the policy and law of the land, too many older women and members of their family networks will have insufficient resources to provide a quality home environment for themselves (Sussman, 1976).

The environmental dimensions that create isolation from family must be considered in the context of the supports that are available to reinforce the social connectedness between children of whatever age and elderly parents. The lack of family financial and service incentives for providing care to older women was a reality in 1981 that in the future could be reversed by federal policies, largely because of the high costs of institutionalization and out-of-home services. To the extent that those policies and the lack of noninstitutional alternatives keep the older woman removed from the family and place the relatives in a position of being unable to cover the cost of arrangements that integrate rather than estrange her, these environmental isolators are very significant.

ISOLATION IN WORK AND LEISURE ROLES

Work and leisure networks can be a positive resource for older women to sustain social relationships. These opportunities should be considered separately for cohorts of middle-aged and elderly women because many of the latter never had a work role that would give rise to a job-related peer network. Many also lacked leisure networks because relationships were primarily linked to the family and the homemaker role. This trend is reversing rapidly, however, as more older women work and thus retire from the job force under circumstances similar to men. The degree to which retirement may promote isolation for older women will depend upon their circumstances before they left their jobs. Much of the current evidence for the continuance of friendship patterns following retirement is based on all-male samples. Even these studies do not present consistent findings on the maintenance of friendship patterns.

The limited attention given to women and retirement has tended to focus on those in higher socioeconomic work positions; often they are professionals and well educated by the standards of their cohort. The few studies of female retirees suggest that work is a major focus for many employed wives (Streib & Schneider, 1971; Jacobson, 1974; Atchley, 1976; Fox, 1977). Yet, despite the passage of the Age Discrimination Act in 1967 and the right to continue to work past 65, older women are victims of subtle or direct pressure to remove themselves if employers do not view their age as a hindrance. A woman of 65 who had been employed as a secretary in a large medical school complex reflected on some of the isolators she had experienced during her department's effort to get her to retire:

"Once the Age Discrimination Act was passed, I thought that I could breathe and really relax because I was legitimatized by law to continue to work at the university until I was 70 years old. I might have been very naive, guess I was, considering what happened to me. The series of indirect messages I got about taking advantage of early retirement benefits, then the encouragement I got from the personnel office to apply for Social Security and consider some optional health plan, all seemed to be hints.

"At first I thought that they were simply trying to make sure that I had all of my paper work straight and that they were working for my benefit, but once I told them that I had already studied the various options and how they would leave me financially and that I planned to continue to work, that source of pressure was taken off and I began to get it from the department where I was a secretary/receptionist.

"First it was in the form of one of the administrators asking me if I really felt up to the rough training that all of the secretaries in our department would have to take on the new computerized machines. The implications were that I might not really want to put out all the effort because I was probably going to retire before the entire system got into operation. The fact that all the secretaries were going to have to be working under production quotas come the next year was also supposed to scare me.

"I was the last of my original secretarial work group to actually retire. Most of the other women I had known for 20 years had retired some time ago. I called them to ask what they thought I should do and they said to "get out" because I really didn't need the pressure. The younger secretaries that I worked with were kind, but they couldn't really understand what I was going through while I weighed the alternatives. At their young age, the thought of being pressured to retire had no meaning because they had little investment in their place as a working woman in that particular office.

"Mainly because I wanted the extra time to spend with my children who were returning from several years in Japan, I decided to go ahead and retire. I'm content with that decision for now because I plan to take a part-time job, but I am not happy about the treatment I received there, but if I had made waves I think that I would have been ignored and labelled as an 'old troublemaker.' "

In this particular situation, this pressured retirement largely involved the older woman's being shut off involuntarily from a role she preferred to continue. On that count she was fortunate because her economic and health situation gave her options, but many women lack that security.

The differences between leisure and voluntary networks and the sources of social relationships they offer can be confused easily by those who do not routinely observe older women involved in, or seeking involvement in, one or the other or both. There is little or no consistent indication that relationships based on leisure activity can satisfy the range of needs for emotional intimacy older women feel in isolation. For some, leisure groups simply do not provide the opportunities for meaningful social interactions that are readily available in volunteerism. The community-based voluntary association alternative is one of the major conceptual and programmatic cornerstones of the aging network and its approach to isolation (Estes, 1979).

Significant numbers of older women may find meaningful social connectedness through involvement in volunteer activities. There are literally thousands of volunteer programs operating throughout the United States that are either staffed solely by older women or that run their programs largely through the time and efforts they contribute. The volunteer role is one that traditionally is compatible with older women's previous socialization and is linked to family and nurturer functions.

One of the problems with the volunteer role is the extent to which it sets up situations where older women can be exploited without their realizing it. It should be questioned whether or not older women undertake doing for, and giving to, others because it is expected of them, because they perceive it as the only acceptable alternative, or because in actuality it is the only way they have access to meaningful involvement that the community encourages or supports.

Perhaps the greatest form of isolation emerges from situations where their availability, willingness, and talents are used in volunteer roles to assist others when in reality it is they who need support in the form of financial assistance or income supplements, persons to listen to their problems and become their advocates, or someone to encourage them to take self-helping actions. It is to be wondered how many times older women have attempted to address the needs of others when they faced some of the same problems. For example, they have worked with a deprived child when one of their own grandchildren was suffering emotional neglect from parents but was not geographically accessible, or they helped at a church charity when they needed the assistance they were providing but were too prideful to accept what others offered.

Practitioners should not overgeneralize about what an isolated older woman gains through participation in such programs. It is more important to encourage and support her in assessing her own gains and estimate whether her participation is meeting her needs and expectations. It is important to stress for older women that:

- Volunteer roles are not the only solution for dealing with the lack of social involvements for all because many of them lack the desire to participate in these activities.
- The daily living circumstances of many do not leave them with the energy to be enthusiastic volunteers because they must spend what personal resources they have on their own survival and well-being.
- Volunteer functions may lead to one-way giving that does not contribute to self-satisfaction from helping themselves.

For older women in these circumstances it would appear that another form of voluntary participation might be more realistic. For the lack of a more familiar concept, a better type of volunteerism could be loosely termed self-help. Self-help groups can be organized outside the formal structure of any human service organization and directed toward dealing with a wide spectrum of problems that numbers of older women encounter.

The best-known example is based on self-help for widows, but other types of groups are appearing across the country with other problem foci, including older women who are providing care-giving functions for older spouses or whose husbands are institutionalized, women who have chronic health problems such as diabetes and need support for diet maintenance or compliance with medication regimes, those who are experiencing dislocation because of increasing condominium conversions, and victims of violence and exploitation.

This form of participation also includes the dual role of helping themselves with a specific problem or need that is isolation promoting while at the same time assisting others. The group need not consist only of older women but the fact that there are many problems specific to later life makes it reasonable and valuable to encourage self-help groups in addition to those offering a wide age range and both male and female members.

The problems that give rise to the formation of these groups are also the sources of isolation. A group of peers who share the same problem, are familiar with the accompanying isolation-producing stresses, and are committed to finding solutions can serve as a direct interventive response to some isolators. Volunteer roles do not offer the same intervention potential even though they are important in reducing social and emotional isolation.

At the very least, to provide an understanding of older women, isolation should be viewed in the context of a full life span. To do otherwise is to run the risk of ignoring or misunderstanding the lifelong patterns of socialization, values, and behaviors that make each one's position unique. However, the informed understanding of life span performance is not to be equated with an estimate of current potential. Some isolators may have existed for many years and others may result from current circumstances or status as both old and female. The ability of older women to form new alternatives and behaviors and undertake new challenges is part of their potential. To the extent that growth possibilities are ignored, not understood, or not facilitated by the older women or others in a position to intervene, another form of isolation emerges that may be reinforced by the myths and stereotypes of being old and female.

This discussion points out the range of isolators that might impact on segments of the older female population and that should be the focal point for intervention. The analysis further reflects an orientation toward older women outside of the formal helping systems or services. The next section describes cases of women brought into the helping network through contacts with age-specific and problem-specific agencies. It suggests how, in the process of receiving interventions, these women not only continued to experience isolators and become more estranged but how new problems emerged through the helping process.

SOMETHING WRONG IN THE HELPING PROCESS

A major research endeavor would be required to empirically validate the long-range outcomes and consequences of the clinical services and programmatic resources that are being offered daily to senior citizens throughout the nation. Too many interventive programs are offered routinely without benefit of objective evaluation of their outcomes. Few evaluations attempt to specifically examine outcomes for target groups of older women. Therefore, many of the critics of these services rely on subjective judgments by the clients and practitioners directly involved to determine their effectiveness. Several cases are summarized from that standpoint. These cases are fairly representative of some of the difficulties in providing interventive services to older women who have complex personal needs and critical limitations in the way of environmental resources.

Helen Winters

She was a thin, wispy woman, 67 years old. Her white, wavy hair framed a bony and fragile looking face. She would appear younger than her years were it not for the anxious, lost, and frightened expression that seemed to be a permanent aspect of her appearance: her face reflected her critical circumstance. Information in her social history showed she had spent a lifetime listening to others and doing their bidding. As she grew older, one source of domination was exchanged for another.

Helen was a woman whose life's boundaries had been very narrow. She never traveled more than a hundred miles from her birthplace. She never held a job and never lived independently. Her only contact with a wider world was through television, which she watched incessantly. As a child, Helen had polio, which resulted in a permanent weakness in one leg that caused her to limp and lose her balance fairly easily. After the polio, she developed severe headaches and had trouble concentrating. Her family physician felt that school was an unnecessary distraction and encouraged the family to end her formal education after the fifth grade. Since she was not involved in school, her time was spent living in her parents' home, cooking, cleaning, and doing other domestic chores. She had no friends, was never encouraged to make them, and was not close to any family member.

When she was 35, Helen married her sister's ex-husband and for the first time moved out of her father's house. However, her life continued in the same way. She cooked and cleaned for her husband, rarely saw anyone else, and left the house only to shop with him. She never learned to drive or use public transportation. She never had children or joined a church. Her life revolved around her husband and the maintenance of their small house.

Helen's husband died after an extended chronic illness and she found herself totally alone with almost no income or resources for self-help. At this point she became connected, for the first time, with a social service agency. Under the advice and pressure of a social worker, she entered a nursing home, although she had no chronic ailment serious enough to warrant this placement. With proper support and training she could easily have maintained herself in the community. At this stage in her life, listening to the advice and directions of others was a long-established pattern.

Helen finally reached a point where her situation, created by others' decisions, was becoming intolerable. She had suffered through the adjustment period of the nursing home only to realize that she could not survive in that environment; lingering there against her wishes, she developed a severe depression. She described her daily responses in the home:

"I couldn't stop crying. . . . No matter what I did or where I was, the tears just kept coming from my eyes. I thought that there weren't so many tears in one soul. Even when my husband died, I didn't cry so much, and I miss him. I miss him so much."

It took time for her depression to be reduced and longer for her to form a sense of trust with the social worker. Once that person made a concentrated effort to support her in making personal decisions, for perhaps the first time, Helen set about deciding for herself what she wanted to do. When the worker asked her what goals she had for herself she said: she wanted to leave the nursing home, she wanted to live in a place of her own where she could have some privacy and quiet, and she wanted to meet nice people.

Helen's depression was seen in terms of illness by her doctor and the nursing staff at the home. She was referred for treatment at a psychiatric unit, where she was hospitalized, medicated, and faced the possibility of shock treatment if she failed to become less depressed. The prognosis was for a short stay in the hospital so she could be returned as quickly as possible to the familiar nursing home environment.

A number of inappropriate interventions were imposed on Helen. The original nursing home placement was not warranted by any medical or psychiatric problem. It was selected because it was available and because Helen did not protest, nor did anyone else. Once in the nursing home she displayed symptoms that medical and nursing staff reacted to as psychiatric without taking into account the information provided by the social worker. Once Helen was in the state hospital, another worker was able to support her effort to verbalize preferences and wants but the system had insufficient flexibility and resources to offer any alternative but a return to the nursing home. Alternative intervention might include:

- A different type of placement such as senior citizen housing or a semi-independent group home would have worked either the first or second time.

- Advocacy efforts could have given Helen support to protest the first nursing home placement. An advocate, possibly attached to the aging network, could have helped her make her needs known to others.

- Training in self-management and independent living skills could have capitalized on her strong motivation to do something. Unfortunately, the professional functions of generating alternatives and then providing the supports necessary to help her learn how to perform under those environmental demands were not available.

- Better linkage to, and greater exploration of, possible family resources could have ascertained whether relatives could offer short-term housing while noninstitutional alternatives were sought.

Coral Foster

Coral was a handsome black woman whose high cheekbones, strong nose, and beautiful ruddy brown skin clearly show her Indian heritage. She was large, still muscular and strong despite her 75 years, and carried herself with great dignity. Coral had 12 grown children, more than 30 grandchildren, and numerous great-grandchildren, although she could not keep their names and ages straight. She considered them ''gifts from the Lord'''and felt fortunate to have such a large family.

Coral, who came from a small rural community in Mississippi, had a special and wonderful relationship with the Lord, whom she regarded as a personal friend and adviser. She had been living alone, but across the street from a grandchild, when her behavior became a matter of concern to the minister of her little church and to her family. Her husband had died a year earlier and although she had taken his death well, she had started missing him greatly in the past few months. She wept a great deal for him but in the process of mourning found that she had lost more than just a husband.

"It seemed as if the Lord weren't listening to me any more," she said. "I couldn't bear to live without the Lord, but he seemed to have left me. I feel like I lost my soul."

Coral's difficulty was complicated by the strong concern and involvement of her large family. They were constantly surrounding her, day and night. She needed to be able to find space for herself in the middle of profuse and disorganized comfort from her kin. Her routine functions in her role as homemaker for herself were being taken over by her granddaughters. The children took her from doctor to doctor, insisting that she be given pills to "fix her up," but did not provide her an opportunity to select which physician to see or, more important, the right to refuse to go. With each new doctor came more medication and since many relatives were making sure that she was taking them from previous and current physicians, no one was clear about what ones she was on or how much she was consuming. It was medication overdose at a dangerous level that left her with pronounced confusion, disorientation, crying spells, and lack of appetite.

Coral finally was taken to a hospital emergency room accompanied by two cars of family members. Fortunately, one granddaughter studying to be a nurse's aid packed grandmother's slippers, medications, and Bible in the event that she had to be admitted to the hospital, which did occur immediately following the preliminary examination. Medical intervention steps were instituted immediately but the medical social work plan did not attempt to assess her situation in relation to the extended family. Important intervention possibilities were missed, for example:

1. Coral had one major isolator operating: her grief. She needed privacy and personal space to progress through the stages of the process she had long delayed to protect her family. When she began to manifest overt grief, her family moved in to "protect her from herself," which encouraged self-isolation. Under a different interventive approach she might have been able to get sufficient support from a medical social worker to enable her to tell her family to give her a chance to work out her grief. Coral might have been able to evaluate whether or not she wanted to join a widow-to-widow group. If an effort had been made to involve the pastor, he could have talked with key family members and his suggestions would be accepted more readily because of his close ties with them.

2. Her pattern of touring physicians' offices needed to end. Family members were perpetuating the cycle and Coral was going along with their decisions. Had a mental health professional been associated with the first physician she encountered, early intervention could have been directed toward developing an alternative schedule of family involvement that would complement Coral's need for less rather than more attention. The key family members might have been able to gain insight into the double bind in which they were placing Coral and that she could not resist. On one hand, the adult children verbally credited their mother with being as "strong as a rock and able to do everything," but on the other hand, were responding to her as though she were "weak and able to do nothing."

3. She would not have become an inadvertent drug abuser if she had not accumulated 10 types of medication. With only one or two medicines she could have monitored herself and had little or no problem with compliance. Had a problem developed, the most qualified family member could have been designated to help Coral monitor herself and keep other family members informed about her ability to stay on the schedule to relieve their tensions.

Anna Roth

The most striking thing about Anna was her sparkling brown eyes. She was a heavy, florid woman of about 72 with curly golden hair done up in a casual old-fashioned style. She dressed in colorful, loose robes that looked attractive on her round, rather shapeless body. Her skin was covered with a multitude of fine scars from many surgical procedures to remove small skin tumors that came from a carcinoma that had plagued her for years. Anna also was being treated for uterine cancer and a variety of other illnesses such as hypertension and an inner ear disorder that left her with a limited sense of balance. Her medical problems were among those common to older women but some of her health problems dated back to early midlife.

In conversation, Anna gave the feeling of complex independence to the point where, during a brief meeting, a practitioner might assume that she had no need of professional help. She was a witty woman who loved to laugh, was clever and funny, and had definite style. Anna considered herself a professional writer. At one time she showed great promise and had written for magazines. She also had published several novels, now forgotten by most people. Her writing career was considered a frivolous waste of time by her husband's family, who felt she had been neglectful of her children and, more importantly, of her husband's career as a physician.

"They told me that it was as important to be a doctor's wife as it was to be a doctor," she said, laughing, and "that I was fortunate to have a doctor for a husband. They told me that the way I dressed, entertained, and conducted myself would impact greatly on his career. We married when I was only 17, and his family was furious, they didn't think I was good enough to be a doctor's wife. Of course he was never home. He was out doing important work 20 out of 24 hours, all for me, he said. Everything was for me and the kids so that we would have all the luxuries.

"Yet he was furious when I hired a maid, so that I could have more time for writing. A maid was all right in itself, but the time that it gave me was supposed to be spent on anything but myself. He never approved of my clothes; he never approved of my friends. He called them leeches and useless. He never spent any time with the kids. I don't know what happened between my children and myself. Somewhere along the line a great resentment was built up, but I don't have the energy to worry about it now."

Anna's situation was one of sustained stress, not an immediate crisis. At that moment she did not have to make a decision as to whether to continue living alone or find an alternative where she could get better intervention and perhaps preventive care for her deteriorated physical condition. She seemed to have been obsessed for some time with the fear of entering a nursing home that was both repugnant and unacceptable to her.

Anna's situation was different from Coral's. Anna had succeeded in cutting herself off entirely from her family to the extent that they were not aware of her condition. She felt that they would not care if they knew and pride would not allow her to risk testing their feelings. Her financial situation was more than adequate so she did not face an economic isolator. Her isolators were the fear and anger that had been present for more than 10 years and were increasing as she tried to defend herself against the prospect of a nursing home and of dying without her family. She had no faith in psychiatrists because of a long history of seeing a series of her husband's psychiatric colleagues with no perception of personal benefit.

A practitioner interested in giving therapy to older women might be eager to work with this woman. Her potential for change was strong in relation to her behaviors, her relationship deficits, and her perceptions of her present and future. If she were a client, the following procedures could be considered:

1. Let Anna state her own problems and through this process let her define goals for herself. For the practitioner to superimpose a definition of her real problems would be likely to turn her away from therapy and reinforce Anna's perception of an inhibiting therapeutic relationship.
2. Select a behavioral program to help Anna overcome her near phobic reaction about a nursing home, an attitude that seemed to include all types of alternative settings, even those where she would have almost total independence.
3. Encourage—actively, if necessary—her explorations of alternatives in the community that might be acceptable to her need for independence while also meeting her health care requirements.
4. Suggest that she use her writing skills to facilitate her emotional exploration of her family's rejection and what actions she really wanted to take to mend these broken bonds. This exploration might form the basis for possible family interventions to rebuild links with her children and their families.

These suggestions of possible intervention alternatives support the notion that individual, family, and group arrangements all can be considered potentially viable. None of the three cases point to possible use of couples counseling as a form of family therapy. However, such therapy should be added to the list of what may be beneficial for other older women. In cases where it is applied, the marital counselor will need to have some understanding of the midlife and late life stages of the marriage cycle and try to reframe the process of establishing goals to ensure that appropriate objectives are set for the older couple, with at least equal input from the wife.

The three cases suggest the possibility of practitioner efforts being directed toward the family. In two cases, the intention to reorganize the family was related to specific problems: finding more distant kinship sources to give Helen a housing situation while a community-based arrangement was found, and inducing numerous members of Coral's family to conform to a less protective and less disorganized series of helping activities. For Anna, the possibility of more extensive family therapy could be pursued, under the right conditions, to resolve longstanding conflict.

Other general intervention issues also emerged from these cases. Every older woman has contributed to other human beings and this can be reinforced as a positive while at the same time she can be encouraged to maintain or develop some self-interest in moving toward her potential. That concept must be operationalized for each woman, and these three cases suggest the differences in what that might mean. The older woman has the right, however, not to be blamed if she does not act to develop her self-potential. The clinical intervenor's function is not to blame her but to help her find and understand her realistic potential, given her functional capacities and personal preferences.

Older women derive much value from integrating memories of their past as they involve significant others and events. Very careful assessment is required before a practitioner evaluates ''hanging onto the past'' as a negative for the older woman. What may be most meaningful for a woman in the present and future will be built on that past life style and those relationships.

Encouraging independence is an important goal that is easy to lose sight of if women are very frail and/or ill. There are many types of dependency that tend to be easily confused in the process of establishing goals. Socioeconomic, developmental crisis-related, nonreciprocal role, neurotic, and culturally supported dependencies have distinguishable meanings and behaviors (Clark, 1972). Older women can be in a difficult struggle to be independent without losing support and personal dignity from those they love. The practitioner may have to take the lead in bringing this issue into focus within the context of helping, but should critically examine personal beliefs and values about dependency in order to avoid extending subjective bias to the older women. The balance between dependency and independency in the helping relationship can be hard to identify.

These suggestions reflect the principles supported by feminist-oriented therapy and clinical gerontology, and by the potential of an intergrated perspective. Practitioners should consistently challenge the existence of ageism and sexism biases that create double jeopardy for older women and increase the likelihood that they will be caught in webs of stereotypes and myths. The intervention perspective that was discussed advocates self-determination as essential and suggests that professional intervention is not necessarily more effective than self-help, but the two in combination may well be preferable to professional intervention alone.

Finally, it is proposed that isolation is almost a synonym for being forgotten, female, and alone. The need for better continuing educational opportunities for the range of intervenors who can be of help to older women is fairly clear, but it is less clear how this need is to be recognized among diverse professional groups and then become financially feasible during a period when the costs of training are increasing, the resources to pay for it are decreasing, and practitioners and their agencies are being pulled into a very conservative philosophy of helping.

CONCLUSION

All of the major human service systems need to be better coordinated for the elderly. (Figure 3-2 shows a social resource system for women in late life.) Confirming through empirical research which systems need to be coordinated most extensively to meet particular needs of various subgroups of the elderly is a task yet

Figure 3-2 Late Life Women and the Social Resource System

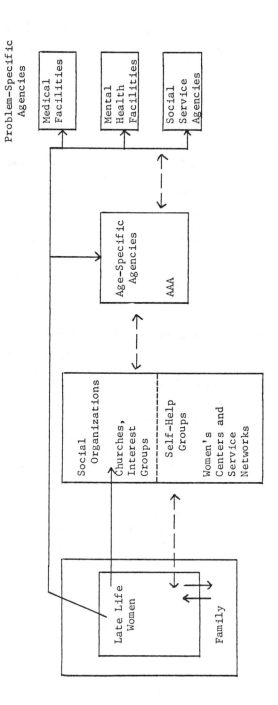

The late life woman is in direct contact with family and community organizations for assistance with social, medical, and mental health problems related to aging needs. These providers, however, often ignore or are unaware of how their planning and responses reflect social stereotypes concerning her needs. Women's groups have yet to become involved in issues concerning older women. There is limited or no interagency planning for special needs of women.

to be accomplished in human service planning. Finding ways to develop some links between services for women and services to the elderly is important. It has not been possible to identify through field research or literature review a model that gives step-by-step suggestions on how this might be accomplished. At the mezzo level of intervention the goal is program development. In communities with both services, many of these could be packaged to facilitate resource coordination.

Less bureaucratic arrangements could be cost efficient and straightforward enough to be workable. For instance, senior health and social centers could contract with gynecological services to offer help that is needed by many older women who are clients of the aging network. There also could be better joint outreach and consultation whereby a center that is oriented toward younger women would be able to extend reasonable services to older ones because it would have gerontological expertise. This might help avoid some of the inappropriate "passing on the older women clients" from one system to another.

In the long run, societal changes that give older women a better place in the social structure require major macrolevel reform. National social policies will have to develop special consideration of older women. To bring about these results there must be advocacy that is well planned and well targeted. As both the women's and the senior citizen political advocacy movements become more effective, perhaps they can be coordinated on behalf of older women. There are preliminary indications that leaders in both movements would like to begin the necessary dialogue but there remains a major unanswered question: How can the silent majority of older women be organized to become a vocal self-interest group with the power of unity behind efforts for social change.

REFERENCES

Arling, G. Resistance to isolation among elderly widows. *International Journal of Aging and Human Development,* 1976, *7,* 67-86.

Atchley, R.C. Dimensions of widowhood in later life. *Gerontologist,* 1975, *15,* 176-178.

Atchley, R.C. *The sociology of retirement.* New York: Halsted Press, 1976.

Barfield, R.E., & Morgan, J.M. Trends in satisfaction with retirement. *Gerontologist,* 1978, *18,* 19-23.

Bart, P. The emotional and social status of the older woman. In N.P. Tragor (Ed.), *No longer young: The older women in America.* Ann Arbor, Mich.: University of Michigan, Institute of Gerontology, 1975.

Berardo, F.M. Survivorship and social isolation: The case of the aged widower. *Family Coordinator,* 1970, *19,* 11-25.

Blau, Z. Structured constraints on friendship in old age. *American Sociological Review,* 1961, *26,* 429-438.

Blieszner, R., & Szinovacz, M. *Women's adjustment to retirement.* Paper presented at the annual meeting of the Gerontological Society, Washington, D.C., November 1979.

Blood, R.O., & Wolfe, D.M. *Husbands and wives: The dynamics of married life.* New York: Free Press, 1960.

Brody, E.M. "Women in the Middle" and family help to older people. *Gerontologist,* 1981, *21,* 471-480.

Cantor, M.H. Neighbors and friends: An overlooked resource in the informal support system. *Research on Aging,* 1979, *1,* 435-463.

Clark, M. Cultural values and dependency in later life. In D.O. Cowgill & L.D. Holmes (Eds.), *Aging and modernization.* New York: Appleton-Century-Crofts, 1972.

Dancy, J., Jr. *The black elderly:* A guide for practitioners. Ann Arbor, Mich.: University of Michigan, Institute of Gerontology, 1977.

Dono, J.E., Falber, C.M., Kail, B.L., Letwak, E., Sherman, R.H., & Siegel, D. Primary groups in old age structure and function. *Research on Aging,* 1979, *1,* 403-433.

Estes, C.R. *The aging enterprise.* San Francisco: Jossey-Bass, Inc., 1979.

Federal Council on Aging. *National policy concerns for older women: Commitment to a better life.* Washington, D.C.: U.S. Government Printing Office, 1977 (Stock No. 052-003-00150-1).

Fox, J.H. Effects on retirement and former worklife on women's adaptation in old age. *Journal of Gerontology,* 1977, *32,* 196-202.

Gove, W., & Hughes, M. Possible causes of the apparent sex differences in physical health: An empirical investigation. *American Sociological Review,* 1979, *44,* 126-146.

Gubrium, J. Being single in old age. *International Journal of Aging and Human Development,* 1975, *6,* 29-41.

Hess, B. Sex roles, friendship and life course. *Research on Aging,* 1979, *1,* 495-509.

Holden, K.C. Public pensions for nonworking wives: Policy choice and equity questions. *Research on Aging,* 1979a, *1,* 65-82.

Holden, K.C. Spouse and survivor benefits: Distribution among older women. *Research on Aging,* 1979b, *1,* 301-318.

Jacobson, D. Rejection of the retiree role: A study of female industrial workers in their 50's. *Human Relations,* 1974, *27,* 477-492.

Johnson, A. Sex differentials in coronary heart disease: The explanatory role of primary risk factors. *Journal of Health and Social Behavior,* 1977, *18,* 46-54.

Kerschner, P.A., & Tiberi, D.M. Health and older women: A look at the knowledge base. *Journal of Gerontological Nursing,* 1978, *4,* 11-15.

Lopata, H.Z. *Women as widows: Support systems.* New York: Elsevier, 1979.

Lowenthal, M.F., & Robinson, B. Social networks and social relations. In R.H. Binstock & E. Shanas (Eds.), *Handbook of aging and the social sciences.* New York: Van Nostrand Reinhold Company, 1976, 432-456.

Matthews, S.H. *The social world of old women: Management of self identity.* Beverly Hills, Calif.: SAGE Publications, 1979.

National Institute on Aging and National Institute of Mental Health. *Report on conference on the older woman: Continuities and discontinuities,* M. Mylander (Ed.). Bethesda, Md.: National Institute on Aging, 1978.

Ortmeyer, L. Female's natural advantage? Or, the unhealthy environment of males? The status of sex mortality differentials. *Women and Health,* 1979, *4,* 121-133.

Pelegrina, I. Ambulatory care of aging women: A gynecologist's point of view. *Clinical Obstetrics and Gynecology,* 1977, *20,* 177-181.

Retherford, R. Tobacco smoking and sex ratios in the United States. *Social Biology,* 1974, 28-38.

Retherford, R. *The changing sex differential in mortality*. Westport, Conn.: Greenwood Press, 1975.

Schein, L. A hard-to-reach population: "Shopping bag women." *Journal of Gerontological Social Work,* 1979, *2*, 29-41.

Seltzer, M.M. The older woman, fact, fantasies and fiction. *Research on Aging,* 1979, *1*(2), 139.

Sommers, T. *Older women and health care: Strategy for survival*. Gray Paper #3, prepared under auspices of Older Women's League Educational Fund, Oakland, Calif., January 1980.

Streib, G.F., & Schneider, C.J. *Retirement in American society: Impact and process*. Ithaca, N.Y.: Cornell University Press, 1971.

Sussman, M.B. The family life of old people. In R.H. Binstock & E. Shanas (Eds.), *Handbook of aging and the social sciences*. New York: Van Nostrand Reinhold, 1976, pp. 218-243.

Turner, B. The self-concepts of older women. *Research on Aging,* 1979, *1*, 464-480.

Uhlenberg, P. Older women: The growing challenge to design constructive roles. *The Gerontologist,* 1979, *19*, 236-241.

Verbrugge, L. Females and illness: Recent trends in sex differences in the United States. *Journal of Health and Social Behavior,* 1976, *17*, 387-403.

Waldron, I. Why do women live longer than men? *Journal of Human Stress,* 1976a, Part I, *2*, 2-13.

Waldron, I. Why do women live longer than men? *Journal of Human Stress,* 1976b, Part II, *2*, 19-30.

Womanpower. Committee on Women's Issues (newsletter). Washington, D.C.: National Association of Social Workers, April 1980, pp. 1-6.

Chapter 4

Service Delivery Issues for Older Veterans

INTRODUCTION

In approaching the task of looking at the isolators that affect elderly men and exploring how they might be different from those faced by older women, only a relatively few differences emerged. Retirement is the single most mentioned potential isolator for men that is different from women in the present cohort of the elderly, but this pattern may be less true among future cohorts.

There is mixed research evidence that retirement is universally seen as an isolator, particularly where the job is menial and gives limited personal satisfaction and where the individual who once faced a dreary job can look to increased satisfaction from other pursuits. On the other hand, some differences between older men and women could be regarded as positives for men in that they insulate many of them from potential isolation. Older men are more likely to be married through their later life than are women, are less likely to spend their later years in a nursing home, and unlikely to lose their pensions or other benefits because their entitlements are connected to some previous work role or other activities in later life.

How these entitlements benefit older men and disadvantage older women was reviewed in Chapter 3 on older women. In this consideration, it became apparent that many older and elderly men have access to a health system and benefits available to few older women (Lyngh, 1980). This system is sponsored by the Veterans Administration. Veteran status is potentially very important to an increasing number of men as they reach later life. Therefore it seemed valuable to direct this analysis of older men toward their veteran status and the care system that serves them.

In the cohort of men now in their 60s and early 70s, a large percentage served in World War II. It is perhaps the most common life experience shared among men of this era. Only 2.1 percent of service personnel in WW II and the Korean conflict were women. The impact of that service and its personal meaning may be lost or forgotten by the majority of men during the postmilitary period, but it can reemerge as important when linked to the possibility of older veterans' using the VA system to meet growing medical needs associated with the aging process. This would be particularly true if veterans were to develop chronic conditions in the face of dwindling private resources or if other third party entitlements proved inadequate to meet continuing care needs.

In addition to the majority of older men for whom military status is not of primary importance during middle years, there is a subgroup for whom their veteran experience is vital. Their veteran status and their service delivery system continue to be important to men who have maintained a lifelong military career and those who for one reason or another did not develop postmilitary family and/or career roles that would produce stabilizing factors following their military experience.

Because of long-standing functional deficits and few alternative roles and relationships, these individuals have maintained their need for connectedness with the veterans' service system. For many, even though their military experiences have long since faded from daily memory, their continuing reliance on the system for needed services or life supports has formed a dependency on and an identity with that network of human services. As this subgroup approaches a period of increasing service needs, its members are likely to increase their already strong dependency on the system for continuing care.

The veterans' service system is in a position to have an adequate estimate of the care needs of career military personnel and of veterans long dependent on it, but it is more difficult to anticipate the needs of the larger group, such as those exposed to atomic testing or other contaminants. However, the majority of immediate new service demands will come from men who in later life for the first time develop needs for the system's services. All of these subgroups together create a potential to overload a major service system that has both age-specific and problem-specific components that often are difficult to integrate for the treatment of old veterans.

Individuals who have been relying almost exclusively on private resources and may now need to turn to the VA system may be faced with a complex system of eligibility requirements that they do not fully understand. Professionals not connected to the system, yet who work with older veterans receiving its services, frequently lack an understanding of eligibility requirements. They are unable to properly advise the veterans and/or their families properly on benefits for which they may be eligible. This lack of professional understanding may be related to the isolation of this system from other service providers in the community.

The system often relies on inpatient care rather than community-based services to help elderly veterans stay out of institutions and, through its own system isolation, inhibits clients from combining community and VA benefits. The VA thus would appear to be encouraging dependence on inpatient care and discouraging clients from staying within their community and taking advantage of what they are entitled to from several systems. Thus the decision to focus on the veteran and the VA system was made because: (a) those who long have been dependent on the VA may be very isolated from community resources, (b) there is a possibility of extensive overloading of the system with older men when existing community services cannot provide all the needed care, and, more importantly, (c) the VA has an untapped potential for assuming leadership in planning coordinated community service delivery to a significant percentage of the older male population both now and in the future.

CHARACTERISTICS OF THE VETERAN POPULATION

Veterans now comprise almost half of the male population over 20 years of age. By 1990, veterans 65 and older will constitute more than half of the elderly population, and by 1995 they will exceed 60 percent of the total above-65 population (Veterans Administration, 1977). In the foreseeable future, the VA system will confront increased demands from older veterans for treatment and supportive services. Concern about that increase in service utilization is predicted on the assumption that certain factors are operative:

1. Veterans have reduced economic resources to meet copayments required by alternatives and there is a larger fraction of economically eligible clients.
2. Widowed, divorced, and single veterans in an increasing proportion will have an increased need for nursing home care and domiciliation.
3. Veterans admitted because of lack of in-home supports that therefore limit placement possibilities will require prolonged hospitalization.
4. Veterans with terminal illness will have an increased use of facilities that may extend over long periods.
5. Veterans will have an increased need for ambulatory services (Veterans Administration, 1977).

In general the characteristics of the veteran population resemble closely those of the total male population. Almost 80 percent of men 65 and over live in families, 78 percent are married, and 20.5 percent are in the labor force. At age 65, men have an average life expectancy of 13.4 years. The vast majority of older males, and thus the vast majority of veterans, are well enough to participate in a wide variety of activities, are reasonably economically secure, and maintain social ties with family and friends (Veterans Administration, 1977; Office of Human Development Services, undated).

Veterans who use the VA system do vary in some ways from those who do not. Applicants for hospital admission tend to be older than nonapplicants; 52 percent of applicants are married, compared to 80 percent of nonapplicants. Veterans hospitalized in VA facilities, compared to those who used all or at least some non-VA facilities, had lower incomes, were more likely to be non-Caucasian, less likely to have private medical insurance, had less education, were more likely to be disabled, and were more likely to have worsening personal finances (National Academy of Sciences, 1977). (Isolators for this group are depicted in Figure 4-1.)

Seventy percent of veterans served by the VA have nonservice-connected disabilities. For some, use of VA facilities came only after they had exhausted other resources. For most veterans the VA system "represents a catastrophic or last resort source of care" (Veterans Administration, 1977). A factor to consider is

---

Figure 4-1 Isolators That Affect Veterans

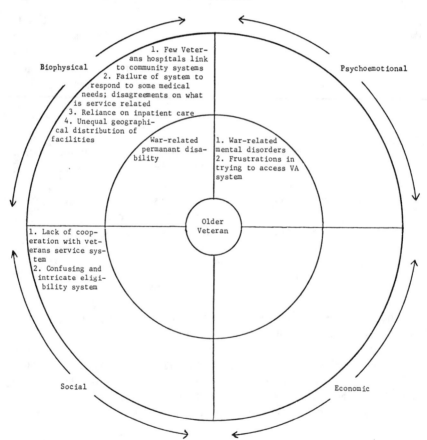

The inner circle contains isolators as they are manifested in the personal lives of older veterans, the outer circle those that abound in the environment.

that the service demands of older veterans tend to come in surges, whereas those of the total elder population are on a smoother upward increase. For the most part older veterans' needs are the same as those for elders in the general population since most involve the chronic diseases of aging rather than combat-related medical needs.

Since veterans comprise such a large and increasing proportion of the male population 65 and over, it would seem unwise to plan for the short-range and long-range service needs of older men without considering the VA service network and the potential to develop new programs to meet current and future need. A major planning objective for older veterans should be to help them make use of community programs in addition to or instead of the specific veteran programs, and not to make the VA system an isolated source of geriatric care.

ELIGIBILITY AND WAYS OF PROVIDING SERVICES

One of the questions that impacts most directly on the emerging geriatric cohorts of older veterans involves eligibility priorities. Congressional mandates state that top priority be given to those with service-connected disabilities and lower priority to those without (National Academy of Sciences, 1977). The question of how these priorities will affect the ever-increasing medical needs of the WW II cohort remains to be seen. As eligibility is defined, older veterans seeking treatment for a service-connected condition are eligible to receive any service available in a VA facility, or if not available there, the agency will pay the costs of having it provided in a non-VA facility. The older veterans thus are helped to move into another service delivery system.

Any veterans who received a medical discharge can be treated for the condition for which they received a medical discharge. Unlimited treatment of a medical condition that began during a tour of active duty is available to veterans at any time after their discharge with a disability rating. Their claims are adjudicated by a board of review, and a disability rating ranging up to 100 percent (or beyond in cases involving serious multiple problems) is awarded on the basis of the permanence and severity of the condition. Veterans with high disability ratings for service-connected conditions also are eligible for care for nonservice-connected health problems. Entitled veterans under 65 without a service disability are eligible for hospital care and most other types of care (except dental) if they certify that they are unable to pay. There is no means test—all entitled veterans over 65 are eligible without certifying inability to pay.

The procedures for providing services to older veterans involve:

1. Direct provision of services: older veterans go directly to a VA medical complex or residential institution where health care is provided. For example, the veterans make outpatient visits to a medical rehabilitation clinic.

2 Purchase of services: The older veterans receive treatment from a non-VA provider through a contract negotiated by the agency or the VA pays one selected by the veteran. For example, veterans who live outside the immediate geographical area of the VA facility may receive home health care services from an agency in their community.
3. Grants to states: Veterans receiving care in a state-sponsored facility will be provided with a grant to cover that cost. For example, a veteran may be receiving care in a state mental hospital (National Academy of Sciences, 1977).

Hospitalization (surgical, medical, dental, or psychiatric), nursing home care, domiciliary care, outpatient medical care, and inpatient dental care all are available for those with a service-connected disability. Additional qualifications are introduced for each service when it is required for a problem that is not associated with a service-connected disability. In this situation the requirements are the same for hospitalization and nursing home care: (a) the veteran is receiving compensation for disability or is entitled to it but is receiving retirement pay instead, or (b) a health condition is associated with and aggravating a service-connected disability, or (c) hospitalization is for care related to a service-connected disability, or (d) care is provided if the patient is willing and services are available for nonservice-connected disability.

Domiciliary care requirements include veterans who: (a) are receiving compensation for permanent disability, or (b) have tuberculosis, or (c) have a neuropsychiatric disorder, cannot earn a living, and have no means of support.

There are numerous circumstances where outpatient medical care is provided: (a) when the condition is associated with and aggravating a service-connected disability, (b) when it is necessary to prepare a veteran for hospital treatment, (c) to complete treatment incidental to hospital care when needed, (d) to eliminate the need for hospital care later, (e) if the veteran is entitled to vocational rehabilitation training, (f) if the veteran has a service-connected disability rating of 50 percent or more, or (g) if the veteran is receiving additional compensation because of being housebound or in need of regular attendance.

The requirements for veterans with no service-connected disability vary from those who do. Theirs are the ones that most determine distribution of medical care since 70 percent of all treatments are provided for those without service-connected disabilities. The same four conditions cover eligibility for both hospital and nursing home care. The veterans must: (a) be 65 years and older, or (b) be a Medal of Honor winner, or (c) state under oath that they are unable to pay expenses, or (d) be receiving a pension. The requirements for domiciliary care involve two conditions: if the veteran served (a) during a wartime era, or (b) after January 31, 1959, and is unable to pay. The major variation between the two groups is that the nonservice-connected veterans are not eligible for vocational rehabilitation training or a percentage disability rating (National Academy of Sciences, 1977).

Despite all of these different requirements, which remain either completely foreign or somewhat confusing to practitioners not connected to the VA system, almost all applicants receive some care. The largest category of service that is denied involves outpatient dental care. Of major importance in this discussion is the point that once veterans reach 65, they are eligible for health care irrespective of their financial status. However, access to care readily available to older veterans does not extend to their dependents (except in cases of total disability), which leaves most older spouses without eligibility.

EXISTING SERVICES IMPORTANT TO OLDER VETERANS

The long-term care needs, both current and projected, are filled by a few specific services that become increasingly important as older veterans age and reach a period of chronic impairments and therefore are at risk of institutionalization. The range of services includes both the institutional-based and the noninstitutional. The nursing home care units (NHCUs) at VA medical complexes (85 units in 171 facilities), the community contract nursing home program that involves both skilled and intermediate levels of care, and the Hospital-Based Home Health Care Program are among the most important and commonly available NHCUs. (These services and their relationship to community resources are depicted in Figure 4-2.)

Each of the 85 NHCUs has some unique features. They vary in number of beds, staffing patterns, waiting lists, and program offerings. In general, these are 24-hour inpatient units providing for veterans who do not require acute hospital care but do need skilled nursing with related medical and health services. Programs emphasize the rehabilitation of each patient but that potential is highly varied in any program. The nursing home care units maintain various types and degrees of service autonomy but are required to comply with the medical policies of the VA complexes to which they are attached. Various levels of care are provided according to the veterans' needs, the capabilities of the unit, and the number of patients that can be treated in any given category.

Screening committees play an important role in the initial and continuing decision making for treatment plans. Admission procedures require medical history, a recent medical examination, a physician's referral, recent test results from standardized procedures including x-ray and EKG, current mental status evaluation, and social and nursing assessments. The NHCU screening committee makes general recommendations on admissions (to admit, cancel, or defer for additional information) that often are referred to higher hospital medical personnel. If a veteran is accepted, a critical point comes if the individual is admitted immediately or placed on the waiting list. Many facilities have long waiting lists, indicating a

Figure 4-2 Older Veterans and the Social Resource System

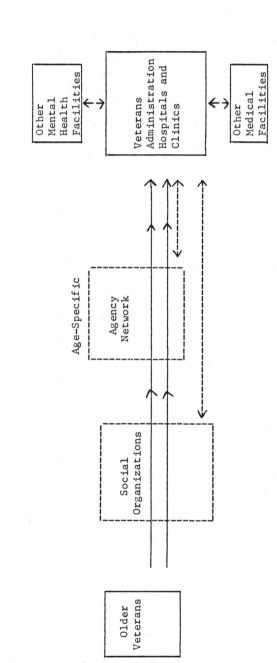

Older veterans with problems they cannot resolve make limited use of community organizations and have little or no communication with VA system. Other problem-specific agencies have limited contact with VA.

need for more beds. The waiting period can be a difficult time for both the veterans and the family or community caregivers.

The nursing home care units provide a number of treatments such as corrective therapy, educational therapy, and social services. Corrective therapists assist patients with physical and/or mental disabilities through the use of medically prescribed physical exercise. The treatment goals are to prevent and/or correct deformities and to maintain or improve physical status, sense of well-being, body image, and self realization with the ultimate goals of returning the patients to maximum physical, mental, and social functioning for living in the community. Corrective therapists use the following modalities to accomplish these patient care goals (Veterans Administration Medical Center, undated):

1. range of motion exercises
2. heavy resistive exercises
3. general conditioning exercises for geriatric patients
4. exercise programs to release aggression and guilt feelings
5. coordination exercises
6. therapeutic swimming for the elderly

Therapists prescribe educational activities to provide opportunities for constructive thinking and progressive reasoning. Educational therapy is becoming increasingly important in the treatment program for long-term geriatric residents.

Manual arts therapists use industrial arts modalities such as metalworking, woodworking, electrical working, graphic and applied arts, and agriculture to stimulate patients emotionally and vocationally. Residents are encouraged to attain intermediate goals and successes that are meaningful to them in terms of contemporary socioeconomic values (Veterans Administration, 1969).

Physical therapists are concerned with the prevention of deformity and the treatment of disease, injury, and disability, with the objective of rehabilitating the patients. They use therapeutic exercises, massages, mechanical devices, and therapeutic agents that employ physical and other properties to rehabilitate patients.

The social services element carries out both inhospital and community liaison activities. The social worker serves on the admission screening committee, takes responsibility for socialization groups, compiles social histories, and works on discharge planning (Department of Medicine and Surgery, 1980). Patients who make progress in rehabilitation can be transferred off the unit to a state veterans home, a community-based nursing home, a residential group, or a family setting.

Those seeking admission to the nursing home care unit may have to wait as much as two or three years so the social worker also must attend to some of the immediate needs of these veterans and their families. This staff member also works with the unit's health team, providing information about the social needs and interests of the individuals; attempts to introduce patients to the range of therapies and activities available through the recreation and occupational therapy departments; and provides individual counseling as a major function. The social worker may carry out liaison activities with outside community agencies such as senior citizen transportation or specialized medical services.

Patient advocacy also is important. Some veterans are afraid to speak to staff members directly about their problems or complaints so they use the social worker as the intermediary. Problems about relationships with staff, roommates, or stolen property, complaints about the food, etc., all may need social worker input to resolve. Some veterans may require help to resolve marital problems. If a patient is drawing a pension and there must be a change in the benefits, the social worker can process the revision. In some cases, the social services staff member also can initiate an appeal process for veterans who are declared incompetent, and may request hearings. The worker can visit family members to calm patients' fears about the well-being of relatives they do not see and talk over adjustment problems with them. The social worker may help patients be readmitted during the 30-day bed-holding period if a community placement does not work out, assist with funeral plans, and work along with the guardian if one is required to handle the legal and personal interests of those who are legally incompetent.

The St. Louis VA facility has a nursing home unit that is fairly typical in terms of the types of patients who reside there and of some of the activities available. The NHCU has 27 WW I veterans, 63 from WW II, and 3 from the Korean conflict. Thirty-eight of them are rated as inpatients because of poor physical health, 22 are there primarily because of mental health problems, and 33 have combined physical and mental problems. About a third of the patients have no social network and a third have a history of alcohol-related problems. Sixty-eight percent do not have spouses and two-thirds have financial need. Forty have an erratic job record with high unemployment since discharge from the military.

Social activities away from the nursing home are an important aspect of programming. One example of the type of activities that can be arranged is described in the following account of a Veterans Day party arranged for nursing home residents.

A VA PARTY AT THE VFW

The Veterans of Foreign Wars (VFW) of Dupo, an Illinois town across the Mississippi River from St. Louis, and its Auxiliary invited 25 of the 93 residents of the nursing home care unit to a supper to celebrate Veterans Day at the VFW Hall.

A flurry of last-minute problems always seemed to characterize the unit when a number of veterans were going out to the community. Procedures always needed to be clarified. This time it was a question from the nursing staff, which said there was no doctor's order to take the patients out, and a last-minute search for drivers for the vans.

Victor, a double amputee, wanted to ride in the front of the van; he loves to go out and was particularly excited about this visit. To see Victor that day would provide a sharp contrast to his usual behavior of sitting in his wheelchair showing little interest in anything or anyone. Victor wore his special tie and jacket; he dresses up only for outside events.

The VFW Hall was decorated and a sense of ceremony pervaded the occasion. On Veterans Day, any hall in a small town can bring recollections of special places for each veteran. Many of the men wore their service caps in honor of the special event that returned them to an organization of which they had been members in earlier years. Those who wore their hats seemed to be demonstrating a feeling of pride that their organization had made the invitation. They were particularly excited that the invitation was for dinner, for good food was particularly important to them.

At the VFW Hall, they were greeted by the officers of the post and were treated to food and drink (even a beer if they wanted), music, and dancing with women's auxiliary members who also had cooked and served the dinner. All in all, it was an evening much like those many had spent in previous years, which made it particularly pleasant.

The party provided an opportunity to view socialization patterns among the men at the nursing home. They appeared to have a close caring relationship among themselves that was demonstrated in the ready assistance those who were able provided to those who were physically impaired in moving into and out of the van. Small friendship groups were maintained even at the party. Indeed, one man had decided to accept the invitation only if his close friend could go.

While the Veterans Day outing was a special occasion to be enjoyed, the everyday socialization activities also were important. In this nursing home care unit, two socialization groups were formed, one for veterans of WW I and the other for those of WW II. The primary reason for developing the two therapeutic groups is related to their differences, such as a wide age differential. The WW I veterans attempt to describe how isolated they feel as a result of having outlived all important family members and friends. They consider themselves different from the WW II men and that the younger veterans do not speak the same language, which implies differences in attitudes, beliefs, and values.

These differences can be better seen in several vignettes:

Dane Madden

Dane Madden is 91 years old and has survived all who were close to him. Although he had been married and widowed three times, he had no children. His only outside contacts are with a niece who visits him occasionally and a young chiropractor who invites Dane to his home once in a while. Theirs is a father-son type of relationship that is very rewarding to Dane. He sees most of the younger residents in the unit as different from himself; he identifies them as having psychiatric problems and can find no common ground on which to build a friendship.

Dane was sent to Harp, the corrective therapist for the unit, and got along with him very well. At first, the staff was optimistic that a relationship would be formed to help involve Dane but this never happened. He told a staff member that Harp seemed to have his own problems and Dane said he felt used by the therapist.

This elderly man, despite his isolation from others important in his past, remains selective in his choice of friends. He maintains this pattern with staff and other patients. He has excellent long-term memory but regularly forgets where he is and will ask staff members to assist him. They have put up signs to help direct him to his room. However, he remembers why streets in St. Louis were named and tells a favorite story about the civic protest that arose when a street name was changed in honor of the first St. Louis GI who was killed in WW II. Events with special meaning from his past, including college experiences, are shared with anyone he finds acceptable and willing to listen.

Gus Kookle

Gus Kookle is 90 years old and the survivor of a life of heavy drinking. He is essentially alone, having long ago broken all ties with family members—he is not sure any are still living. He never married and thus never developed his own family. He grew up in a midwest city and held various political jobs. He worked for the city as a park raker and commented how great it was for him and his buddies to always be able to park the truck near a tavern.

He is very dissatisfied with his placement at NHCU. He has been there for seven years and still makes connections with the old "flophouse" where he had lived. That 18-room residential hotel continues to be his perceived home and where his pals reside. He hates the food he has to eat three times a day. Gus wants to return to his former residence so he continues to maintain telephone contact with the manager, who does come to visit him. His constant request to the social worker is to help him telephone the hotel manager to come and take him home. This does not seem possible since the hotel has no air conditioning and Gus cannot tolerate the heat, but even when the staff repeats these facts, they do not change his desire. He wants freedom that is not available to him in the NHCU and, despite an agreeable overall behavior on the unit, he clings to his goal: to go back to the hotel.

Kyle Hankin

Kyle Hankin is an 87-year-old white male. He held various factory jobs throughout his life. He has a niece who occasionally visits and takes him out to eat. He has never been married and likes to joke about how he avoided all the ladies in his younger days. He is quite alert mentally and enjoys staying in the home. Kyle has adapted to the unit in a way fairly characteristic of a man who has entered the institutional setting from an environment in which he had made little personal investment. Nothing about his important social relationship with his niece seems to have been disrupted. His history indicates that the VA was the system to which he usually turned when he had a need.

Bert Otter

Bert Otter is a 58-year-old white male with a history of schizophrenia since WW II. He was married once and divorced 10 years ago but has two children with whom he has important relationships. He has a daughter who is a scientist who visits every two weeks, but these are not an adequate compensation for the loyalty he wants from his son.

At approximately five-year intervals, Bert's mental condition worsens so that he must be placed on inpatient psychiatric care. Fortunately, his periods of dysfunction are at significantly long intervals and are treated rapidly so he is able to return soon to the unit. He was taken to the VA inpatient psychiatric unit recently when he became somewhat aggressive physically and upset over his relationship with his son. He has told the social worker that he wants a teacher to help him learn to work with veterans. During his periods of remission he helps escort patients to therapy sessions. It is to be wondered whether a man such as Bert could develop his desire to be more helpful to his peers beyond pushing a wheelchair.

Glen Alexander

Glen Alexander is a 55-year-old divorced white male who suffers from multiple sclerosis. He was a journalist in a major east coast city, is highly intelligent, and yearns for an opportunity for stimulating conversation. Glen had exhausted most of his personal financial resources for private medical care for MS before moving to the VA home. His costly treatment has exhausted his financial flexibility and his only resource is the VA.

He is very active in the WW II discussion group on the unit. Glen and the other well-educated member of that group find that differences in educational backgrounds make communication with others unsatisfactory. Unless someone talks with him at his level, he declines to open up with group members. He likes to talk about journalism and politics. He reads *The New York Times* three times a week and has been able to obtain it because a staff member has made a point of picking it up out of personal concern. He is confined to a wheelchair and has no potential for physical rehabilitation. He has a sense of little or no control over his life. He seeks control over something, usually the staff, with his demanding behavior. If the food is bad or if something else upsets him, he becomes very angry and frequently behaves quite aggressively.

Sandy Beggett

Sandy Beggett is a 60-year-old white male who suffers from a neuromuscular disease that causes many types of dysfunction but his inability to control his bladder is the worst problem. A retired military career officer, he is highly educated. He never worked in any nonmilitary job. His condition is a constant source of concern. His immobility outside the institutional setting is connected to his embarrassment over his bladder problem.

Sandy has several sisters and one brother. Before moving to the unit he lived with his sister and his mother, for whom he cared until her death. He attempted to return to live with his sister but while that was an important experience, it lasted only 10 days and he then returned to the unit. He feels he was placing too much burden on her. His unwillingness to talk about those problems indicates a sense of further frustration over his limitations. He is very religious and goes to Mass at the facility at least four times a week. His meaningful participation in this experience seems to be enhanced by a close relationship with the Catholic chaplain.

Fred Menlott

Fred Menlott is a 60-year-old black male with a chronic heart problem and arthritis but he is ambulatory and takes frequent walks throughout the hospital grounds. He lived and worked all his life in a southern Illinois community with his mother, whom he cared for until he was admitted to the nursing home. She still lives in their home, in a poverty and high-crime neighborhood, where he sometimes visits. He watches television and reads; for the most part, his activities on the unit involve little interaction with other patients. The one exception is with a white male patient who is dying of cancer. He is close to only one staff person and displays a general mistrust of most people in his environment.

While there are differences within the WW I and WW II groups, largely because of educational and interest differences, there are significant other variances between the two. The WW I veterans are the last survivors of their immediate family group. They thus have no family connectedness that could be described as intimate. Their interests lie in reminiscences of the past, their problems are primarily physical, and they look to their immediate environment for fulfillment of social needs. The opportunities to find meaningful involvements are closely connected to whatever ones exist in the environment. The WW II veterans include those with primary mental and primary physical disorders. Many still are quite involved with family and with concerns in the larger world outside of the VA system. For some veterans, family connections are limited to interactions initiated by the relatives. There appears to be greater demand among the WW II veterans for personal attention from staff for need fulfillment.

The therapeutic goals of these two groups differ considerably. For the WW I group, it involves an emphasis on getting the three or four older veterans to share past experiences with each other. This supplies them with their most meaningful exchanges. However, all would seem to prefer to have the staff group leader as a one-to-one listener. The WW II group is intended to facilitate problem solving and build more supports among the younger men. Relationship building can be a most difficult therapeutic task when a veteran's life is not enriched by close peer communication. That becomes even more difficult in a situation where intimacy is the exception rather than the norm.

COMMUNITY NURSING HOME CARE

The VA has introduced a system of community (contract) skilled and intermediate nursing home care for veterans. The contracting approach was initiated in 1976 with enactment of P.L. 94-581, the Veterans Omnibus Health Care Act. In programs authorized by this legislation, the VA enters into a contract relationship with nursing homes licensed by the states and in compliance with the certification standards set for participation in a state Medicaid program. Veterans are assessed to determine the need for the level of care before being placed.

To ensure quality of care, the VA undertakes an additional certification before approving a nursing home for veterans. These standards emphasize additional nursing service requirements, including greater supervision by a licensed professional nurse, full-time coverage on each eight-hour rotation by a licensed professional or practical nurse, and backup coverage during staff absences. Efforts are made to select a setting where the veteran will have access to rehabilitation, activity, and social services.

VA inspection teams are composed of a physician, nurse, social worker, dietician, safety engineer, and medical administrator. Contract nursing homes must be inspected every two years by the VA. The contracting policy has expanded the range of long-term care resources that can be offered and thus coordinated by the VA without the cost of building additional nursing home beds at its facilities. While this arrangement has proved satisfactory overall, it is less than adequate in areas where the availability of nursing home beds is scarce and/or the majority of homes do not accept Medicaid payment and therefore are not licensed under the state Medicaid program.

HOME CARE SERVICES

Another service important to older veterans is hospital-based home care service (Veterans Administration Hospitals, 1974). The VA hospitals maintain their own home care teams and rely on a core of professionals, including physicians, nurses, social workers, dieticians, physical therapists, and other specialists. Services are provided through referral at the time a veteran is hospitalized in a VA medical facility.

As with other home health programs outside the VA system, home care services cannot be provided unless the patient meets certain requirements: assurance that there is a person in the home willing to participate in the care, assurance that intensive care no longer is needed and that outpatient care is feasible, and assurance that the patient be nonambulatory or have other special conditions such as a terminal illness or be currently ambulatory but soon to become nonwalking because of a specific disease process.

Two requirements limit accessibility to VA-sponsored home care: (1) if the veteran is not treated in a VA hospital, the service is not available; and (2) if the patient resides more than 30 minutes or 30 miles from the serving hospital, an alternative source of non-VA connected home care may need to be sought. As of 1976, the program was available in 30 VA hospitals (Veterans Administration, 1977).

GERIATRIC RESEARCH, EDUCATION, AND CLINICAL CENTERS

Geriatric Research, Education, and Clinical Activity Centers (GRECC) were conceived by the VA in 1973. The agency first requested funding for the GRECC program in 1975. In that same year, the Office of Extended Care was created to give focus to the diverse range of long-term care programs offered in the VA system (U.S. Senate Report, 1980).

Each of the eight GRECCs established by 1981 obviously pursues a broad geriatrics program but each focuses on a different set of priorities. In general, the existing GRECCs were designed to encompass three areas: research, education, and clinical activities. The research is designed to focus on basic and clinical investigation with an aging focus; the educational component includes the development of knowledge, attitudes, and skills related to geriatrics at undergraduate, graduate, and continuing education levels; and the clinical care element involves the development of small inpatient and outpatient demonstration units.

The research of some GRECCs assigns priority to biomedical and psychiatric/ psychological areas while others direct most emphasis to issues of a more direct service and care nature. The variations may be attributed to such factors as the priorities of a facility medical director, the staff members who are part of the unit, the budget of an individual GRECC, and the interrelationships and linkages between the GRECC and other units in the complex in terms of resource sharing, clinical services, and research participation.

Legislation (P.L. 96-330, the Veterans Administration Health Care Amendments, 1980) mandates the establishment of up to 15 such centers at VA health care facilities. The requirements for sponsorship of a center are specified in that legislation to ensure that the facility's organization, personnel resources, and educational institutional linkages required to meet the goals of a GRECC are in operation. There must be arrangement with an accredited medical school that provides education and training in geriatrics. Medical school residents receive training in geriatrics by rotation through the GRECC and the components of the medical facility where older veterans are served, i.e., the nursing home care unit and the extended care unit of the complex and its domiciliary entities. These settings provide residents with the opportunity to receive in-depth training in diagnosis and treatment of chronic illness.

There must be additional teaching relationships with nursing and allied health programs and the GRECC may be used for comparable geriatric training. Research assumes a position of importance in these new centers and continues in those already established. The goals of multidisciplinary research are to engage in health care research that is of significance to the elderly veteran population. The establishment of these centers places the VA in a potential leadership position in the advancement of knowledge about the aging process and service development for the elderly in the United States. However, current funding cuts have slowed the timetable to increase the number of centers.

The VA strategy to develop GRECCs is one of the most important steps to date in dealing with current and future needs of older veterans. A national committee was to be formed under the authority of the Chief Medical Director with a representative membership of experts who are not federal employees but who have demonstrated interest and expertise in the fields of gerontology and geriatrics. It was to include at least one representative of a national veterans service organization. This committee was to have major responsibility for evaluating the progress of the GRECCs and determine the extent to which the centers' activities are facilitating the expansion and upgrading of clinical services, professional staff, and the general knowledge required to better serve elderly veterans.

Title III of P.L. 96-330 specifies that this committee will (a) assess the VA's capability to provide high-quality geriatric, extended, and other health care services to eligible older veterans, taking into consideration the likely demand from older veterans, and (b) assess the current and projected needs of eligible older veterans for geriatric, extended care, and other health care services.

This assessment was to come in a formal report to be presented to the VA Administrator through the Chief Medical Director by April 1, 1983. This report was to encompass evaluations of the activities of each of the GRECCs as well as provide recommendations for other programs and services that might be needed for meeting elder veterans' health care demands (Veterans Administration Health Care Amendments of 1980). However, budgetary limitations have required that planning activities be reconsidered; the full developmental program is contingent upon federal support.

The legislation offers each GRECC the opportunity to develop a research, education, and training mission that is appropriate for the particular elderly veteran population it serves. To maximize the potential of a GRECC to accomplish this challenging task, an additional advisory component could be instituted to increase community awareness of the center's activities, identify local resources that can be valuable to the various educational and clinical activities of its staff, and increase the extent to which the GRECC and other gerontological programs can interrelate for mutually beneficial ends. This means that, given the requirement for formal teaching relationships between the VA site where the GRECC is located and close-by academic institutions, it seems worthwhile to build a relationship that facilitates cooperative exchange in medical and related health care research activities. It may be possible for both the teaching institutions and the GRECC to cooperate in joint research projects for training institutes.

It also is important for the GRECCs and community-based service organizations to develop channels of communication and cooperative activities. The centers could assume a leadership role in facilitating a more active exchange between the various sectors of the VA complex and community agencies that may have common interests and concerns for client populations that include older veterans.

For example, at one GRECC is a research psychologist interested in the area of alcoholism and aging. In the metropolitan area where the center is located there is a growing concern about the need of the elderly alcoholic population to receive better services but the community lacks expertise and information about such problems. As the VA complex has a long history of treating older alcoholics in its chemical dependency program, the community and the GRECC could make specific efforts to share information, develop a plan for joint service connections between locally based resources and VA services, and cooperate in the design of a model program that would add to the strength of the VA offerings through making resources available in the area.

St. Louis was designated as one of the eight VA sites for a GRECC between 1975 and 1977. The others were Bedford, Mass.; Little Rock, Ark.; Los Angeles; Minneapolis; Palo Alto, Calif.; Seattle/American Lake, Wash.; and Sepulveda, Calif. The St. Louis GRECC recruited staff with interdisciplinary backgrounds, examined clinical program roles it could assume, and planned for its future as a major geriatric knowledge and research center for the entire St. Louis VA medical complex. However, the expansion of a clinic depends on a steady increase in its operating budget. Present funding patterns indicate that growth in the staff at the St. Louis GRECC will proceed slowly, if at all.

This GRECC sponsors an exercise rehabilitation program that focuses on treating patients with pulmonary conditions through a regular system of exercise, monitoring, and counseling. To some extent, this program remains autonomous from the other sections of the complex that are involved in rehabilitative medicine. Its patients are carefully screened to match the sampling needs of the biomedical and therapeutic research requirements of the program. The mean age of those participating in this program is late midlife, with high medical risks that are likely to increase as they age.

The GRECC personnel and other specialists who staff the cardiopulmonary rehabilitation program are interested in exploring structural and service expansions of the rehabilitation effort in order to increase service capacity and to provide more comprehensive care to those who qualify. Patients receive their exercise therapy on a scheduled basis. While they are at the center, few other services are provided and many of these clients are left without activities once they have completed the routine program (especially those who are dependent upon others to transport them to the GRECC and may not be available to take them home immediately after the therapy). The staff was analyzing the feasibility of introducing a multiservice day therapy component as an adjunct to the rehabilitation program that could be used by center patients receiving other treatments.

One model had a socialization and service coordination service focus along the lines of a limited social-health day treatment center. It emphasized that:

1. A service coordination component would enable patients to receive all of the treatments such as physical/occupational therapy, nutrition counseling, and psychological and therapeutic counseling in a single day.
2. Socialization and occupational therapies built into the program would use group therapy and a specialized effort to meet individual needs. The latter program would require the addition of a clinical psychologist or social worker with skills in group process techniques and in providing individual counseling and service coordination.
3. An expanded program would receive input from the occupational and/or vocational therapy components of service available in the complex.

Staff members involved in the rehabilitation program were concerned about what type of routine the patients maintain during the days they do not visit the exercise clinic. A number of these clients live rather isolated and inactive daily routines that are interrupted only when they join the program. This daily living pattern may be counterproductive to the patient's needs. Long periods of inactivity and isolation within the home on a daily basis can encourage sedentary behavior and eating, smoking, and drinking activities that are harmful and likely to generate general lethargy and negative self-image. If the patient's spouse works or if the veteran lives alone, problems in the daily routine may be even more dysfunctional because there is no other person to give encouragement to positive habits and behaviors or to give supportive assistance in behavior monitoring.

The ideal conceptualization of an intensified day program would have a center these patients could visit several days a week for socialization, counseling, and other peer group programs. However, the lack of economic resources for covering the costs of a program and the absence of a transportation system for these patients constitute a barrier to the development of a more comprehensive day care program. Many of the patients must depend on others to transport them, often long distances, since the catchment area for this hospital is quite large. There is no VA-sponsored transportation system that could carry the patients to and from their homes.

The range of therapies and activities for individualized treatment plans that must be coordinated through the day program were divided between two major medical treatment settings that were some distance apart. The GRECC is in the far southern end of the metro county and many of the outpatient clinics are in the city. Only a shuttle bus connects the two facilities and may not be appropriate for the type of patients the program would serve.

In planning broader day rehabilitation services, the center faced the questions of how persons could access the program and how cooperative arrangements could be made with components needed for the patients but operated by units not affiliated with or directly linked to the GRECC. The clinic's specialized treatment emphasis also precluded the use of supportive service from community agencies that are nearer to the patients' homes. The staff was not in a position either to link patients to the potential resources with the overall VA medical complex or to facilitate their involvement in community-based programs that provide some of the needed socialization functions that could be supportive to the center's rehabilitation goals.

These difficulties are illustrative of the problems faced by all VA geriatric facilities in trying to plan more extensive noninstitutional services for older veterans. Since the problems faced by an individual GRECC are likely to be unique, each center must plan which services it can provide, what ones are available in the VA institution and the surrounding community, then find aspects of those two components that seem the most amenable to cooperative efforts to institute and evaluate innovative programs.

VETERANS ORGANIZATIONS' INFLUENCE OVER PROGRAMS

To understand the forces that affect the development of services to older veterans it is necessary to analyze national organizational structures and political activities that influence congressional decisions and VA service priorities. To a large extent, these national political and policy formulation efforts are independent of the bureaucracies of the local VA medical complexes and the local levels of veterans organizations. At the national level are the three most influential groups:

1. The Veterans Administration is the organization that administers all facets of services to veterans and develops and implements policies that emerge from federal legislation.
2. The House and Senate Committees on Veterans Affairs give leadership to the development of legislation and appropriations impacting on services and

benefits to veterans. The House committee has been most involved in protecting the traditional veterans programs against inflation and innovation while the Senate committee has tended toward supporting more innovative programs and advancing programs and benefits to Vietnam veterans.

3. The major lobbying groups promote the legislative interests and concerns of all veterans. The American Legion, Veterans of Foreign Wars, and Disabled American Veterans have sufficient strength in membership and active leadership from veterans of WW II to have significant impact on legislation of concern to veterans (Keller, 1980).

The American Legion is the largest veterans organization with 2.7 million members and a very active women's auxiliary of a million, many of whom are the spouses of older veterans. It supports three registered lobbyists in Washington and can mount a major effort on behalf of veterans legislation despite the fact that it is characterized by a complex local, regional, and national structure. The Veterans of Foreign Wars is smaller than the Legion, with 1.8 million members and an auxiliary of 620,000. The Disabled American Veterans has 620,000 members with service-connected disabilities and is attracting a rapidly growing representation from the Vietnam cohort.

Two organizations with a major interest in Vietnam veterans are the Vietnam Veterans of America and American Veterans of World War II, Korea, and Vietnam (Keller, 1980). Combined, they have influence on the development of specialized programs for older veterans and on the VA system's organizational structure and functions to meet these needs. For example, the legislation to develop the GRECCs and to establish a national level evaluation committee ensures that at least one of these service organizations is represented on this panel. This representation can help assure that the GRECCs' activities are made known and assessed by the organizations that represent older/elderly veterans.

There appear to be two reasons for concern about the continuation of adequate financial support for programs that are particularly beneficial for elderly veterans. First, there may be a shift in lobbying emphasis away from elderly veterans and, second, there may be a deemphasis of special programs for veterans as opposed to those for the general population. These trends result from the following factors:

1. The unique priorities of veterans of different eras, as are most apparent in a contrast between the World War II and Vietnam cohorts, may shift lobbying pressure toward greater program priorities to younger veterans as they become more influential in these organizations.
2. There are fewer congressmen who are themselves veterans. Those who are veterans are more likely to have served during the Korean or Vietnam conflicts and thus do not identify with older veterans' circumstances.

3. There is a general trend toward fiscally conservative legislation that may lessen support for generous appropriations to the Veterans Administration and/or lead to increased scrutiny by the General Accounting Office (GAO) for better cost-efficient monitoring of VA expenditures.

These factors may influence the actual appropriations for the GRECCs that were authorized in Title III of P.L. 96-330 at $10 million for 1981 and $85 million for fiscal years 1982, 1983, and 1984. To ensure that the GRECCs can implement their legislative mandate, these multiple lobbying forces will need to have some consensus about the priority to be given to the upgrading of geriatric services.

CONCLUSION

There are many diverse and complex characteristics of the veterans service system. The fluctuating needs of various cohorts make VA planning at the local and national levels very difficult. The overall system recognizes the need to develop an increased capacity for meeting the needs of older veterans, but such planning may go by the wayside unless there is a demand on the system. The wave of WW II veterans will not diminish for several decades so actions to meet their needs must be implemented quickly. The system's response should not short-change the older veteran group nor place its needs in competition with younger cohorts.

Some merging of existing programs within facilities may prove cost effective. These intrasystem mergers should make existing efforts more responsive to the needs of older veterans who now use the system or who might seek its services in the future. As a community lacks medical expertise in geriatrics, it might be possible to link the VA's medical and surgical expertise to the general health care system in the locality.

Community facilities already are used through payments under fee-for-service contracts. While this offers an opportunity for linkage of an encapsulated VA service system with other service efforts, it does not provide a forum or opportunity for joint planning and consideration of how better to link programs. The GRECCs offer an excellent potential forum for this cooperation. What seems to be needed is for community workers inside the VA system to make greater contact with local facilities and for local agencies to follow that same approach.

As the VA system moves away from increasing its emphasis on inpatient care as its response to the long-term needs of older veterans, it becomes important for the agency to have connections with and make more direct use of community resources. If there are gaps between the VA and other important resources that continue to remain unfilled, the older veterans will not derive the maximum benefits to which they are entitled.

REFERENCES

Department of Medicine and Surgery. *Professional services: Social work service,* Part XII. Washington, D.C.: Veterans Administration, June 1980.

Keller, B. How a unique lobby force protects over $21 billion in vast veterans' programs. *The Congressional Quarterly,* June 14, 1980, pp. 1627-1634.

Lyngh, R.E. Rates and income limitations increased in pension and parents' DIC. *The American Legion Bulletin,* National Veterans Affairs and Rehabilitation Commission, May 5, 1980.

National Academy of Sciences. *Health care for American veterans.* Report of the Committee on Health Care Resources. In the Veterans Administration, Assembly of Life Sciences, National Research Council, Washington, D.C., May 1977.

Office of Human Development Services. *Facts about older Americans 1979.* U.S. Department of Health and Human Services, HHS Publication No. 80-20006, undated.

U.S. Senate Report No. 96-747, 96th Cong., 2nd Sess. Reprinted in *U.S. Code Cong. & Ad. News, 1980, 2463.*

Veterans Administration. *Medical care of veterans.* Washington, D.C.: U.S. Government Printing Office, 1967.

Veterans Administration. *Rehabilitation therapists in the Veterans Administration,* VA Pamphlet No. 10-106. Washington, D.C., August 1969.

Veterans Administration. *The aging veteran: Present and future medical needs.* Washington, D.C.: Veterans Administration, October 1977.

Veterans Administration Health Care Amendments of 1980, P.L. 96-330, Title III—Geriatric Research and Care, and Title IV—Miscellaneous Amendments, 94 Stat. 1048-1051, August 26, 1980.

Veterans Administration Hospitals. *Hospital-based home care.* St. Louis: Veterans Administration, December 20, 1974.

Veterans Administration Medical Center. *Rehabilitation medical service guide.* St. Louis: Veterans Administration, undated.

Chapter 5

The Rural Elderly of Tolivar and Folk County

INTRODUCTION

"Rural elderly" seems to be a straightforward term to many but in reality there is much confusion and disagreement about how to define that population in the United States. There are two general approaches to describing this segment as a distinct subgroup of the aged population. The first is the demographic approach, which focuses on population size and community type, the second is the qualitative approach, which takes into account personal characteristics of individuals and groups in relation to a subcultural status.

The former approach identifies elderly persons residing in particular communities and the latter their personal characteristics regardless of their current residence (Adams, 1975). The demographic approach is the one used most often in gerontological literature, perhaps because there is no agreed-upon set of characteristics that define elderly people as rural. Demographic definitions are related to census statistics and frequently apply a maximum population size of 2,500 as a numerical cutoff for defining rural areas, provided the areas are not within a Standard Metropolitan Statistical Area. The population of a rural town as classified in the literature is under 10,000 persons (Powers, Keith, & Joudy, 1975).

There is great diversity among the rural aged and no single or simple profile of characteristics can be applied to them in the nation as a whole, its various regional areas, or even within states. Some states with significant rural populations have attempted to formulate a "rural service strategy." These plans sometimes focus on such difficult questions as distribution of services to clusters of rural aged in areas without services, balancing the demands between urban inner city and rural sectors, and development of policies for monitoring the effectiveness of innovative rural programs.

Differences between states are so great that applying the strategy of one to another's needs should be done with caution. Differences among rural communities within a state also vary according to history, economic and social factors, and citizens' attitudes about human service needs and provision. Each state and region should develop its own data from comprehensive community-by-community information upon which to plan for services for the elderly. Practitioners should use these data to establish familiarity with the rural individuals and communities in their geographic regions (Coward, 1979; Schooler, 1975; Rathbone-McCuan, 1981).

This chapter analyzes one rural community in Missouri where the authors conducted an assessment of the needs of the isolated elderly and made recommendations for addressing them through proposed new services and modifications of existing programs. The focus is on the isolated elderly in Folk County and its county seat of Tolivar. The trial-and-error approach provided some experiences upon which to suggest general guidelines for evaluating the needs of isolated rural elderly. Figure 5-1 indicates the aspects of a community analysis relevant to the isolated elderly. It encompasses the following information areas:

1. the community's social and economic history
2. current community conditions, including demographic and economic information
3. community values regarding acceptance of social responsibility to provide formal services
4. community acceptance of needy individuals who are dependent on external resources
5. community willingness to move beyond its boundaries to develop additional resources to meet local needs

All of these factors contribute to the presence and quality of community resources available to meet the needs of its residents. History, current demographic and economic conditions, and attitudes are relevant to individuals' behavior and influence their understanding of the available social supports. These factors also help determine the willingness of individuals to use these services, to demand more social supports and resources, and/or to do without and struggle alone in the absence of help.

The analysis of community assistance is particularly relevant when dealing with the isolated elderly since that group's very existence and its size are related to the availability of social supports and their utilization. While this general relationship is not unique to rural communities, it becomes more at issue when physical distance makes resource access a greater problem for the elderly so that even more is demanded of the locality to facilitate the linkage between individual and resource. When the problems of physical distance are combined with a higher social valuing of independence and self-reliance (as may often be the case in rural communities) the unique problem of such areas emerges.

Figure 5-1 Understanding Community Responses to Residents in Need

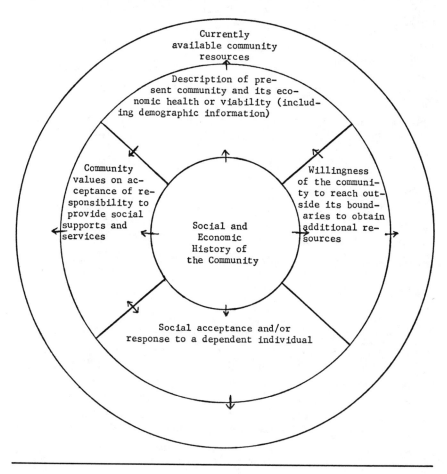

DESCRIPTION OF TOLIVAR, FOLK COUNTY, AND THE RESIDENTS

The characteristics of the town, county, and population and the historical and current social and economic factors set the background. Tolivar is a town in southern Missouri that is unknown outside its region. Its political and economic influences are important within the region but it is not one of the stronger geopolitical areas of rural Missouri. A state representative commented that most of the representatives from St. Louis and Kansas City did not even know of its existence until they had been in politics for a while. It may be categorized as an area of rural Missouri with a modest array of services. Other rural areas have far fewer resources but have capitalized on the expansion of human services more than Tolivar and Folk County. From the standpoint of the rural elderly in Missouri and their service needs, it is neither the best nor worst area because it has some resources that other communities lack.

Its history, while interesting, is not particularly noteworthy. Few historians have bothered to study its growth and change since the early nineteenth century. The greatest understanding of its past is available from residents who pride themselves on their intimate knowledge of the area's development. The history of southern Missouri's growth is reflective of both Tolivar and Folk County. For instance:

> Before the 1830s the combination of Indian tribes and the surrounding mountains kept the area unpopulated. Timber, game, and water resources were an incentive to settlers from the Appalachian states to migrate to the area. By 1855 the current county formation was in place, but the only commercial investment in the area was related to lead and zinc mining. The post-Civil War period gave birth to strong conservative Republican politics, a brief timber industry boom, the expansion of the railroad, and the emergence of wealthy and influential families who were to continue to exert major influences on the county and town. During the first half of the twentieth century economic development progressed slowly in the region. Clothing, sporting goods, and lumber became the focus of small industrial manufacturing after WW II. Between 1950 and 1970 there was a period of outmigration to urban areas and not until 1970 did the population begin to increase. Many of the immigrants are retirees in search of an ideal retirement area. These new clusters have placed demands on community facilities and public utilities of town and county government (Extension Division, 1974, & 1975).

The population of Folk County is about 32,000 and the largest town in the county has about 7,500. Some 16 percent of the population is 65 and older and in parts of the area the elderly represent 25 percent of the total population. The population density of Folk County is 39.1 persons per square mile but in some sectors drops to 28.7, as compared to 69.3 for the state. The area contains a somewhat larger proportion of aged than might be expected from statewide statistics. This overrepresentation is expected to continue throughout the next decade and to increase at a faster pace than younger age categories. The youth dependency ratio for the area is less than the overall state and the aged dependency ratio is greater.

The racial composition of the area is almost 99 percent white, so a nonwhite elderly person is rare. The high percentage of the aged contributes to the fact that there are three times the number of one-person households as there are of those with six or more. There are housing problems of various kinds that impact directly on the elderly such as deteriorated farm residences that cannot be repaired adequately but will not be abandoned and/or the lack of small apartment facilities to accommodate those living alone and needing space appropriate to their situations. In Folk County and Tolivar, transportation consists of private vehicles supplemented with erratic in-town taxi service and limited bus service in only a small section of the county.

A one-mile walk in Tolivar's residential neighborhoods contrasts sharply with a comparable walk outside the town limits. The sense of in-town neighborhoods fades quickly into a country and farm landscape. Visually, Tolivar resembles many other small midwestern towns in Missouri, Illinois, and Iowa. Commercial buildings and residential housing are designed in a pattern that moves out in neat geometric rectangles from the courthouse at the center of town. There is traffic and noise around the courthouse from 6 a.m. to 6 p.m. six days a week. On the seventh day, the traffic, people, and their activities shift from the economic and business focuses to the religious life. Several large parking lots at the Baptist Church overflow on Sunday mornings with hundreds of worshipers. By comparison, attendance at Sunday Mass is small because the Catholic church membership is not large. However, any local church becomes an important place for Sunday gathering.

The quietness of evening in-town generates a common question by urban visitors as to where people go and how they spend their time. The noise of day seems to be silenced. The newspaper, funeral home, jail, and the cafes around the courthouse offer only infrequent signs of life that provide a drastic comparison to an urban neighborhood. This quiet and relaxed pattern is broken during the summer by tourists who retreat from the city's heat and frenzy to the numerous lakes and recreation facilities dispersed throughout southern Missouri. These visitors, however, do not alter or enter into the day-to-day community life of most residents. Tourism is tolerated because the vacationers spend money at local businesses.

There are two light industries that provide the major job sources in the area, employing more women than men. Their executives play major leadership roles in the community's political and social life. There are a surprising number of very wealthy individuals in Tolivar. They are distinguished by their long family residential history there and are highly respected. In general, the residents are slow to approve local taxes for human services such as public health, mental health, or education but the support of one or several leading families increases the acceptability of such programs.

There is a wide spectrum of life styles among the elderly residents, including active farmers, retired farmers still living on their farms or in town, lifelong local citizens, and urbanites recently retired to the rural area living either in the town or on a farm. All individuals described in the following cases live in Folk County and in or near Tolivar, the majority having been in the area for many years. Lifelong Tolivar residents like the quietness and simplicity of their town. It would be incorrect, however, to assume that all of the town's elderly are charmed by and totally satisfied with the community. Many have negative feelings about the changing social and economic fabric. Some were and continue to be ambitious, valuing their economic resources as a base for high social status that, based on their advancing age, is not assured; for some, it assures they will lose status once they retire or become widowed.

The ideals of the elderly Tolivarians, such as self-sufficiency and independence, reduce the acceptability of help from outside the family or from an informal helping network unless people are in a crisis. The elderly are accustomed to doing things by themselves and for themselves. To the extent that material matters have been important to individuals in their earlier life, these priorities continue in late life whether or not the financial means for obtaining luxuries are available. The key for individuals and family is social status or good name in the community and is very important in later life.

Many of the delightful qualities of Tolivar as a place to live may become obstacles to the well-being of the elderly residents to the extent that these characteristics keep them isolated from the kinds of services they need and locked into the kinds of life styles they have attempted to maintain. (Isolators that affect the rural elderly are shown in Figure 5-2.) The severely impaired elderly generally have a dilemma almost impossible to resolve—the pursuit of lifelong goals of self-sufficiency, independence, and autonomy that are hampered by their personal circumstances and the realities of resources not available. Fortunately, many of the sources of formal helping and those who serve as leaders in planning social and medical services are familiar with the uniqueness of many people's situation and apply their understanding in the larger context of formal and informal resources. The elderly who must be helped by professionals who have no knowledge about them as individuals tend to reject that assistance.

The local shortage of professional and/or supportive health and social services forces the elderly to travel long geographical and psychological distances to receive help. This discourages both the elderly and local professionals from looking at resources too far away unless there is an emergency. The professionals know that even short distances can be prohibitive. The elderly who no longer can drive or lack a driving spouse are forced to adjust their transportation needs to the schedules of others. If they have maintained good relationships, especially with the younger females in the multigenerational family who can drive, they are likely to be transported.

Figure 5-2 Isolators That Affect the Rural Elderly

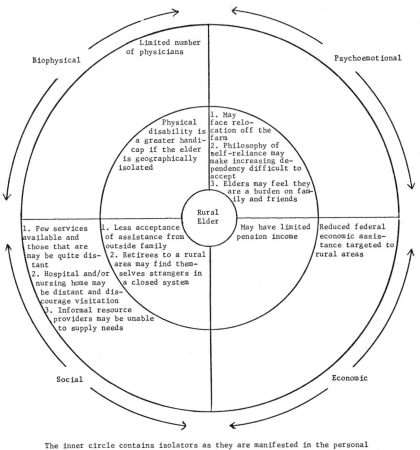

The inner circle contains isolators as they are manifested in the personal
lives of rural elders, the outer circle those that exist in the environment.

Yet this transportation dependency results in the loss of many opportunities and
the personal choice of where and when to go for many needs outside the home.
Elderly who lack transportation are acutely aware of their dependency on family,
friends, and neighbors. Only limited public resources for personal transportation
are available through the Older American Transportation Service, brought into the
county under the auspices of the Community Action Corporation. However, the
agency van rides are not acceptable to all those in need of transportation because
they are public, so getting around becomes a dependency not easily accepted by
those with pride over lifelong self-sufficiency.

Some of those who have the benefit of informal helping resources may tend to look to those sources for more help than can be offered conveniently. Some families resist their elderly members using public transportation because they regard it as a stigma. Fortunately, most informal helping sources can make judgments about when professional assistance is required, especially in crisis periods. Other problems can and do arise when their decisions do not reflect sensitivity to the elderly persons' preferences and/or past history of connection with formal helping sources.

The implicit and explicit influence of family feuds (longstanding inter-generational and intragenerational conflicts) can prevent relatives being a source of help or affect the elderly person's willingness to accept the assistance. For most of the elderly in the area there is significant reliance on informal social supports but some vary from that pattern—the recently relocated who do not have access to the informal networks available to lifelong residents. These new residents are the most isolated group of elders in Tolivar.

The Medical Social Worker

A medical social worker having extensive contact with many of the elderly in both the town and the county described in an interview how the formal/informal sources usually combine to provide assistance.

"When I first came to the community I was 'the big-city social worker' and very used to the existence of a formal multiservice network that did not work together; agencies did not know that other resources existed in the community because there were too many. There, many agencies rarely worked together because of resource competition, red tape, eligibility issues, client service unit quotas. . . . I expected that in Tolivar there would be a formal network separated from the informal, but found that people rely on the informal network first and then the formal. These must work together or else people won't get services.

"There are simply not enough formal resources, so to expand what is available requires getting the informal and formal linked, building better linkage among the formal sources, and improving the efficiency of the various professional re-sources. We need to explore better ways to work with the informal parts of the community. Getting that informal part together to help individuals and get it to work in the way I would desire is sometimes impossible because no professional can control that . . . it offers a lot of help to many elderly in Tolivar.

"People, particularly the elderly, don't like asking for help. I think that attitude extends to both the informal and formal sources of support. I know that many of my clients simply won't ask their willing friends, family, or neighbors for assistance until there is absolutely no alternative. That may be one of the reasons why early health intervention is so difficult and makes prevention nearly impossible. Not asking for help serves to keep people's behavior consistent with their values but it stands in the way of their receiving help.

"That pattern of not asking is truer for social service than medical services. A greater number of older people seem willing to come to the physician at the early stages of a physical problem than to a social worker for a social problem. When the elderly person's situation involves both medical and social problems, there are times when the medical intervention being offered is seriously reduced in overall effectiveness because the social factors stand in the way and people do not want anything done about those areas of their lives. Putting the social intervention into a health context does seem to increase the acceptability of some intervention, but there is still resistance.

"Another characteristic is the way that people don't, yet do, follow up with professionals they see. Problems may be talked over once or sometimes twice and some intervention is suggested, but never followed up on again. I cannot count the times when I ended up learning about what happened in a particular situation either at the grocery store or when I went out to eat. People will stop and share outcomes to their problems because they felt that I cared enough about them as people even though they probably thought there was not a whole lot I could do to help them.

"The rural elderly don't usually have the expectation that a social worker is going to do a lot for them . . . they just have the assurance that somebody cares. I guess it is rather provincial practice . . . the art of caring as compared to emphasis on the outcome. The trust factor seems to be built not so much on what you actually do for them but how you care about them. The caring is what they sense and this gives a potential base for developing trust. They don't judge you on the solutions you can find to their problems . . . many of them don't believe in solutions and maybe they are right."

The views expressed by this social worker are congruent with those of many of the social intervenors who have practiced in rural areas with at-risk populations (Ginsberg, 1976). The possibilities for providing services to elderly rural persons depends on the ability to establish interpersonal relationships of the sort that encourages them either to accept offers of assistance or to seek them when they perceive themselves in need of assistance. Knowledge of the community and its resources—and what is not available—also becomes part of effective helping.

CASE HISTORIES IN FOLK COUNTY

Some of the elderly persons mentioned by citizen leaders and professionals in interviews as examples of the rural isolated elderly are described next. Their current life circumstances vary and they differ in the types and extent to which they experience isolators. However, some environmental isolators have a powerful impact on many elderly and are related to forces outside Tolivar and Folk County.

Louise Seddy

Meeting Louise was an experience of the sort many people will never have, but few who do will ever forget her. Almost every professional consulted agreed that she is a lifelong farm dweller who became at risk because of her life style in her later years. Her actual legal age was once a matter of much concern for service eligibility reasons but Louise regarded it as no great problem. She knew that she once had had a birth certificate but was convinced the county clerk, elected in the 1930s, "took off with it." She assigned her own birthday as December 25 because she always received a card or two around that date. To her the year 1899 sounded right for her year of birth; if so, she was 81 in 1980.

It still makes no sense to her why the county Department of Family Services worker, "the welfare worker," made a big fuss about something as unimportant as when Louise Seddy was born. She has always been around Folk County and thinks she will be there a while longer. She has one or two reasons for wanting to keep going. Her 12 cats and countless kittens don't like strangers. The home health agency will not visit her house any more. After months of sending workers to her farm to perform chores and having her run them off, the agency has given up for the time being. Louise refused to get rid of any of the cats, disregarded all warnings about her poor sanitation conditions, and refused to move into town during the winter even though her well froze and she had no source of water other than what people brought to her.

During the first six months of 1980, she lived in and out of the nursing home in Tolivar. However, while she was there, Louise continued to be the center of community concern. Some service providers felt she should be declared legally incompetent because she could not care for herself or her farm and was unwilling to move off the property permanently. Other professionals were unwilling to see this happen and were fighting against a declaration of legal incompetence because it would destroy her will to live. She agreed to go to the nursing home for brief periods because she believed she would return to the farm. The physician was one of the major forces preventing a formal competency hearing.

However, the rapidly growing pressures of her disabilities and endangering conditions were becoming too great for the network of formal and informal helping sources. If Louise returned to the farm, it was likely that, for her protection, the sheriff might take her back to the nursing home even if it meant getting a legal order. Her physician anticipated that her reaction to this loss of autonomy would be devastating. For years, her daily routine had been to feed the cats, draw water, keep busy with all those who wanted to help her, and fight with neighbors who became angry when she threw the bodies of her dead cats into their yards. Institutionalization would destroy her life routine.

The helpers in her network viewed her as isolated but she did not express that opinion. They believed she could not make it through another winter but she was sure she could because she had made it through all previous ones. She thought she may become ill if she had to live permanently in the nursing home.

This case illustrates the potential threat to the independence of a solitary life style that can result from actions of concern by agency personnel. Service providers agreed on what isolation represented in Louise's situation but did not agree on solutions. This elderly lady had her cats and her farm and did not feel a need for anything more. Her physician and several other persons understood her position. Providing service to ensure a client's safety should not mean taking away the individual's right to choose, even if that person is old, in a vulnerable condition, and has choices that are at odds with the views of others.

Oscar Smalt

According to Oscar, who was 76 years old, he was making it just fine. The way he dealt with his widowed circumstance (six months) may be like other widowers in Tolivar and Folk County. He lived alone but his daughter and son-in-law were of great help before and after his wife's death. They had to travel from Kansas City, 250 miles away, which often made travel impossible in bad weather. Oscar felt they worried too much about him and he did not want to be a burden. During the first weeks after his wife died he was very sad and said he did not care whether he lived or died.

His daughter and son-in-law took him to Doctor Finch and he received a complete examination, the first since his retirement. The physician talked with him about not eating properly and about taking his medications. He did not know how to cook and had not worried about taking medicines on schedule when his wife was alive because she reminded him about them.

The social worker at the Finch Medical Clinic talked with him after his physical examination and wanted to help. She enrolled him in Meals-on-Wheels and called the ladies' group at the church to have someone go to his home to clean. Oscar felt that was like having a stranger enter his house who wanted to know all his business. He remembered his daughter's asking him what foods he thought he could prepare for himself. He found he did not like soup and TV dinners and did not remember to look at the weekly schedule his daughter had written for him to follow. The social worker set up an arrangement to call and remind him about preparing lunch. He discontinued Meals-on-Wheels because he did not like to eat alone but forgot to inform his daughter or the social worker. Meals at the Baker Cafe were better, and he thought it the best place to eat in Tolivar. His wife had taught one of the young waitresses to bake pies. He felt it was good to see people when he ate because they all greeted him. Some he did not know by name and knew his wife had been upset at his forgetfulness. She used to say, "Oscar, it isn't friendly not to speak to folks by name."

Oscar has found an acceptable social resource in the cafe. As long as he can afford the expense of eating out and is able to get about, it would seem a much-needed social outlet. It is to be wondered whether a nutrition site, if it also offered social activities, would not be an attractive opportunity for Oscar.

Cora Carter

Cora was 78 years old and lived alone. Her nearest neighbors, the Dayne sisters, were retired school teachers. Because her telephone was not working, Cora one afternoon hiked three miles down the road to the sisters' home to ask them to take her to town to see a doctor because she had a bad rash all over her back. She wore several wool sweaters, even during the summer, and had been in the strong heat. The sisters agreed to take her and called their doctor to tell him that they were bringing Cora. The doctor agreed to wait at the clinic until they could drive the 20 miles. The sisters were afraid to drive at dusk but, because Cora was their friend and this was a medical emergency, they did the favor.

Shortly after that, Cora's niece, who usually was responsible for transporting Cora to her own doctor, learned of the situation and became very upset. The sisters described the severe pressure the niece began to put on Cora, telling her that she (the niece) could not walk around always feeling guilty if Cora was in a real emergency situation and could get no help. For a while Cora and her niece had a real battle going. Ultimately, Cora called the Dayne sisters and said she was going to move into a new nursing home in the town where her niece lived. The sisters remarked that they would have been willing to continue to take her to their doctor, shopping, or whatever she might have needed, but since neither she nor her niece asked them, they felt they could not butt into a family matter.

This case produces a sense of tragedy. Here was a woman who could take a three-mile walk while in severe discomfort and could fulfill her own daily needs. However, her niece's influence promoted the inappropriate nursing home placement. Cora had a supportive network of neighbors but that help was never incorporated into a service plan for her.

Sam Berry

Sam was 91 and blind. No one was sure how long he had been a resident of Folk County. He lived with his unmarried daughter, Ella, and his 50-year-old retarded nonverbal son, Jake, in a cabin that had a dirt floor and no actual windows. There was no plumbing or heating, and the three used plastic feed sacks for their makeshift bedding. The family was serviced by the county poverty agency. Its link, however tenuous, was through Ella, with whom the agency had communicated for three years. She was the major caregiver to her father and rarely left their property. Through trust built up over time, the agency was able to provide her clothing, food, and special items. Despite the major problems in the condition of the cabin, the agency did not have the resources to fix it up.

The agency spent much time trying to identify what could be done to help this family, which was totally unconnected to the community. The property could be used as collateral for a low-interest housing loan; however, the staff members recognized the family's fear of debt and that if they were to push the issue with Sam they would lose even minimal contact with Ella.

Larry and Elizabeth Mead

Larry, age 63, and Elizabeth, 62, moved to Tolivar after he sold his plastics manufacturing company in California. Larry had decided several years before retiring that he wanted to go into light farming. The move uprooted Elizabeth from her two adopted sons from a previous marriage. Almost immediately after arriving in the area, she began to develop a series of medical problems for which she had no prior history. Larry was very happy on his farm and had no apparent need to develop friends. He had retired to Folk County to get away from people and to be a farmer. Elizabeth greatly disliked the area and said she wanted nothing to do with the local social networks.

They were on-paper members of the Methodist church. Their minister repeatedly attempted to make home visits and encouraged Elizabeth to become involved in the church activities but neither gave any indication of wanting to do so or to be in need of the minister's assistance. They relied for help on the realtor who sold them the farm and contacted him for any major need or advice. However, the realtor felt unable to help the Meads so his response was to contact the minister, whose offers of help were rejected.

In this case, a retirement move to a new community represented an uprooting that was successful for Larry but for Elizabeth meant a loss of contact with other family members and familiar surroundings. They did not integrate themselves into the new community. Perhaps their withdrawal and rejection of opportunities for social interaction was voluntary, but they did reach out to one person they trusted who felt unable to help—the realtor. Elizabeth experienced a void created by estrangement from family but rejected the minister's encouragement of social involvement in the church. Elizabeth needed consistent support to mobilize herself to develop new friendships.

Walter Baker

The public health nurse of Folk County was interviewed regarding what she considered to be the difference between serving the isolated elderly who lived in Tolivar and those who resided on the farms farther from town. She said she thought the terrible conditions of a few farm residents in the county would never be tolerated in Tolivar. She retold a veteran nursing story:

"Every Wednesday last winter I went to Walter Baker's farm to dress the draining ulcer on his left leg. The only access he had to the house, the one I also had to use, was through the backyard, which was also the pig pen. One side of the original feeding area had fallen down so the pigs had taken over all of the backyard. The time I remember best was when I went there last February. Walter had somehow managed to continue to feed the pigs a healthy mix of slop. During the previous week, the yard had frozen over and the food he had last thrown to them from the back door, which was about as far as he could hobble, was frozen over. The pigs were rooting around trying to dig through the ice.

"When I entered the yard, the pigs started milling around me. I had the thought of the biggest sow rushing and knocking me down to the ice. As I moved toward the house I kept trying to push the pigs away. That trip across the yard was even worse because I had visions of Walter in the house without adequate heat. All of a sudden Walter threw the door open and said, 'Howdy Mrs. Seber, I just made a fresh pot of coffee. I was awaitin' you. I got a letter from Freddie, my grandson, yesterday and he did real good in college.'

"Later, after I finished with his dressing, I told Walter the conditions outside were really bad and that he could get a bad infection from that mess and I would have to take some action if he didn't. I thought about the consequences and those were worse because, without treatment through the winter, he could have lost that leg.

"I decided I would try to see Walter through until spring and that if something didn't change I'd have to take steps to get those pigs removed from the property. Walter kept saying that Freddie would fix the fence in early spring when he came to visit. Much to my surprise, the fence got fixed and Walter's leg finally healed."

In this situation, the nurse's decision to wait before she took steps to protect Walter worked in his favor. Often the practitioner's sense of urgency is far greater than the client's and becomes the motivation to take action. Well-meaning but untimely, inappropriate, or unnecessary action can have very destructive consequences for the aged.

The isolators illustrated in these cases are representative of those that confront the aged in rural areas: physical distance from neighbors and services, values and beliefs that make asking for and receiving help not acceptable, interpersonal problems that estrange the individuals from family and/or helper, lack of financial resources, the community's lack of understanding of the needs of the elderly, relocation from lifelong residence and family, and loss of physical vigor and family members. The continued existence of these isolators cannot be separated from the absence or inadequacy of community support systems, both formal and informal, that can mitigate such circumstances and events.

THE COMMUNITY AS THE ENVIRONMENT FOR INTERVENTION

The question of how to provide services to the isolated rural elderly such as those just described cannot be explored adequately without an understanding of the formal resources available for intervention (Figure 5-3). In Tolivar, the impact of the age-specific network was minimal. In fact, the Southwest Area Agency on Aging (AAA), the network designated as the organization to be the centralized coordination, planning, and service development unit for Folk County and Tolivar, was relatively unknown to many of the isolated elderly and was not linked to most of the health and social service agencies available to serve the general adult population in the county.

The Southwest Area Agency's central office is in a metropolitan area and its designated multicounty service area is large. The agency has an assigned representative in Folk County who is not known to the major intervenors in the area, without meaningful connections to the elderly leadership stucture, and without a base for advocating for the elderly within the agency's organizational structure.

The limitations of this staff person's role may be representative of other practitioners who are sent out from a central urban coordinating agency to perform advocacy, community organization, information, and referral service in an area with which they are not familiar, that has limited formal resources for the elderly, and is characterized by resentment toward the control exerted by an out-of-their-county entity. Persons working in Tolivar-based agencies admired the efforts of the Southwest staff person because they considered him a concerned person who was doing his best to get to know the community's needs. However, they were far less satisfied with his agency.

The lack of comprehensive assistance for Tolivar's elderly citizens reflects the unequal status of all forms of human services for the rural as compared to the urban elderly (Berry, 1978; Gerrard, 1978; Noll, 1978; Taietz, 1975; Tsutras, 1978). Some federal legislation seeks to rectify the nationwide discrimination against the rural aged. The Rural Policy Development Act of 1977 is intended to benefit the rural elderly directly (Adams, 1978). The 1978 Amendments to the Older Americans Act established a new formula weighted in favor of rural communities in states with high proportions of rural elderly. These states must spend 105 percent on the aged clustered in such areas. This legislation may be an important force to equalize the financial resource distribution to rural aged (Nelson, 1980).

However, the distribution of these funds still is closely linked to the discretion of area agencies. The Southwest Area Agency on Aging serves a number of counties that have clusters of isolated rural elders who are socially and economically disadvantaged. Its structure provides an opportunity for citizens from Tolivar and Folk County to serve on its advisory board. In the past, Tolivar residents had not maximized this opportunity. On the contrary, the most articulate and well-

Figure 5-3 The Rural Elderly and the Social Resource System

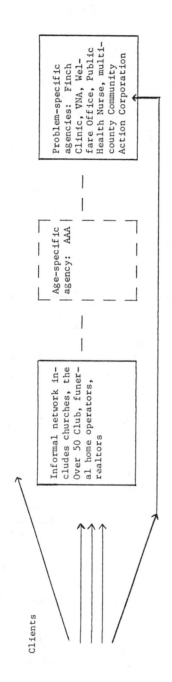

Clients

Problems arise with individuals who are not part of an existing network. For some, this is not a problem, they have made the choice to live alone.

Informal network includes churches, the Over 50 Club, funeral home operators, realtors

The real weakness of the system seems to lie here. There is no functioning age-specific agency to facilitate movement from social networks to problem-specific agencies. While some clients do receive services from the latter type of agencies, many go without because they lack awareness of the assistance or their beliefs inhibit their use.

Age-specific agency: AAA

Problem-specific agencies: Finch Clinic, VNA, Welfare Office, Public Health Nurse, multi-county Community Action Corporation

There are inadequacies both in the number of problem-specific services and in their coordination and cooperation.

informed persons there had not actively sought participation as a vehicle for local needs advocacy.

Committee membership on the advisory structure of the area agency was regarded as a social activity for an elite group of well-intended senior citizens who were willing to volunteer their time. When the politics of area agency resource distribution in rural America are either not understood or not taken seriously, the potential force of citizen input to improve conditions for isolated elders will not be realized. Education for skills in self-advocacy continues to be a neglected issue that reinforces environmental isolation and resource inequities.

Taking into account the unsatisfactory and unacceptable status of age-specific services in Tolivar and Folk County, the elderly who are at risk because of their isolation will be helped largely through the efforts of problem-specific agencies or formal resources that are directing assistance to the general adult population. In Folk County, the problem-specific service agencies are the major resources now available and it is to them that the elderly must turn.

The health and social intervention strategies that fit this rural area must rely on introducing appropriate gerontological expertise into systems that are geared to serve all adults with certain types of problems. The general service agencies also are the major sources of help to younger adults with problems such as alcoholism, intrafamily violence, and chronic unemployment. These formal entities, combined with a small array of age-specific sources, are what now exists to provide information, referral, and linkage to the available health and intervention sources. Whether or not they are adequate, these agencies comprise the sources beyond family, friends, and neighbors from which intervention for the elderly must be forthcoming.

In this community, ministers and morticians are two of the most important sources of outreach, referral, linkage, and clinical intervention. The role of the minister is more recognized as important but the mortician's functions are overlooked even though they are crucial to some isolated elderly.

Twenty to 25 percent of the congregations of the two largest Protestant churches in Tolivar are 60 years and older. The two have different approaches to meeting the needs of their elderly members. The Baptist church, the larger of the two and with a membership more than triple that of the Methodist, has a social group of senior members known as Never Too Old that meets monthly for dinner with attendance of 70 to 100 older persons, the majority of whom do not have major ambulation problems. The Extension Department of the Sunday school has 30 members who visit the homes of those who are housebound, read the Bible, and together study the religious material upon which the weekly sermon is based. There are 38 deacons responsible for visiting and identifying the needs of the 500 families who comprise the congregation (13.2 families per deacon).

The Methodist church maintains a similar home visitation effort but its network is much less structured. The minister assumes much of the responsibility for

keeping in touch with older members. He feels the pull and tug of two responsibilities. On the one hand, the elderly, especially those alone or with restricted
mobility, need the personal social contacts afforded by his home visiting. On the
other hand, there are strong competing demands for his time from a range of church
and community activities, particularly with the youth.

When asked what those who live alone discuss during his visitations, he
commented that the topics seemed to range widely, depending upon the health and
degree of functioning. The less impaired focused on lighter topics such as church
governance, the community, or daily living problems affecting the family. Those
living alone and without close family often talked about death, funeral arrangements, and recollections of past events that had special meaning. He relies
extensively on the active assistance of several retired members in the congregation
whom he respects greatly. Both churches make a major, seemingly effective,
effort to personalize their relationships with elderly members.

Church membership plays an important role in the lives of older persons in
Tolivar and Folk County. Active and long-term membership appears to palliate
isolation for many of the rural elderly. Of all of those interviewed in this community, it was the ministers who seemed to have the greatest sense of the social and
emotional aspects of isolation as defined here. Personal involvement in church
functions, hearing the social concerns of fellow parishioners, contacts with ministers, and the sense of being long-time members of a congregation are but a few of
the wide range of feelings the elderly expressed about their relationship with these
rural community institutions. The general attitude on the role and value of church
membership could be summed up in such comments as:

"I think I would not have lived through my last illness without the prayers and
loving concern of my ministers and the families of the church."

"If you don't belong to a church, play golf, and like to fish, Tolivar is no place
to be if you are old."

"I feel respected by the young people because I know the Bible and I can quote
its passages as well as the minister."

"Since I moved into town from the farm I think that I would have gone crazy if I
didn't have my church activities to keep me busy."

On the surface, the town's funeral homes appear to be places the elderly wish to
avoid, but none can forever. The funeral directors deal with the range of crises
associated with death. Their role is important to the elderly, who rely extensively
on them when there is a death in the family.

Elderly persons, especially widows, turn to these individuals for more than
funeral arrangements. As in urban communities, funeral directors frequently are
involved in giving important advice on matters ranging from the simple to the
complex because (a) deceased husbands told their widows little or nothing about

financial matters, (b) difficulties arise about the availability of funds for burial through insurance, (c) the widow must handle the couple's estate, and (d) the older people have a high level of trust and respect for these men as key community figures.

Many of the elderly women do not know the local bankers well, beyond a mere hello on the street or at church, and have few or no business transactions with them. There is hardly an elderly widow in Tolivar who does not know the Douglas brothers, who are both the most influential financiers and also the patriarchs of the community and who continue to wield much influence at their advanced ages of 86 and 89. Men of such high esteem are known to elderly widows as the "bankers," but, particularly for older women from a farm and from low to upper-lower socioeconomic status, approaching the Douglas brothers or others of their status usually is more than they will attempt without supportive directives to do so.

These women have a similar lack of familiarity with legal resources. The funeral directors become legal interpreters, confidants, and important sources of referral and reinforcement to take the many steps required to protect these women's resources. Lone rural elderly women are prime targets for fraud and con games that do occur in rural communities but rarely are spoken about because the victimization may never come to anyone else's attention.

Interviews helped clarify the different circumstances the elderly face when a family member dies. How these contribute to isolation is not clear, but it is an area to which intervenors must give greater attention if they are concerned with the social, emotional, and physical health factors associated with grief. The pattern of rapid sequential death in family deals a heavy blow to the elderly. The usual pattern of death rate in an immediate family is one every seven to nine years. However, it is not uncommon for the multigenerations of immediate family to lose several members in a short time.

As a case in point: three generations of Clarkson women died within seven months. Great-grandmother, great-aunt, and infant great-great-granddaughter all were buried from the same funeral home. Tragedy rocked this four-generation family, touching all of its individuals and generations. The eldest male Clarkson responded by announcing a zealous intention to keep the family together, his wife became disillusioned with her faith and briefly removed herself from close and long-established church involvement, and the young Clarkson couple moved from Folk County to the West Coast. This family experienced isolation reactions both from within and in relation to the community.

Elders living on a farm, especially widows, must confront decisions about whether or not to remain on homesteads that may be too much for them to manage. That difficult decision can be avoided if the couple moves into town before the death of either spouse but this is not done often. The elderly make great efforts to retain the farm as a residence, many times at great personal and economic costs. They may discuss these decisions with the funeral directors but the latter simply listen because to do otherwise would be overstepping their professional bounds both as defined personally and as perceived by the community.

The economics of burial are a major financial concern to some of the elderly, especially those with limited resources. It is not uncommon for an elderly man, woman, or couple to make trips to the funeral director's office to pay monthly premiums on a death/burial policy. It is very important, to at least a few of the elderly in Folk County, to have the financial arrangements adequately covered in advance of death. Burial costs there range from $500 to $5,000, with $2,000 the average. Folk County does not have a regular policy for handling pauper burials. To be buried under such circumstances is public disgrace to some surviving family members, and the aged fear they will be remembered with dishonor. Social Security and pension coverage usually do not provide enough to cover the cost of the average funeral.

The mental health concerns of the rural elderly are known to clergy, funeral directors, physicians, and other health intervenors. Some elderly persons with psychiatric problems receive no help at all from professional sources trained in mental health or social intervention. In Tolivar, there are a few elderly individuals and their families whose disorganization is so pervasive and chronic that they require a highly disproportionate amount of help from mental or other health sources but this assistance often is uncoordinated among a multiplicity of formal and informal sources. These community service providers often are in the best position to know the full range of helping sources that can be useful or acceptable even though they are not in a position to offer coordination.

The limited number of service sources in Tolivar make a remarkable effort to avoid having the elderly feel dependent when seeking and receiving help. The fear of stigma is so strong among some of the elderly that they never reach out for assistance. A person with expertise in community organization for older persons could initiate collaboration involving appropriate caregiving organizations and informal sources. A coordination strategy is needed to reach more elderly during those periods when social, economic, and physical isolators are locking them into the process of isolation.

VIEWS OF HEALTH AND SOCIAL INTERVENTION SOURCES

Practitioners familiar with the analysis of service delivery networks in small communities are aware that it takes little time, if they listen and ask the right questions, to learn what people perceive to be the most influential sources of care and intervention. In Tolivar, one of the most consistently identified sources of knowledge and information about problems of the isolated elderly is the Finch Medical Clinic. There the elderly can be linked to comprehensive and coordinated medical, health, and social services. The clinic's capacity for wide-ranging ambulatory care is strengthened by the availability of its x-ray and laboratory facilities, physical therapy, medical social work, counseling, pharmacy liaison, and computerized medical data systems—all onsite.

Some of the individuals described earlier as examples of isolated elderly or at risk of isolation are patients at the Finch Clinic. Older couples, several elderly women together, and occasionally an aged man or woman alone can be found in the waiting room at peak hours when there is a constant hum of activity. There always are individual reasons why they visit the clinic but elderly patients enjoy the sociability and personalized conversation with the clinic staff and with other older persons. The physician and medical social worker set the pattern of interaction with the aged patients, and all other clinic staff members and employees are expected to behave toward the elderly in ways that reinforce individualized personal concern.

The major health problems affecting the 600-plus persons 65 years and older in this clinic practice (one-fourth to one-third of the overall patient load) are arthritis, diabetes, heart, hypertension, obesity, chronic respiratory problems, and arteriosclerosis. A high percentage of the older men are farmers with ulcers. The physician noted that the extent of the emotional condition of some of these men was influenced by the degree of stress over higher or lower beef prices. Obesity is a major problem for the women over 55. This often is related to a complex set of behaviors that go beyond the narrow definition of medical concerns so these patients may be referred to the social worker for additional assessment and counseling.

The Finch Clinic serves as a training and field research site affiliate for a rural behavioral health research and training project being conducted by Washington University of St. Louis. In its early stages, the project's predominant orientation was on the emotional and social factors that interacted with the health problems of rural children and younger adults. This priority has been expanded, in large part because of the high proportion of elderly patients that Dr. Finch has referred to the behavioral health specialist trainees assigned to the clinic.

From a review of caseload information on the patients whom the staff considered seriously isolated, it is clear that social, emotional, and economic isolators impact on their health behaviors. The increased emphasis on the individual's responsibility for health maintenance and care (introduced into the Finch Clinic through its affiliation with the Washington University project) is compatible with the values of self-sufficiency and personal control. Yet only a minority of the elderly patients have behavioral health histories that reflect consistent disease avoidance practices, appropriate utilization patterns of service, or compliance with prescribed regimes. Their longstanding health-related patterns are the result of a very complex cluster of attitudes and beliefs, roles and social norms, and individual and environmental factors.

The lack of a knowledge base about the health behavior of the rural elderly makes it impossible to document how their patterns of isolation—or the degree to which they are isolated—influence their health behaviors. There is great need for investigations into the different sources of health care of the rural elderly, the organizational structures of the settings where they receive such intervention, the range of health beliefs among them, and the regimes requiring aged persons to alter important aspects of their life styles in order to promote the prevention of illness or further deterioration of existing conditions.

When the physician was asked what he felt was the most important factor in providing good health care to his elderly patients, he stressed the importance of continued social and physical activity. Retirement is not the solution for many elderly in this community. According to Dr. Finch's observations of his isolated patients, retirement consistently tends to promote a feeling of dependence and worthlessness. Retirement has no long-range acceptability to many farmers or small-town businessmen nor their wives. Some elderly retirees make an adequate adjustment to retirement but they must be able to find some substitute activities to enjoy.

The Foster Grandparent Program operating in Folk County under the administrative auspices of the Multicounty Office of the Regional Community Action Corporation is one example of a highly acceptable source of alternative activity. The role a foster grandparent can play was observed at the Good Samaritan Boys Ranch. This is a residential program for delinquent boys and is considered in rural Missouri to be a model of therapeutic activity. It has successfully used three elderly persons from the Foster Grandparent Program in key roles. Their involvement is strong evidence of the value of multigenerational family surrogate living and support in a therapeutic environment for young, socially at-risk youth. The results of this small experiment have been so positive that the board of directors of the ranch is seeking funds to add living facilities for up to 10 senior citizens. If the money can be raised, it will provide a model alternative living arrangement for the elderly in the county who are seeking a socially active life style.

Both the physician and the chief medical social worker at the Finch Medical Clinic were asked what resource Tolivar and Folk County needed to better meet the health and social needs of the isolated elderly. The physician spoke about the numerous social problems stemming from the fact that there was no hospital within a reasonable distance of the community:

1. Emergency medical service needs are not just physical. There is a major amount of trauma associated with an elderly person who must be rushed to an emergency room 50 miles away. The medical dangers are more obvious. The long distance and what occurs medically to the patient during the ambulance trip can be the actual cause of death.
2. The complexities of transporting elderly persons to another town for medical screening and testing that requires the facilities of a hospital are great, especially for those who have serious mobility problems and must depend on

children, families, or friends to transport them. Many times the elderly person either will put off going or just not go unless there is an emergency. This makes it difficult to provide some types of preventive care or to treat chronic conditions.

3. The burden of having an elderly family member in a hospital 50 miles away makes visitation difficult. If one member of an aged couple in the 70s or 80s falls ill and must be hospitalized outside Folk County, it is difficult, if not impossible, for the spouse to get to the facility for regular visits. Many older couples lack the financial resources to rent a motel room and stay in the city even for a few days, let alone for an extended period. The resultant inability for regular visits is a type of emotional isolation that can affect the condition of the ill spouse.

The physician regarded the development of a hospital in the county as essential if anything was to be done to reduce such recurring isolating circumstances.

The medical social worker offered equally important suggestions as to the types of interorganizational linkages, service programs, and community organizational efforts that could be undertaken in Tolivar and Folk County to reduce some of the isolation problems of the elderly:

1. There is a great need for better coordination of all the various health and social services that elderly patients utilize. Since there are only a few key formal service providers, it should be possible to develop individualized coordination and case management. For example, the sources of social services, mental health treatment, and medical care should be coordinated. In a community of this size, unlike an urban area, all the sources of formal services are identifiable. There needs to be better coordination among the few physicians in the county in terms of scheduling emergency and night/weekend coverage. There also should be more coordination in the family because members often will go to different physicians and the entire group or the aged couple may need joint counseling to deal with care and treatment issues.

2. The community has not been creative in fostering contributory social roles for the elderly. There are only a few traditional volunteer roles, especially for older women, and they do not really capitalize on these persons' tremendous potential to give to and receive from others. One program has been proposed to involve older men and women as volunteers in an abuse shelter program for young women and their children.

Several agencies offer home health care services in Folk County. Taken together, they provide skilled nursing on a regular basis from 8 a.m. to 6 p.m. daily, with weekend, holiday, and evening care available upon request. Physical therapies are provided by the home health care agency but medical social work is not available. Nursing personnel provide nutrition counseling as part of their health care function. Two agencies receive referrals from physician, family, friends, self, hospitals, nursing homes, and other sources.

For the elderly to receive skilled nursing services, there must be a written directive and supervision from a physician. The acceptability of home health care services among the elderly is difficult to assess as there are no data regarding clients' satisfaction or unmet needs. Even though the benefits of home health care have been evaluated informally, medical and social practitioners believe there is no question about the need and the role these service sources play in supporting both the formal and informal aspects of noninstitutional long-term care for the elderly in Tolivar. This observation is strongly supported by research that indicates the need for rural home health care of all types (Hayslip, Ritter, Oltman, & McDonnell, 1980).

A major value in expanding and coordinating the home health care services in Folk County is the extent to which they can extend the physician's capacity to work with the isolated rural elderly. Here, as in many other counties in Missouri, and perhaps throughout the United States where there are high concentrations of the rural elderly coupled with physician shortages, the lack of doctors and support medical personnel is the major barrier to better health care. To the degree that quantitative and qualitative improvement can take place in the home health care services, the capacity of the physician to work with the homebound physically at-risk elderly will improve.

While some rural physicians still make home visits, this is disappearing rapidly because of low reimbursement from third party sources, the overwhelming daily office visit schedule, and the increasing mean age of the private practice doctors who provide the majority of primary health care. In Tolivar and Folk County the physician-patient ratio is 1 to 4,072 and in some parts of the region the nearest doctor's office is 50 miles away. The community has been unsuccessful in recruiting and retaining new physicians who will make a long-term professional commitment to practice in the rural area.

Residents and professionals both have positive attitudes about the few nursing homes in their communities. The facilities in Tolivar offer a positive influence in the provision of long-term care to the elderly but this generalization is not characteristic of nursing homes in all rural areas in Missouri. Many factors contribute to the quality of leadership provided by administrators whose nursing homes become very important and visible sources of long-term care. The administrator of the Tolivar Nursing Home is highly qualified, having had training in clinical social work and with the county's Department of Family Services.

This nursing home is licensed as an intermediate care facility. Most residents are from Folk or surrounding counties. However, a few newcomers to the community from Kansas City moved their elderly parents into the home. The mean age of residents is 82, and 74 percent are female. The home serves as the only source of Meals-on-Wheels for the elderly in town. The facility took on this responsibility because no other agency had a dietitian and was willing to support the service. The administrator believes another agency could do a much better job of meeting the communitywide need but no others have expressed an interest. The program is important to the discharge planning program because the small percentage of residents who do return home usually need meal preparation support.

The unequal distribution of Medicare funds to urban and rural elderly has been noted. Despite the fact that it is designed to offer all of the elderly equal coverage in medical services and hospital care, in reality older persons in urban areas receive about 40 percent more in Medicare benefits than do their rural counterparts (Clark, 1978). The nursing home administrator spoke at length about the differential rate-setting procedure for Medicaid reimbursement in Missouri for urban vs. rural locations. He said that of course the practices favor urban nursing homes, which can document higher costs, but he does not believe those expenses actually are greater. He attributes this pattern to the lack of political organization that characterizes all health and human service providers in rural Missouri. The fact that rural communities such as Tolivar cannot attract geriatric health specialists probably is another factor. When asked about future planning for long-term care in Tolivar and Folk County, he said:

> I think that all of us in this area who work with the elderly realize that there is a lot of potential to build a better system of long-term care in this county. However, there are a lot of barriers that are not easy to resolve. The first thing that we must do is to recruit more physicians to this community. Everybody, especially our own local doctors, will agree on this. Without additional medical backup I am not in a position to expand the size and scope of the services we deliver. I think that I'm already receiving the maximum possible cooperation from the private physicians we have in this community. There is so much agreement among all of us that we need additional doctors.
>
> The impact of the rural health initiative on this area has really been minimal. The motivation of these young doctors is short lived. They come into the area for several years, put their time in, then leave. Few if any of those that have come to this part of the state have made any real investment in developing a practice that will benefit the residents of Folk County.
>
> People, especially the old people, are very resistant to go to those clinics supported by the federal program. They complain strongly because they never know if they will be seen by the same doctor. I can foresee no viable way of involving them in the planning that I'd like to undertake for this county.

The current concepts of long-term care and the reimbursement structure that supports it is very dependent upon the medical model. . . . The
physician must be the team leader and so I try to use my limited staff
resources to facilitate what little physician time I have to the benefits of
the patients. I have seen one definite payoff of this as we have been able
to do active rehabilitation with some of our patients.

CONCLUSION

In looking at the service offerings in Folk County in terms of the interventive
model presented in Chapter 3, the problems in the present system can be discerned.
In this community, the first problem is the number of isolated elderly who do not
belong to any of the social participation organizations. It is within these groups that
basic socialization needs can be met. In this rural community, however, the bulk of
these informal organizations are organized at the churches for their members. For
the individual who is not associated with any particular church, this important
source is unavailable. There is a distinct impression that the churches make a rather
limited effort to reach out to nonmembers to meet socialization needs, particularly
if they are of low socioeconomic status.

The churches in this community would seem to be the guardians not only of a
religious code but also of a self-defined acceptable life style and set of personal
values. This would make it difficult for their members to be truly accepting, in
other than a missionary sense, to individuals without long-standing church connections. The senior center that exists outside of church sponsorship is known as an
elitist group and thus is not available as an optional source of socialization to fill the
gap for many persons who are not connected with churches.

A valuable informal source in this community would appear to be a sense of
neighborly help. However, since individuals in the town seem unconnected with
formal agencies, their help can be dead-ended when problems become too difficult. Cora Carter, who was getting help from neighbors to remain in the community, might have been able to continue her independent life style had someone been
available to discuss her needs with her niece. For while on the surface Cora was at
risk and isolated, she seemed to be deriving much satisfaction from her connection
to her own land and home. To remove her, reluctantly, from those familiar
surroundings was to create isolation of another sort.

Other individuals would seem to be able to use specific problem-related services. Elizabeth Mead required professional outreach and counseling to deal with
her isolation and psychosomatic symptoms. As a couple, the Meads might be able
to communicate more effectively about her incompatible feeling toward farm life if
they could have received marital counseling. Unfortunately, the minister representing the informal helping network was unable to link the couple and a counsel-

ing source. Their requests for help circulated between realtor and minister rather than reaching a specific agency.

On the other hand, Louise Seddy, Sam Berry, and, to a certain extent, Walter Baker, were connected to agencies that provided specific supportive services but they were not benefitting from social participation opportunities through formal sources. A complicating factor for both Louise Seddy and Sam Berry was their life styles, which were viewed as deviant by many older citizens. There is a suggestion, in both cases, that to increase the probability of their acceptance by others, they would have to significantly alter their way of living. However, these patterns may be so deeply ingrained and/or the separateness from others so cherished that change is unlikely. Perhaps a more realistic intervention goal for such individuals is to start by coordinating services that meet basic needs and, over time, encourage access to appropriate social participating opportunities beyond their own informal network.

The discussion of service delivery in Chapter 2 included suggestions for roles within the age-specific agency. Such an entity was viewed as a specific link between isolated individuals and the problem-specific agencies. A major function of this vital link was to provide outreach to clients in need, to make available information on clients in need to the problem-specific agency, and to create an awareness of the services of those agencies among the informal networks and potential consumers. In this illustration, these functions—and the ability of the age-specific agency to perform them—are all but missing. Informal helpers such as the realtor and the funeral director could listen, advise, or speak to another informal helper such as a minister, but they all lacked a relationship to the problem-specific agencies that could deal with issues that could not be solved at the informal support level.

While the regional AAA had designated a worker for this particular area, that person's identity was not even known in the community. The Community Action Corporation did seem to be performing some age-specific functions but in a piecemeal fashion. What is needed from either of these organizations is an effort to help develop a system of linkages for services to the elderly. This organizational effort would have two focuses to deal with this community's problems. The first should be directed toward establishing a linkage from the informal network to the problem-specific agencies, the second toward establishing a case coordination or case management system among the problem-specific helpers and agencies.

In this community, the first focal effort—linkage between informal networks and problem-specific agencies—might best be accomplished by a community organizer from either AAA or the Community Action Corporation. The organizer's efforts would be directed toward interesting the already established informal helping groups (e.g., churches, Over 50 Club) to establish a citizens council. The involvement of community members could be built on the tradition of volunteerism and neighborly help that already existed there.

By organizing around representatives from several existing organizations, it would be possible to avoid having this effort labeled or linked to a specific group, thereby making it less acceptable by others. It would be toward this group that the problem-specific agencies could present information on the type of help available and try to convince these community representatives that acceptance of these services was legitimate.

These representatives would be expected to carry the information back to their respective organizations. To maximize the probability of generating acceptance of social services, the representatives should be well-respected members of the community. This group would be in an excellent position to analyze, discuss, and prioritize the needs of the elderly. It also would be in a good position to spell out the problems its members see in service delivery. This information could be fed back to problem-specific agencies.

In actuality, it is quite difficult to feed the information gathered by a citizen group back to a scattering of problem-specific helpers and agencies. The need for some organization among such service providers is clear. This could be accomplished by having one agency designated as case manager or by creating a council composed of representatives of the community's problem-specific agencies. Since this town has a clinic that combines both medical and social service providers, it may be an ideal site for this function for a number of reasons.

First, one of the problems for the elderly (in this and other communities) is that more than one doctor prescribes medication for a client so some coordination among physicians is necessary. The private physicians are less likely to work through a nonmedical facility for case management or consultation. Since the clinic also offers social services, it also could use this case coordination function to make the private physicians more aware of the impact of unmet social needs on physical functioning and encourage the doctors to refer patients for social assistance by acting as a model in the delivery of combined services. In the case of Louise Seddy, where the physician is fighting a lonely battle to preserve her independence, this goal might be enhanced if a worker were in continuing contact with her to help mediate the conflict with her neighbors so that she would be less isolated from this potential support system.

Second, there appears to be a need for medical inpatient facilities in the community. This need was being addressed through efforts to obtain a new Folk County hospital. However, there should be a communitywide priority to introduce a strong social work center in the hospital that reaches out into the community. A community planning group to promote the development of such a center would stimulate an increased awareness of: (a) the special at-risk groups that have both social and health needs, and (b) the establishment of intervention approaches that meet more than medical needs but are acceptable because they are connected to a medical facility and that could offer more crisis resources.

In summary, this rural Missouri area involves a town and a county in which residents value self-reliance and independence. There is a reluctance to intrude in personal or family matters; however, neighborly concern for others is widespread. A dependence on churches for social support is appropriate for some but other activity sponsorship is needed. Better communication and coordination among all aspects of the formal network and between the formal and informal is needed to help the most isolated aged.

The absence of coordination and information exchange about the isolated serves to keep them in that state. During a period when the resources to provide special health and social programs in rural areas is disappearing rapidly, communities must experiment with ways of (a) ensuring that human resource distribution through state-controlled block grant approaches serves to provide equal resources to rural areas, (b) providing greater representation of small rural communities on advisory and decision-making boards, and (c) channeling community concern about the isolated rural elderly into appropriate interventions.

REFERENCES

Adams, D.L. Who are the rural aged? In R.C. Atchley & T.O. Byerts (Eds.), *Rural Environments and Aging.* Washington, D.C.: Gerontological Society, 1975.

Adams, S. Wiping out gaps, overlaps, conflicts. *Perspective on Aging,* 1978, *2*(1), 25-26.

Berry, J. The silent minority often unserved. *Perspective on Aging,* 1978, *2*(1), 24, 32.

Clark, D. Too much promised, too little done. *Perspective on Aging,* 1978, *2*(1), 9-10.

Coward, R.T. Planning community services for the rural elderly: Implications from research. *Gerontologist,* 1979, *19*, 275-282.

Extension Division. *Ozark gateway regional profile,* Edition MP-360. Columbia, Mo.: University of Missouri-Columbia, Extension Division, 1974, p. 5

Extension Division. *Lakes country regional profile,* Edition MP-366. Columbia, Mo.: University of Missouri-Columbia, Extension Division, 1975, p. 5.

Gerrard, L. The most disadvantaged. *Perspective on Aging,* 1978, *2*(1), 2, 10.

Ginsberg, L.H. *Social work in rural communities.* New York: Council on Social Work Education, February 1976.

Hayslip, B., Ritter, M.L., Oltman, R.M., & McDonnell, C. Home care services and the rural elderly. *Gerontologist,* 1980, *20*, 193-199.

Nelson, G. Social services to the urban and rural aged: The experience of area agencies on aging. *Gerontologist,* 1980, *20*, 200-207.

Noll, P. An alphabet soup of agencies fail. *Perspective on Aging,* 1978, *2*(1), 19-23.

Powers, E.A., Keith, P., & Joudy, W. Family relationships and friendships. In R.C. Atchley & T.O. Byerts (Eds.), *Rural environments and aging.* Washington, D.C.: Gerontological Society, 1975.

Rathbone-McCuan, E. Integrated health and mental health planning for the rural elderly. In P.K. Kim & C.P. Wilson (Eds.), *Toward rural gerontology.* Washington, D.C.: University Press of America, 1981.

Schooler, K.K. A comparison of rural and nonrural elderly on selected variables. In R.C. Atchley & T.O. Byerts (Eds.), *Rural environments and aging*. Washington, D.C.: Gerontological Society, 1975.

Taietz, P. Community facilities and social services. In R.C. Atchley & T.O. Byerts (Eds.), *Rural environments and aging*. Washington, D.C.: Gerontological Society, 1975.

Tsutras, F. Congressional rural caucus. *Perspective on Aging*, 1978, 2(1), 5; 37.

Chapter 6

The Isolated Black Elderly

INTRODUCTION

The next focus is on the social and psychological dimensions of isolation that influence the lives of inner city black elders. Although much of this analysis may apply equally well to black elders living in rural or semirural environments, most of the information base was gathered from urban samples. The analysis of intervention strategies to meet human needs associated with conditions of isolation emphasizes the role of the black church, primarily because:

1. Most formal health and social service organizations have limited linkages to it.
2. Health and social services practitioners often ignore or misunderstand its role in the lives of their black elderly clients.
3. It exerts a significant influence in preventing social isolation.
4. It is a cornerstone in the urban neighborhoods where many black elders live.

The role of the church as a resource to meet social and emotional needs of black elders is considered with an understanding of: (a) the church's limits in dealing with the serious health, economic, transportation, and housing needs of large numbers of urban black elders, (b) its contemporary and historical traditions of maintaining an organizational structure and function differently from other community institutions, and (c) the dynamic and dramatic changes it has undergone over many decades.

The discussion involves the complexities of both the structure and the functions of this community resource that is, unto itself, somewhat isolated from other formal organizations serving the elderly. This is achieved through sharing the results of practice experience and those of black colleagues because it is a neglected area, as well as through exploring the church as an underdeveloped component of the resource network available to these elders because community agencies have ignored and/or misunderstood its potential significance.

Specific isolators analyzed include the separation of black elders from the extended family because of mobility linked to job seeking (of self or children), lack of information about available services, and a complex cluster of factors that influence their attempts to utilize existing community services and programs. Utilization patterns are influenced by a history of real and suspected discriminatory practices as well as agencies' failure to take into account cultural differences in planning and providing services. The intention is to provide guidelines for the development of a better partnership between the black church and health and social service intervenors to meet the social and emotional needs of these elderly.

PROFILE OF THE BLACK ELDER

Many issues must be taken into account when describing the isolated status of urban black elders. Figure 6-1 depicts major factors which lead to isolation in the lives of America's elderly blacks. The published literature available from the middle to late 1970s frequently is based on 1970 census data that seemingly undercounted their numbers. Census data provide sociodemographic information on the black elderly but are not sufficient to make a meaningful analysis of their life styles. Life style variables do influence patterns of isolation and adaptation to isolators. The 1980 census data, unavailable at the time of writing, was expected to do little to alter the problem of undercounting or add new insights into the uniqueness of the life style of the black elder. In advance of the census data, minority group advocates had a low level of satisfaction concerning its quality. An adequate description of the patterns of social and psychological isolation of the black elderly requires more than survey data. On the other hand, the statistical information that describes their socioeconomic status as compared to older whites consistently reveals differences between the two groups.

Black elders are more economically disadvantaged than their white counterparts. According to the results of a National Council on Aging (NCOA) survey, the median income for black elders (both as unrelated individuals and as family units) was two-thirds that of whites. The most economically disadvantaged of all were elderly black females who lived alone. In 1975, of those 65 or older, 13.4 percent of whites and 36.3 percent of blacks were below the poverty level (NCOA, 1978). If those near the poverty level (125 percent of the poverty level income) were considered, these percentages would rise to 23 percent for white and 51.6 percent for black elders, with older females comprising the largest group among both whites and blacks (NCOA, 1978).

Low income affects isolation patterns among a significant proportion of all elders. Any poor older persons not able to provide for themselves adequate

Figure 6-1 Isolators That Impact on Black Elders

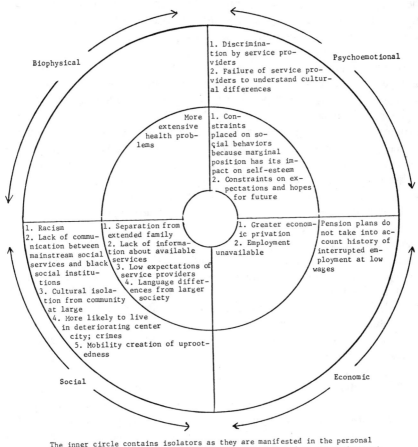

Biophysical

Psychoemotional

1. Discrimina-
tion by service pro-
viders
2. Failure of service providers to understand cultural differences

More
extensive
health prob-
lems

1. Con-
straints
placed on so-
çial behaviors
because marginal
position has its im-
pact on self-esteem
2. Constraints on ex-
pectations and hopes
for future

1. Racism
2. Lack of commu-
nication between
mainstream social
services and black
social institu-
tions
3. Cultural isola-
tion from community
at large
4. More likely to live
in deteriorating center
city; crimes
5. Mobility creation of uprootedness

1. Separation from
extended family
2. Lack of informa-
tion about available
services
3. Low expectations of
service providers
4. Language differ-
ences from larger
society

1. Greater econom-
ic privation
2. Employment
unavailable

Pension plans do
not take into ac-
count history of
interrupted em-
ployment at low
wages

Social

Economic

The inner circle contains isolators as they are manifested in the personal
lives of black elders, the outer circle those that abound in the environment.

housing, transportation, diet, health care, personal safety, and recreation needs
will have their well-being affected. Fewer black elders own their own homes as
compared to whites (57 percent vs. 71 percent), and a larger percentage of the
black elderly live in deteriorating central cities. More black elders reported crime
was a serious problem (41 percent) than for all elders (23 percent) (NCOA, 1978).
They often are confined to deteriorating living quarters and unable, because of
risks to person and property, to move freely within crime-ridden neighborhoods
where they are easy targets. Even in their residence they may be easy prey,
regardless of the meagerness of their resources.

Black elders often are survivors of lifelong poverty. Their membership in a resource-depleted community environment over several generations suggests that their coping styles may have a fixed quality passed down from generation to generation because new styles do not prove relevant to conditions continuously across generations and that there are unchanging low levels of expectations of supportive environmental resources.

Multigenerations of black clients express mistrust of social and health service providers and thus wish to avoid encounters. If younger generations do not escape the harsh conditions of their poverty, they may have little to offer the elderly to supplement their material needs (Herzog, 1966). This important point—the lack of resources among younger generations to give to older blacks—is conveniently avoided in economic and social service policy formulation. Among the most deprived segment of the poor, individuals' own survival may occupy so much of their energies that they can spare little concern for a dependent elder. Even when that older person can make a contribution to family management (i.e., in the care of children) or to family income (such as Social Security monies), there still may be a drain on family resources.

A practitioner working with black elderly clients probably will find that extreme poverty is the overriding issue in their isolation. The individual health or social service practitioner might be able to do little to alleviate that problem except to assist the elderly or their families to apply for any benefits to which they may be entitled, if this has not been done already. Even if these benefits are not sufficient to maintain the elderly comfortably, little more can be done to improve their financial status if no other sources are available. When the practitioner focuses exclusively on financial needs, the intervention strategy may be the same for both black and white aged clients.

The frustration of a practitioner's not being able to change the system for needy clients is a common problem, even though professional literature underplays this situation. However, economic isolators are not the only problem areas. Factors such as language use, family relationships and style, and social resources become important when the practitioner deals with social and emotional needs. Then barriers of age, poverty, and race take on special significance as the variables that impact on problem resolution or that minimize the consequences of those problems become more complex.

While the number of blacks over 65 has increased dramatically since 1900, there still is a substantially higher proportion of white elders as compared to total white population (11 percent) than there are older blacks compared to the total black population (7.4 percent) (NCOA, 1978). This differential can be explained by whites' more favorable life expectancy and the current higher birth rate among blacks (NCOA, 1978). These trends suggest that the lower life expectancy rates of the black elderly as a special subgroup will continue into the future and remain a statistical fact denoting societal injustice.

Nonwhite elders have a lower median age at death (66.4 for males and 74.2 for females) than older whites (72.5 for males and 80.2 for females). However, this difference does not suggest that all blacks die sooner than whites, since expectation of additional years left at age 65 is the same for both white and nonwhite males and only slightly higher for white females (17.6 vs. 16.8 for nonwhites). Nonwhites are more likely to rate their health as poor (18 percent) than whites (8 percent) and are more likely to experience mobility limitations (23.7 percent vs. 17.0 percent) (NCOA, 1978).

In an analysis of urban elders, Sauer (1977) found no substantial differences in mean morale scores but the determinants of morale varied between groups of older blacks and whites. For both groups, high morale was related to better health and to participation in many solitary activities. Higher morale for elderly whites also depended on greater frequency of interaction with family. The morale variable, while frequently investigated by gerontologists, is operationalized from theoretical frameworks not grounded in subcultural or minority considerations.

This information on socioeconomics and health in both black and white elders demonstrates the disadvantage in being old and black. A double jeopardy hypothesis has been advanced to account for this differential. The hypothesis, proposed by the National Urban League in 1964 (Dowd & Bengtson, 1978), states that there is a cumulative effect of two forms of discrimination—race and age. (A triple jeopardy hypothesis might be suggested since black elderly females seem to be more disadvantaged than any other group.) To substantiate this hypothesis, Dowd and Bengtson (1978) report income declines of 36 percent for white and 55 percent for black elders. They also report that health scores decline 9 percent for white elders and 13 percent for blacks.

To the extent that the double jeopardy hypothesis is verifiable, it has implications for the development of social programs, policies, and personal intervention efforts. To accept the fact the black elderly experience problems differently or more intensely because of the additional impact of racial discrimination is to suggest that perhaps public provision of resources should be handled differently for them. To provide different resources, such as medical services, housing, and financial needs, much more specific information would be needed on how the double jeopardy operates. If the black elder's income is reduced by a larger percentage than a white's, it is necessary to understand the consequences of that cut on overall functioning, i.e., decision making, coping behaviors, morale, and social interaction patterns.

Without understanding these dynamics, it is impossible to define the extent and nature of appropriate changes in Social Security, pensions, or other economic resources. However, the planning of major national social policies should be grounded in a knowledge of the black experience and should be weighed in such a way as to ensure equity within the system. In this way, social policy modification can be based on multiple variables rather than on race as the single condition for major reform. This of course would increase the complexity of policy decision making because it would have to take into account needs that are unique to specific subgroups rather than to fashion a simpler policy based on the stereotypic needs of a traditional concept of the mainstream elderly.

While differences in health and financial measures do support the double jeopardy hypothesis, this is not necessarily true of other variables. Indeed, on such variables as interaction with relatives and life satisfaction (tranquility and optimism) Dowd and Bengtson (1978) found a reduction in ethnic variation over time. It is on this evidence that age can be seen as a leveler. This would suggest that it is unwise to try to explain all problems of elders exclusively by ethnic or racial differences; to do so ignores "variation across ethnic boundaries and within ethnic categories" (Dowd & Bengtson, 1978). Solutions to double jeopardy problems must be approached from comprehensive knowledge, taking into account differentials in racial subgroups of aged.

A clearly racial isolator is discrimination by institutions and service providers. This discrimination is a present reality and has had a historical influence on the lives of all black elders. They carry memories of the lynchings and race riots of the earlier 1900s and of the public stereotypes and of white society's general attitude toward them (Bardo, 1974). Given this historical background, it is understandable that older blacks expect less from the social institutions designed to meet the needs of the elderly and would be disinclined to press for greater need fulfillment through utilization of these services (Dancy, 1977).

It also must be recognized that in the historical context of the black culture, certain norms developed apart from those of the white mainstream. For example, cultural variations included differences in educational and language patterns, which of course varied within the black community depending on socioeconomic status and place of residence (urban-rural, north-south). The most marked cultural divergence affected the very poor black elders in urban northern cities who had migrated from southern rural areas. They more frequently lack basic reading and writing skills to the extent that communication with community agencies may be hampered, particularly when an agency depends on written communication to inform the public of services (Dancy, 1977).

Not only may literacy rates be low in some areas but also the black elder may place greater importance on oral communication for reasons other than inability to read and write (Dancy, 1977). It is obvious that if information on available programming were to be disseminated through written communication it would not reach those who could not read it or who were inclined to ignore that form of exchange. The process of information dissemination for preventive and interventive functions also is relevant in the application of mass media and outreach to the elderly, e.g., radio communication and information for the elderly.

Another language difficulty involves the different sentence structure and pronunciation that characterizes the nonstandard English used by poor and less-well-educated blacks. This language differential can be traced back to the arrival from Africa of black slaves from many tribes speaking numerous languages. Since no organized attempt was made to teach them English, they developed among themselves a "creolized English" as a common language base (Dancy, 1977).

When the language differential takes the form of a unique use of words, the problem becomes even more difficult. An excellent example of this is the illustration provided by Dancy (1977) in which an elderly black, a resident in a state mental hospital, repeatedly asked for "cat's heads" rather than the food he was given. The staff perceived this as additional evidence of his psychiatric illness. Over time it was discovered that "cat's heads" referred to biscuits and molasses. The black elderly may have difficulty understanding service providers and agencies; in turn, the personnel of those institutions may have difficulty comprehending their requests, needs, and reticence or failure to make use of health and social services.

Within the black community, great emphasis is placed on the extended kinship system. The importance of being a part of a family and community network makes isolation from that network particularly painful for the elderly. This extended family concept is rooted in community traditions that include those carried from Africa. In the more recent past, extended family relationships have been a coping mechanism that ensured survival in light of limited access to community services (Dancy, 1977). Within that familiar network, the black elderly feel a freedom of expression and association that would not be possible if they were to be placed in an institution or participate in a service program that did not provide that sense of community that is defined in terms of the presence of other blacks.

Many of the black elders now living in large cities migrated from the rural south in search of jobs in their younger years. Although only 52 percent of all blacks now live in the South, many of the elders in northern urban areas have roots there (Dancy, 1977). Southern black cultural patterns, which include their own variants on religion, food, language, and life style, may increase the elders' feeling of isolation or difference from the surrounding milieu. This separation from an extended family network can coexist with their being apart from children, who in turn have migrated to other areas or even neighboring suburbs in search of better living. Where there is separation from the nuclear or extended family, the likelihood of isolation will increase rather than diminish.

Thus, urban black elders may find themselves isolated from kin and from the life and surroundings they knew as children and young adults without even the closeness of immediate family to compensate. These isolators are not common to all older blacks nor are they always the most important ones. But when the isolation among the white elderly that can result from such other factors as low income, age discrimination, or poor mental or physical health is combined with the specific isolators that may affect black elders, the greater vulnerability of the latter must be recognized and taken into account in developing intervention alternatives.

Isolators reflect a unique cultural heritage important to blacks but it is not clear how they have been addressed in service planning. Planners tend to debate alternative strategies on the basis of personal political ideology. One major question in the debate is whether separate services may be required for the black elderly. The call for separate services is manifested in various plans that range from a relatively simple one to provide a few services that are culturally specific to the black elderly to a very complex one for developing completely separate and equally comprehensive programs. White service providers often suggest the approach of offering different services to black elders based on a vague belief that their needs are somehow different from whites. The development of a separate service system often is justified on the basis of testimony of need and injustice but the rationale is not backed by documentation. Offering of separate services assumes that: (a) black elders differ in so many ways from whites that it is not possible for one system to serve both and (b) this is what would be preferred by all older blacks. The merits of strategies at both levels are questionable since they often are not based on input from black elderly service consumers and the knowledge available about such individuals is insufficient as a rationale for implementing separate service structures.

Another important issue is whether or not the services the black elderly utilize should be provided exclusively by black workers. While there are numerous cultural variations that may present serious difficulties for a nonblack practitioner's effective interventions with black clients, is it desirable or feasible to operate from the assumption that only blacks can help blacks? There are potential differences between black worker and black elder that may be of great importance. These may vary from the ones present in the white practitioner/nonwhite client interaction but could be as influential on the outcome of intervention.

For instance, black professionals may have generational and socioeconomic differences that do not promote acceptance and appreciation of the cultural and prior socialization experiences of older black clients. These could have more negative influence on intervention outcomes than a racial difference between worker and client. Some agencies make greater use of paraprofessionals closer in socioeconomic status to the black elderly client as a strategy to overcome these differences. Rather than using social status characteristics as the basis for staff selection, it would seem more important to match workers' qualifications to the tasks and skills required.

In an attempt to resolve the dilemma of how to plan services for the black elderly, some alternatives are worthwhile exploring. The one to be developed here encompasses the role and function of the black church as a resource to meet some of the needs previously specified as related to the social and psychological conditions of isolated black elders. Building a rationale for using the black church in the intervention strategies is supported by the need to ensure that the public health and social service resources reflect individualized client needs and to make certain that those available to the black elderly through informal structures, such as the church, are taken into account in planning.

IMPORTANT COMPONENTS OF THE BLACK CHURCH

To understand how the black church can be used as an important resource for practitioners serving the black elder, it is necessary to consider its position in the community, the role of the black pastor in the lives of the congregation, and the potential status available for each individual through membership in a church.

Much has been written about the black church and the black experience. Some of the underlying themes in these works have been:

1. the patterns of voluntary association and how they support black ethnic identity (Layng, 1978; Babchuk & Thompson, 1962)
2. the extent to which the black church provides a complex counterbalancing force to the bias and self-negating premises of the white society (Frazier, 1964; Williams, 1974)
3. the adaptive functions church membership affords black individuals in relation to both the black and white communities (Logan, 1980; Nelsen & Nelsen, 1975).

This literature, not exclusively devoted to the black elderly, is a valuable background for understanding some of the components of the black church. It has significance for those who want to explore alternative ways to resolve the social and psychological isolation problems among older blacks.

The pastor's responsibilities in the spiritual and secular dimensions of the church have been largely ignored by practitioners who work with elderly black clients. This generalization is made repeatedly by those who have attempted to establish a link with a black church. Many practitioners do not take into account the role of the clergy in the social networks that define the support system available to large numbers of the black elderly. When asked about the important community resources available, they often do not even mention the pastor but agree to that individual's importance if suggested as a resource.

If these perceptions are correct, it is important next to share observations about the primary place members of the clergy may have in the community life of older black Americans. Historically, the clergy have held central roles in the black community. During the era of slavery, preachers also were a mainstay to families struggling to survive in bondage. The study of the rich and dynamic history of these ministers expanded as more scholars began to add to the history of black America (DuBois, 1903; Frazier, 1964; Drake & Cayton, 1970, Banks, 1972; Becker, 1972).

These histories sensitized readers to what the black community's ties to its clerical leadership have meant to its people, probably of all ages. The preacher was a charismatic force who held blacks together during times of crisis and long periods of repression, prejudice, and discrimination. Then, as now, black ministers are educators, spiritual advisers, and representatives of their community empowered to interact with the white community on many important economic and general welfare issues.

On the other hand, the role of black pastors is now in transition. As a group, they have been greatly influenced by the leadership of the Rev. Dr. Martin Luther King, Jr., and countless others who played key roles in the civil rights movement during the 1960s and early 1970s. Today their influence continues, but some may see their roles and responsibilities more closely related to the social and personal needs of their own congregations. (This does not necessarily imply that the black clergy have turned inward, away from social action, any more than have whites. Rather, it implies that the urgency for all members of the clergy to participate in organized change efforts is less than a few years ago when social action and the church were more synchronized.)

The black clergy are in a unique position to help their congregations turn the negatives they face in everyday life into positives. The historical writings suggest a longstanding need among black congregations to have their clergy be the leaders in turning poor circumstances into tolerable ones. For example, in 1981, the black clergy of Atlanta bore the burden of translating murders of black children into a context that offered solace to a terrified and angry community. To summarize the statements of one midwestern black minister interviewed:

> Daily the lives of my people are affected by the forces of racism and discrimination. The children's futures are often limited by inadequate schooling, poor mothers are often degraded by the welfare system, unemployed fathers are demoralized by their inability to provide for their families, and many elders remain unserved by a system of service designed to meet the needs of all elderly. As a church we have limits because not all of life can be made just, but our worship becomes the source of celebration to strengthen ourselves to live each day with pride and dignity.

Black pastors are adept at leading their congregations to adopt a strengthening mental and emotional attitude toward their victimization, i.e., the consequences of racial discrimination and/or social injustice. Concentration on the strengths that can be experienced through spiritual wisdom and religious conviction can offset feelings of hopelessness and frustration. This pattern of entrusting problems unto God can make individuals tolerant of daily struggles. This message is reinforced through sermons, biblical readings, and personal guidance of the minister and other members of the congregation who share in the opportunities for interpersonal support. This personal ministry is directed toward assisting individuals in their struggle with difficult circumstances, conditions, or events and helping them perceive these experiences as challenges to overcome.

Another minister described this as the transformation of what, on the surface, seems intolerable to what is tolerable, if not in fact advantageous, for the betterment of life now or in the future. It prevents individuals from being overwhelmed with defeatism by difficult situations that they cannot easily manipulate by their own actions or those of others.

The extent to which ministers maximize the coping abilities of the congregation varies with their relationship with the congregation as a whole and with its various parts. Programs offered through the churches promote a strong sense of family life as a vehicle for mediating conflict. The church as an important social organization also confers status, provides for leadership development, offers a forum for advocacy for the black community, and creates opportunities for release of tension and for social-recreational activities (Staples, 1976). The messages conveyed through sermons, Bible study, missionary work, and education of youth emphasize pride and dignity. A focus for preaching becomes a search for strength, dignity, unity, and compassion in the midst of burdens, ridicule, divisiveness, and indifference. For the young as well as the old, special opportunities are created in the church that are not available in the white community.

These opportunities are largely manifested by the many roles open to the church members, who regard them as significant even though they often are not even recognized by others. Some of the roles of importance to black elderly congregation members include:

1. *The Caller* who visits those who are ill or homebound because of physical infirmity.
2. *The Mourner* who attends funerals and visits grieving families.
3. *The Deacon* who as a decision maker may have little opportunity to impact on the wider community but is provided a leadership role in the church.
4. *The Fund-Raiser* who helps provide for the needs of others and in turn gains experience in organizing and assisting them.
5. *The Teacher* who passes on what has been learned to the young (a time-honored role for all elders).
6. *The Musician* who provides part of the services and in turn is recognized as a contributor.
7. *The Mothers* who are a select group of females whose place as a nurturing and wise force is formalized. They provide the continuing recognition of these functions long after their own children move away from home.

All of the special roles the elderly play in the church benefit them by providing meaningful social positions and an outlet for creativity and meaningful contributions for which much support and recognition is provided from within the congregation. One elder, Lottie Taylor, was insightful regarding her own role in the church, how it prevented her from becoming isolated, and how it allowed her to contribute to social work—her lifelong passion—in a way that she could not obtain through programs not linked to the church. She perceived that these roles were markedly absent in some of the social programs available to the elderly.

Lottie Taylor

Lottie is a 79-year-old black widow who has two living children, seven grandchildren, and three great-grandchildren. Neither of her children live in the city but two grandchildren reside in the area. One granddaughter and a great-granddaughter live with her. Her social relationships are closely linked to family but she also views her life's meaning as being derived from the church to which she has belonged for 70 years. Her perception of herself includes a strong sense of being an active church member from early childhood and is associated with recollections of it and happy times there.

She describes how church continues to be meaningful and a cornerstone of her life through early adulthood and midlife age as she raised her children, held her family together, buried some of her children, and lost her favorite grandson in Vietnam. She regards that death as the tragedy of her old age because he had been drafted out of law school and never had an opportunity to achieve greatness in his work as a professional black man with rank and prestige in the community. (This must be considered as a major late life crisis for Lottie even though such a label would have little meaning to her.) Her recollections of that time involved her reliance on spiritual strength, symbolized for her as "God's strength to go on living because there were the ones still left to grow up."

During this difficult period, a time when she felt God was hearing her prayers, she was blessed with the opportunity to do missionary work outside the city. She attended a regional denominational conference in a southern state where she had relatives she had not seen for many decades. At this weeklong meeting she saw old family members and was renewed spiritually for her work in her church. She spoke with pride about how, on her return, her ideas for new church activities were received by her minister.

To Lottie, her extended family—numbering more than she can count—is divided into those who came from the South and those who still live there. It was important for her to have renewed the bonds. She believes the youngest generations of her family may return there because it holds possibilities not realized by the younger people in old cities "going to the dogs." She, herself, would not relocate anywhere because of too little time and because of her church.

Radis Farley

The case of Radis Farley contrasts with Lottie's in that he retired early with the intention of doing little with his church and pursuing his hobby of carpentry.

Radis is 63 and lives with his wife in an old and established black neighborhood in the North Side. His connection to the church has been marginal for some years. He described anger some years back at a previous minister "who let the people of the church down." It appears from his discussion that Radis never found much he could do with or for the church other than help it stay out of trouble. He does not espouse a social activitist community role for the church because he feels there are many needy members who are more important. He contends that too many young pastors try to be like Dr. King, and since there will only be one Dr. King, the others should not try.

He was drafted, somewhat unwillingly, by his wife several years ago to do handiwork for elderly church sisters who needed repairs on their homes. Radis now serves as the source of carpentry assistance to other members who cannot afford the home improvements and need odd jobs undertaken. He laughs about the fact that his wife would not let him fix up their house further and that they were too old to build one so he had to find other jobs outside his home. He expresses much pride in the special recognition he has received from helping the elder members in this manner and feels he has grown closer to his church through these contributions.

This role, available to him through the church, provides recognition, status, and opportunity for leadership to members. It suggests ways in which the church can assist black elders who are not involved in socialization programs for the aged. For those who do or could receive social and emotional benefits similar to those of Radis or Lottie, it is important that this linkage be encouraged and/or facilitated. Community service agencies may have little formal connection with black churches as a whole, and practitioners may not recognize them as a resource.

This is important for practitioners to familiarize themselves with this resource. What is being suggested even more, however, is a broader role for the black church. It should reach out beyond its membership and become a resource for those who are isolated and underserved in the community and act as a bridge of understanding between those in need and the agencies capable of serving them. This could be accomplished by expanding the supportive help now given to members to include needy elders who reside near the church but are not parishioners.

Some of the factors that influence the degree to which churches can become a community resource are determined by denominational differences that are reflected in their internal organization in: (a) the leadership structure, (b) the degree of autonomy from the larger denominational hierarchy to which they are affiliated, (c) the stability of the congregation and the church base, (d) the pattern of economic funding, (e) the distribution of resources for the operating budget, and (f) the pattern of connectedness to other churches of the same denomination or other congregations that are compatible in their ideology.

Brown and Walters (1980) suggest that number of members, budget and annual revenue, and staff composition are important factors determining the extent to which a church may involve itself in community affairs. Factors such as these impact on the church as an organization and on the resources available to which the black elders may or may not relate. Black church organizations tend to be heterogeneous. The diversity of both structure and functions precludes many descriptive generalizations about the actual or potential patterns of delivering outreach beyond the actual congregation. When considering the feasibility of such activities among the black churches that were contacted, variables such as denominational ties, leadership structure, and organizational linkages most influenced the response to problems of isolation. For example:

1. Denominational ties: If a church is closely connected to a larger organizational structure in which there may be a national priority on youth leadership development, this may direct it to stress religious educational resources for that age group. If no similar priority were given to religious education of the elderly, individual churches would not have similar incentives to prioritize such teaching. Different churches in the same community and denomination can differ widely on the priority they will give to the elderly, depending upon the attitude of the minister and the congregation. Some churches tend to follow denominational priorities while others question the credulity of any mandate not set by the congregation itself.

2. The leadership structure: The structure of laity and the minister in overall decision making varies widely. The governance traditions may be influenced by the history of the congregation, the presence of more or less conservative orientations, the church's status in the community, the strength of individual leaders, and patterns of conflict and competition. Based on interviews with various congregational representatives, some churches would experience intraorganizational conflicts if a large-scale outreach to nonmember elderly were proposed. Others would find widespread support and little conflict, especially if the economic resources were available without sacrificing other priorities.

3. The degree of linkage to the community: Some churches never have taken a leadership role in the community while others have placed highest priority on being in the forefront in the identification and resolution of community social problems. A diversified pattern of recent community involvement was evident. Some churches had reduced that involvement once the civil rights movement became splintered by differing ideologies. That lessened role was not necessarily desired but sometimes was required because too many

external projects drained finite resources. Some churches elect to have a single focus for community involvement, concentrating their efforts on one project, while others respond to a greater array of external issues that have social and spiritual importance.

In proposing to use black churches in a more intentional and planned manner to meet the needs of the elderly, it is important to look at the unique features of each. A source outside of the congregation may or may not prove an effective catalyst to facilitate an expanded program for elders. The overall conclusion is that an outside stimulus first must become acquainted with a church, e.g., the clergy and its leadership. Building a partnership for increasing outreach to the elderly, whether members or nonmembers, requires thorough consideration of many factors. None of the churches studied were likely to give up congregational autonomy in serving the elderly, even if that function was viewed as appropriate. This would make linkage with community agencies difficult.

UNDERSTANDING THE CHURCH AS A RESOURCE

Readers acquainted with service projects for the elderly sponsored by local churches (or in which they hold membership) might conclude that the factors of structure and function, as important variables in the ability to support community programs, are similar for both blacks and whites. This suggests that in order to understand the potential of the black church to respond to its elders, it is necessary to step back and consider its role (regardless of racial membership) in programming for the elderly. To conceptualize a meaningful strategy, it is important to review some of the general issues that confront the church as a community institution and its ability to make critical choices about current and future responses to the isolated elderly.

Some spokespersons from different lay and clerical sectors point out that the social and emotional isolation experienced by the elderly cannot be addressed by the church effectively if it makes a "religious business as usual" response. They call for a special priority to be given to the church's relationship with the elderly in the form of active outreach and special religious program offerings. They assume that the spiritual components of church life have the capacity to support and enhance the elderly who may be isolated from other dimensions of community life. The type of actions taken to implement a specialized program for the aged will vary among denominations and among churches in the same denomination. They also will vary between churches that are either predominantly or exclusively black or white. Some of the guidelines for action that have been developed by predominantly white religious leaders must be evaluated for their relevance to meeting the isolation needs of elderly blacks.

The role of the black church needs to be considered in relation to what it, as a community institution, may provide as a specialized program for the elderly. The authors have explored these issues but stress that they have many qualifications about what is written here. This includes analysis of previously published materials on the black church as a social institution and its specific relationships to the black elderly. However, this does not provide adequate information on the extent to which any new directions have been adopted by black churches throughout the United States.

To a large extent, any guidelines available to churches treat the elderly as a homogenous group and address the common characteristics of structure rather than differences. Thus, general information now available may have limited applicability to the infinite array of national religious groups that dominate America and the various racial and ethnic groups that comprise denominational membership.

NATIONAL INTERFAITH COALITION GUIDELINES

In recent years the National Interfaith Coalition on Aging has spearheaded the exploration of the spectrum of issues relevant to the church's ministry to the aged. To some extent this group has provided a unifying voice among the major faiths and the multidenominations of Protestantism. As a cross-sectional religious coalition, its cohesive factor is a shared commitment to an overall goal. As a group, it aspires to educate and facilitate sensitivity to the needs of the elderly. It also gives guidance to clergy, churches, and larger denominational leadership structures in responding to the needs of the elderly. The coalition's national conventions have provided a forum in which general positions could be formed and action strategies prepared, debated, revised, and eventually shared with the national religious community.

While many practitioners are unaware of these efforts, their force has been important. They are acknowledged as core content for ministerial preparation used in a National Institute on Mental Health training program for the clergy to improve their ability to work with the social and emotional needs of the elderly (Hands, 1981). They also have been incorporated by various state and local interfaith groups concerned with the elderly (Missouri Interfaith Commission on Aging, 1977; Smith, 1981) who have special needs associated with the developmental changes of life within the context of the church. Some of the major contents of the guidelines are summarized below.

> Data and information about the characteristics, needs, and geographical distribution of the elderly members of the congregation, as well as the elderly in the community where the church is located, are important in planning both membership and outreach programs. The attempt to gain

information from the elderly church member in a comprehensive and systematic manner may provide answers to the question of how adequately the needs of these members are being met by the church.

Steps can be taken to make the church more sensitive and relevant to the aged membership. Expanding the survey outward to elderly in the community, particularly in neighborhoods and areas within geographical proximity to the church, can be helpful if the church wishes to engage in outreach to nonmember elderly.

There are multiple and important educational functions that the church should assume, e.g., preretirement education which facilitates preparation for individuals making transitions and adjustments; religious education which appeals to the interest of older and elderly persons and that stimulates their ability for active learning; and continuing education that creates group learning, supportive self-exploration, and spiritual enhancement. From this latter type of educational opportunity, support and fellowship can be developed that offer elderly persons far more personalized, intimate, and diversified interactional opportunities than may be characteristic of other adult groups in the church popular among younger persons.

The church assumes a cooperative position with other community organizations, therefore it seeks areas of community concern which reflect the type of involvement and goals compatible to the church's commitment. As a congregation develops awareness of issues, needs, and problems, its members can serve to facilitate community education and other efforts to reduce stereotypes and negative attitudes toward the elderly. Worship and religious participation opportunities should be structured to encourage the active participation of elderly persons in important ceremonies and insure an in-depth participation of older individuals compatible to their personal choice and need.

The clergy and entire congregation must be concerned about the needs of those who are chronically ill, dying, and/or suffering bereavement associated with death of family and friends. There should be an effort to reach out beyond the church setting into situations where the elderly and their families are involved with caregiving in a home or an institution. It is appropriate for the church to insure that the nonmobile elderly person is not cut off from opportunities for worship, fellowship, and other meaningful spiritual activity. The attitudes of the congregation toward the elderly should be of concern to the congregation as a whole, with a commitment of resource for enrichment and fellowship. Physical facilities should be assessed to determine their appropriateness for elderly persons, especially those who may require special environmental adaptations because of physical mobility limitations.

Educational opportunities, in the ways and means of providing for the elderly, for clergy, and laity is important and becomes a resource to be developed within the church. These and other efforts are directed toward tapping the resources of older persons and the aged to meet the human needs and spark the potential of all who want to share in the community of the church (National Interfaith Coalition on Aging, 1976).

These suggestions reflect the thinking of a highly aware and concerned religious leadership group that wants the relationship between the church and the elderly to be of major help and value. If a congregation adopts such an action strategy to better serve the elderly, two commitments become central:

1. developing responsibility to individual elderly persons in the form of immediate and personal supportive assistance, guidance with long-range personal planning, transportation, and creation of special groups
2. structuring the internal activities of the church in a way that addresses the needs of the elderly through worship services, religious education and leadership, communications, and information sharing and advocacy

The research to date has not focused on the extent to which guidelines have been discussed throughout the national religious community (i.e., multiple denominational organizations), their content has been critiqued by the clerical community, or their impact on local church activities has not been thoroughly understood. An exploration of these general guidelines, their implications for church-sponsored activity, and attitudes of practitioners are important for both the black and white elderly.

RESPONSES TO ELDERS AND THEIR SPIRITUAL NEEDS

It is difficult to comment on the overall national position of members of the clergy regarding their level of awareness of the aging process and its various physical, psychological, social, and economic dimensions; their priority for meeting the needs of the elderly in their congregation and/or in the larger community; or the needs of older persons they encounter through their ministerial role. Urban members of the clergy who were contacted reflected as much variation in attitudes toward the elderly and the role of the church in meeting their needs as did the clergy from Folk County, as described in Chapter 5, on the rural elderly. Many of the urban clergy, both black and white, knew little about the aging process and few had taken any educational training in gerontology. They varied on the extent to which they felt the church could give leadership to the community on behalf of the elderly, but many mentioned members from their congregations who they perceived to be doing much to help the aging in nonchurch-affiliated groups. Several felt that critical needs of both the young and very old members placed a dual demand on their ministry that had to be balanced because of limited resources.

Based on what these members of the clergy understood to be the reasons for participation of the elderly in the church, the search for fulfillment of spiritual needs ranked very high. This aspect of need fulfillment was noted as important to the elderly in general by both the black and white clergy and was stressed slightly more for black church members. The extent of concern for spiritual needs is of interest as another complex isolator. It is not uncommon for health and social service practitioners to have little or no concern for these spiritual needs because they are outside the role of mainstream clinical tradition or because the experts place their intervention priority in other areas. Practitioners' responses that ignore these factors do not alter these needs. Such needs seem to have much importance to some members of the clergy, who place priority on their personal relationship with elderly members. The clergy rarely considered this spiritual area as a mental health or social service need, per se. Some tended to view other formal services and resources for the elderly as unrelated to spiritual need.

A practitioner who finds an elderly client has a need or desire to discuss, reflect upon, or seek guidance about areas that involve relationship to God, salvation, or life after death will need to evaluate how these may be handled to the optimum benefit of the individual. They may be outside the realm of practitioner comfort and confidence. It then may be necessary to help the older person form a relationship with other professionals skilled in pastoral counseling or associated with the clergy (assuming that these elderly individuals are not involved already with such a person). In attempting to facilitate a connection, the practitioner should approach this step with the same degree of serious attention as any other types of clinical referrals. Too frequently, the issue is dismissed by a simplistic statement that the aged individuals should contact their ministers. The practitioner then assumes this will be done, advice given, and the problem resolved. No thought is given to this as a type of formal referral.

If a referral is made for pastoral counseling, there is a responsibility to follow through to determine whether there is a way to support the older person striving to find affirmation in this aspect of life. For example, the practitioner may be able to serve as a supportive listener if the client wishes to share the personal joys of a religious experience or reflect upon spiritual fulfillment. That role might change if the focus of spiritual well-being shifts to concrete decision making such as leaving one church and seeking participation in another or questioning how to undertake the difficult step of having surgery for a serious illness based on the client's faith in spiritual oversight of that process (or religious beliefs).

It is alarming to note practitioners' responses that reflect a pattern of attempting to prescribe a certain type of spirituality for a client based on their personal religious beliefs and practices. Such behaviors seem to violate the rights of elders, or any clients, to be free of superimposed personal values from the practitioner. There is information to suggest that both the clergy and practitioners assume that the church has a special role in meeting needs, but few have explored what it may offer as an organization. When the church's capacity to meet the needs of the elderly has been evaluated, such studies have been stimulated largely by the clergy, concerned lay leaders, and older members of congregations. In many cases where the two-way relation of church and the elderly has been explored, professionals associated with formal service delivery organizations have been uninvolved in that process, for a variety of reasons such as:

- the hesitancy of professionals to become involved if efforts are directed by a church other than the one in which they hold membership

- the conscious decision of church leaders to maintain autonomy from professionals and formal organizations as they plan the direction they will take

- a lack of channels whereby the service professionals and their organizations and representative church members can come together

Recognition of the conditions that block the integrative efforts between church and other sectors of the community does not imply that this is universal. The history of charity and social welfare is filled with the combined efforts of church and professional service organizations to explore human needs and address human conditions. However, there still is a gap between these resources. One example is the extent to which the church and other organizations do not join to plan communitywide service and helping responses to the elderly. Many times the church adopts an attitude of independence when it initiates efforts to plan for services to groups of people in need. When the philosophy of separation of church from other community welfare efforts prevails, a type of interorganizational isolation does exist and has an impact on the elderly.

At the core of the church's response to older persons, spirituality is important. As a state of being, it seems likely to be connected with the social and emotional aspects of isolation. A greater awareness of this relationship developed through interviews with older blacks and their pastors, but not from practitioners. Based on the total input received on this dimension of isolation, it was concluded that:

- for some elderly, both black and white, the presence of a spiritual need is basic to their own search for personal meaning

- the clergy understand this need more than do practitioners but vary greatly in the extent to which they address this through counseling activities
- there may be cultural differences between elderly blacks and whites about how they express their need for spiritual enrichment (additional research is required to clarify this potential difference)

The response of individual churches to the needs of the elderly can vary along a continuum from no specialized program to a very highly developed ministry. The guidelines from the National Interfaith Coalition contain many useful suggestions about how to develop a comprehensive program. Any member of the clergy can influence a congregation in the direction of a specialized ministry but other factors also will determine how much emphasis is placed on the elderly. Important among these factors are the attitudes of the elderly members and their perceptions of needs and the appropriate functions of the church. However, the program components are not the only vehicle for meeting the spiritual needs that create or prevent isolation.

THE BLACK CHURCH AS A RESOURCE

Practitioners need to consider new options for the role of the black church as a community institution to meet the needs of the elderly. The new options have been hard to define, given the rather simplistic discussion of the role of the church in the lives of older blacks and the confusing historical tradition of its linkage with formalized human service organizations controlled by the larger white community (including the aging service network).

Getting the church, as a community resource, to participate with other human service sources now working with the black elderly and helping it reduce their lack of relationship with these resources is an important concern. Figure 6-2 details the complex web of social service organizations available to the black elderly. If health and social service practitioners wish to explore answers and discover new options, a simplistic analysis of the black church in the lives of the elderly will not be helpful. Discovering new options will require trial and effort at the community level. A variety of perspectives can facilitate the exploratory process.

In all urban communities, the coexistence of social welfare organizations and religious entities (church congregations) is balanced by the presence of religious-affiliated service agencies. Church groups, more than a century ago, established religious service organizations that now are increasingly financed through public funds (in 1973, the government provided one-fourth of all income for Catholic agencies). The dependencies that result are changing the character of religious service organizations (Marty, 1980). Therefore, it is correct to say that these entities do play an important role in providing human service but not that they benefit older blacks.

Figure 6-2 The Black Elder and the Social Resource System

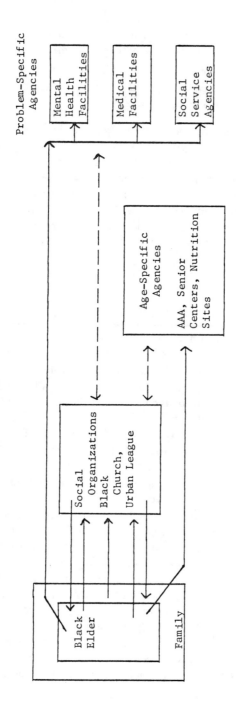

Many blacks facing potentially isolating problems find assistance from black social organizations; some seek help from community age-specific and/or problem-specific agencies. There is no communication or cooperation between formal community agencies and black social organizations.

The division of labor in a religious institution to meet the needs of the elderly is divided between the church and its sectarian human service counterparts. However, these entities have a pattern of mutual ignorance (Davies, 1956) that must be understood in order to enhance each party's role in meeting the seniors' needs. The limited exploration of this coordination suggests few linkages. When they are present, they operate infrequently and informally (Steinitz, 1980). This condition must change if there is to be a more viable involvement of the black church.

From this background, it is possible to envision the development of a two-directional informational system between service providers and pastors of the black churches as a viable vehicle through which an information exchange can be accomplished. This exchange could prove valuable for black elderly church members and nonmembers alike. Nonmembers may be less informed about and/or not disposed to utilize public services than are members. Under this arrangement the practitioner would provide the clergy with information on the services available in the community, such as nutrition centers, activity programs, and whom to contact for further information. Developing this information system certainly would entail more than the mailing of brochures and would include visits to the pastors and invitations for them to attend programs related to the information system resources.

This concept of linkage, while simplistic, is not necessarily an easy objective to attain. The position of the pastors will vary according to their willingness and interest in developing channels of communication with the agencies and the extent to which they perceive the referral function as relevant. The practitioner's approach also may affect the pastor's receptivity, and the likelihood of success is increased if the commitment to achieve a linkage is a high priority. Viewing it as of only secondary importance will reduce the amount of energy devoted to its formation. Steps to be considered in approaching the pastors include:

- obtaining information about each individual church to be contacted in order to avoid generalized perceptions about their organizational structures and the characteristics of the congregations
- arranging an introduction to the pastor through a black elder congregation member
- determining how other members of the clergy or community leaders might help reinforce the importance of the involvement
- presenting concrete examples of how the pastor's personal involvement in the referral process may offer a unique contact with black elders who are not familiar with or trustful of formal agency-sponsored assistance.

In many urban communities, there may be numerous black pastors who could be involved in the information system. If there are too many to contact in person, informal group meetings or educational forums could be used. However, it would be preferable for the practitioner to make a personal effort to establish the pastor's initial interest. Preliminary and continuing contacts between agency representatives and black ministers should be scheduled to ensure that the contacts are neither too rushed nor too intermittent.

The former pattern may promote the feeling that the pastor is being pushed into an arrangement that intrudes on the autonomous functions of the church and the latter may imply that the church's participation is really not all that relevant. Initially, the somewhat wary black ministers may not be eager to be involved. This is to be expected and their hesitation is understandable. For example, some may have had previous encounters with formal human service organizations that have proved exploitative or that ultimately generated no assistance to congregation members at a time when crisis intervention was required.

The clergy vary in the extent to which they assume responsibility for referring the members of their congregations to external agencies, especially if the individuals are beloved and respected members or who mistrust agencies such as the welfare office and mental health center. It is to be hoped that pastors could pass along to their elderly congregation members accurate information and facilitate their acceptance of agencies in the information system that are available and committed to help. The ministers also serve as an important source of potential feedback if the agencies have a negative image and could recommend specific modifications that might make their programs more acceptable among black elders and within their community.

Since many of the black elders who are most isolated do not belong to any church, a long-range goal might be to encourage the members in each church to take an interest in nonmember elders who live in the immediate neighborhood. However, this task cannot be thrust upon a congregation and must be motivated from within. There may be value conflicts and a history of incompatible church and neighborhood relationships that conflict with outreach.

The extent to which members offer volunteer assistance to nonmembers varies from church to church. In congregations where this pattern is well established, outreach projects may be more supported. However, the helping hand to nonmembers may not be welcomed. If the sponsoring church does not represent personal beliefs acceptable to an isolated black elder, who is to say that church-based outreach will be any more acceptable than services available from public agencies. Community suggestions that the church could or should offer a specialized program for the elderly would not necessarily motivate members. Congregations insist on maintaining a degree of autonomy regarding the establishment of church priorities. Similarly, nonmember black elders have the right to avoid outreach efforts from any and all sources.

In assessing the capacity of a church to do volunteer work, especially for nonmember isolated older blacks in the neighborhood, more than good-will must be involved. If cooperative working relationships exist between pastors and the service agency representative, the latter could offer professional guidance. For example, the professional's input could ensure that volunteers did not assume too much responsibility for providing daily service to highly impaired and dependent elders. Consultation might prevent volunteers from being caught by conflicting needs because of their inability to extend services at a time when they are most needed by a black elder to whom they have made a commitment to help. The daily circumstances, living conditions, or behaviors of these elderly may be overwhelming or frightening to a church volunteer without adequate training. Without some preparation, their outreach effort might prove counterproductive by lessening the acceptance of help and by demoralizing themselves.

Financial limitations may preclude a church from sustaining the elderly in the community without input from public agencies. For example, without a contractual arrangement with an area agency on aging, adequate financial resources to support a demanding volunteer program might be beyond the resources of a single congregation. A church that conducts its programming quite informally might find itself constrained and uncomfortable in a continuous relationship with the formal demands of organizations operating with structured bureaucratic demands.

These are examples of the limitations on independent and autonomous volunteer efforts as they attempt to help meet the needs of the isolated black elderly. In spite of these obvious difficulties, it would seem unreasonable for the public services to ignore the potential value and assistance that could be forthcoming from the church. These potential resources include altruistic concern for these isolated elders, respect from the black community as an institution, and continuing service programs for needy members provided in a spirit of kinship.

CONCLUSION

Planning linkage between or among health, social service, or aging network resources and the church to meet the needs of the isolated black elderly lacks a prototype model. No single innovative program that has proved successful in one church can be packaged so it can be replicated in all others. What might be helpful is for each of the major denominations to commit resources to develop a descriptive inventory of the innovative programs of their member churches. Practitioners with expertise on these elders then could evaluate these programs in depth and group them in relation to a typology of urban black churches.

This could provide the leadership structure of individual churches with examples of programs that are within the realm of possibility, given the level of resources of a particular congregation. It is important to provide pastors with project suggestions that are within the range of church resources; it is not helpful to propose what is not feasible. Realistic projects are more likely to gain the enthusiastic attention and cooperation of a pastor who otherwise might be turned off by extensive and elaborate programs that the minister knows are beyond the resources available.

Practitioners wishing to plan programs for the isolated black elderly should not overlook the potential resource that can be found among those individuals themselves. They may be the ones most capable of planning and implementing program ideas that can be of benefit to all older blacks. The black elder leaders (some of whom may be known to the service agencies by their participation in other volunteer activities) are naturals to take on the task of problem solving for this cohort and to develop valid approaches to meet its needs. In the final analysis, it is the strength of the black leadership that is the most underdeveloped resource.

REFERENCES

Babchuk, N., & Thompson, R.V. The voluntary association of Negroes. *American Sociological Review, 1962, 27,* 647-655.

Banks, W.L. *The black church: Its origin, growth, contributions and outlook.* Chicago: Moody Press, 1972.

Bardo, H.R. Attitudes of the black aging. In J. Dorsett-Robinson (Ed.), *Proceedings of the workshop on the black aging and aged and the conference on the black aged and aging.* Carbondale, Ill.: Southern Illinois University, College of Human Resources, 1974.

Becker, W.H. Black church: Manhood and mission. *Journal of the American Academy of Religion.* 1972, 40, 316-333.

Brown, D.R. & Walters, R.W. *Exploring the role of the black church in the community.* Washington, D.C.: Howard University, Institute for Urban Affairs and Research, 1980.

Dancy, J., Jr. *The black elderly: A guide for practitioners.* Ann Arbor, Mich.: University of Michigan, Institute of Gerontology, 1977.

Davies, S.P. The churches and the non-sectarian agencies. In F.E. Johnson (Ed.), *Religion and Social Work.* New York: Harper & Brothers, 1956.

Dowd, J.J., & Bengtson, V.L. Aging in minority populations: An examination of the double jeopardy hypothesis. *Journal of Gerontology, 1978, 33*(3), 427-436.

Drake, S.C., & Cayton, H.R. *Black metropolis: A study of Negro life in America.* New York: Harcourt, Brace & Co., 1970.

Dubois, W.E.B. *The Negro church,* Atlanta University Studies #8. Atlanta: Atlanta University Press, 1903.

Frazier, E. *The Negro church in America.* New York: Scocken Books, Inc., 1964.

Hands, D.R. *Clergy for the aged.* Unpublished presentation at the Second Annual Technical Assistance Workshop for directors of the National Institute on Mental Health Clinical Training Program, Rockville, Md., February 1981.

Herzog, E. Is there a culture of poverty? In H.H. Meissner (Ed.), *Poverty in the affluent society.* New York: Harper & Row, Inc., 1966, pp. 92-102.

Logan, S.M.L. *The black Baptist church: A social psychological study in coping and growth.* Unpublished dissertation, Columbia University, 1980.

Layng, A. Voluntary associations and black ethnic identity. *Phylon*, 1978, pp. 171-179.

Marty, M.E. Social service: Godly and godless. *Social Services Review*, 1980, pp. 463-481.

Missouri Interfaith Commission on Aging. *Programs with the aging: Community, social, religious.* Kirkwood, Mo.: The Messenger Printing Company, 1977.

National Council on the Aging. *Fact book on aging: A profile of America's older population.* Washington, D.C.: National Council on the Aging, Inc., Research and Evaluation Department, 1978.

National Interfaith Coalition on Aging. *Reports from the 1974 and 1975 National Convention.* Athens, Ga.: National Interfaith Coalition (Bulletins I and II), 1976.

Nelsen, H.W., & Nelsen, A.K. *Black church in the sixties.* Lexington, Ky.: The University Press of Kentucky, 1975.

Sauer, W. Morale of the urban aged: A regression analysis by race. *Journal of Gerontology*, 1977, *32*(5), 600-608.

Smith, R. Member of Missouri Interfaith Commission on Aging of the Missouri Council of Churches. Interview, March 1, 1981.

Staples, R. *Introduction to black sociology.* New York: McGraw-Hill Book Company, 1976.

Steinitz, L.Y. *The church within the network of social services to the elderly: Case study of Laketown.* Doctoral dissertation, University of Chicago, School of Social Service Administration, 1980.

Williams, M. *Community in a black Pentecostal church: An anthropological study.* Pittsburgh: University of Pittsburgh Press, 1974.

Chapter 7

The Hispanic Elderly: Cuban, Puerto Rican, and Mexican

INTRODUCTION

The Hispanic community in the United States is an aggregate of several cultures. There has been a tendency to lump the Hispanic elderly from countries of different origins together, then compare them as a single group to other major minority elderly cohorts such as blacks, Pacific Asians, and Native Americans. This tendency has downplayed the important differences and special needs of each minority, promoted politically induced competition between and among these groups, and devalued rather than valued the rich cultural and ethnic identities that characterize the older American population and the contributions of Spanish-speaking elders. It is their special status as unique older people in this culture that gives significance to similarities among subgroups.

As of March 1978, the Hispanic population in the United States was 12,046,000, composed of several distinct ethnic groups. It was estimated that 60 percent are Mexican-American, 15 percent Puerto Rican, 5 percent Cuban, and the remaining 20 percent from Central and South America. Nine percent of the total Hispanic population are 55 years and older. There are differences in the percentage of elderly in each of the subgroups: 7.9 percent of Mexican-Americans, 6.7 percent of Puerto Ricans, and 22.5 percent of Cubans are elderly (U.S. DHHS, 1980). The major similarities among the three Hispanic subgroups are the Spanish language and recent immigrant status (U.S. DHEW, 1979).

Despite the common language base, the very different regional variations create communication barriers. Hispanics in the United States can be as different as Irishmen from Englishmen or Englishmen from Americans (Rothman, 1979). Over the next 25 years, the projected proportionate increase of nonwhite elderly will double that of their white counterparts, and older Hispanics are expected to constitute the most rapidly increasing group of minority aged. Their numbers will force society to begin giving greater consideration to their needs.

The Hispanic elderly are more likely to live with a spouse (60 percent) than alone. Only 10 percent live with their adult children (Woerner, 1979). Factors such as economics, mobility patterns, and housing inadequate for three and four generations under one roof contribute to their problems. Close examination of census data reveals, however, that the stereotypic image of the three-generation Hispanic family no longer is valid. While the multigeneration family unit continues to play an important role, there is no basis for sweeping generalizations about the extended family as a future source of support for these elderly.

For Hispanic families, like the rest of the society, the accelerating demands of modern America have diluted some of the longstanding patterns of support for the elderly. (Figure 7-1 presents isolators that are most important to all Hispanic elders.) The image of extended family caregiving in this community should not be so widely generalized that it blocks recognition of the need for additional sources of support for the elderly and for their adult children. Poverty resulting from lifetime low incomes is an important cause of economic insecurity. The number of elderly Spanish-speaking individuals with incomes below the poverty level is 37.5 percent—more than one out of every three. Only Native Americans have lower average income (Woerner, 1979).

The average older Hispanic has less than 3.3 years of formal education. This has meant inferior job opportunities, lower lifetime earnings, and hence little or no savings, pension plans, or Social Security benefits (Rothman, 1979). Sometimes the elderly remain quite unaware of Social Security eligibility even if they do qualify because information about benefits may never be provided or prepared in a way they understand. Employment options are important for Hispanics even though chronic health problems may prevent some of them from pursuing job or retraining opportunities when they are made available. Early retirement in the 40s often is necessary because of disability and health problems that preclude full-time or even part-time work.

The high percentage of Hispanic elderly who are Roman Catholic (U.S. DHEW, 1979) is an important demographic characteristic, but it does not give adequate insight into the role of the church in the emotional and social lives of these elderly. Little data is available to describe the interrelationship between religious affiliation and social support resources. Strong pronouncements about the central role of religion in the lives of Hispanic elders cannot be empirically documented.

The Mexican-American subgroup has had difficulty choosing a name. The younger, more radical ones call themselves Chicanos, but older individuals seem to prefer Latinos, or the more popular term Hispanic-American. Some families arrived across the border this morning, others have been in what is now the United States continuously for 300 years. Although most immigrants came from Mexico as farm or factory workers, more than 80 percent of them now are urbanized.

This chapter discusses problems of isolation among the urban Hispanic elderly, including Cubans, Puerto Ricans, and Mexican-Americans; however, there is

Figure 7-1 Isolators That Are Most Important for Hispanic Elders

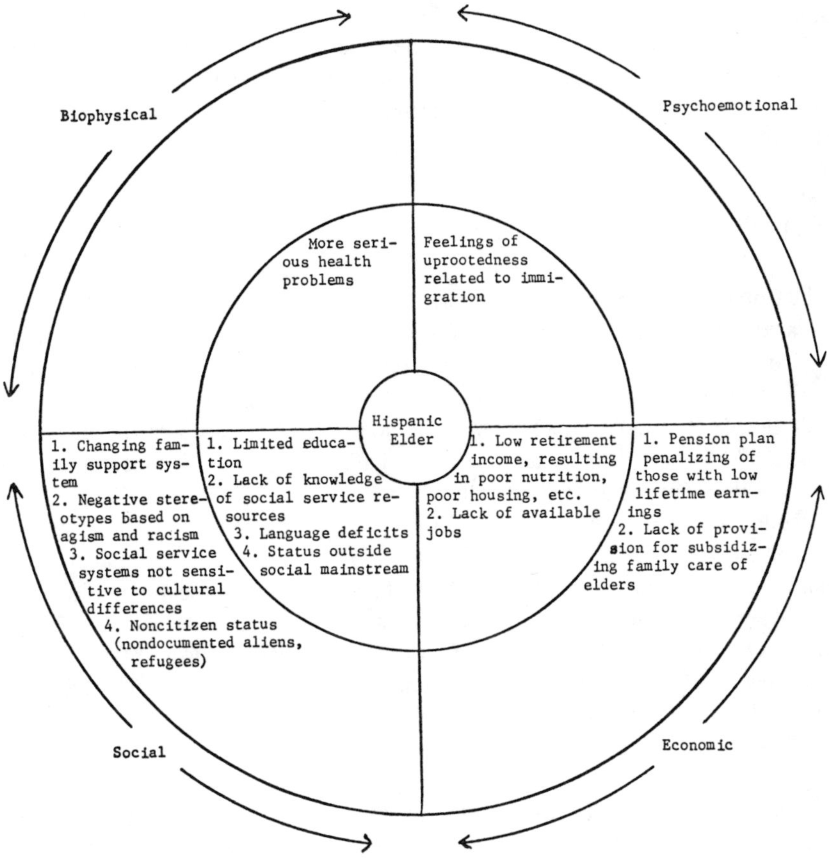

Biophysical

Psychoemotional

More serious health problems

Feelings of uprootedness related to immigration

Hispanic Elder

1. Changing family support system
2. Negative stereotypes based on agism and racism
3. Social service systems not sensitive to cultural differences
4. Noncitizen status (nondocumented aliens, refugees)

1. Limited education
2. Lack of knowledge of social service resources
3. Language deficits
4. Status outside social mainstream

1. Low retirement income, resulting in poor nutrition, poor housing, etc.
2. Lack of available jobs

1. Pension plan penalizing of those with low lifetime earnings
2. Lack of provision for subsidizing family care of elders

Social

Economic

The inner circle contains isolators as they are manifested in the personal lives of Hispanic elders, the outer circle those that abound in the environment.

particular emphasis on Mexican-American seniors, the largest proportion of Hispanic elderly in the United States. First is an overview of Cuban elders in Miami and Dade County, Fla., Puerto Ricans in New York City (East Harlem), and Mexican-Americans in San Mateo County, Calif.

The Mexican-American elderly are the subject of an in-depth discussion of the problems of isolation and intervention strategies, focusing on a pilot community survey conducted in California by the San Mateo County Area Agency on Aging. These persons are compared to the self-reported needs of a group of Hispanic elderly who attended the First Annual San Mateo Minority Elders Conference

(1980). Their participation was an important first step in the preparation of a Spanish-speaking position statement for the 1981 White House Conference on Aging. The success of this first San Mateo conference will set a precedent for future meetings, provided there is sufficient community support. The chapter conclusion addresses the need to develop alternative intervention programs that build on the obvious strengths of the informal helping networks available to these Hispanic seniors in their communities.

THE CUBAN ELDER

The Cuban elderly comprise an important segment of the population that should be considered as a special subgroup in overall planning for older Hispanics. It is estimated that more than 750,000 Cubans have settled in the United States. Most of them—more than half a million—live in the Greater Miami-Dade County area of South Florida (U.S. DHEW, 1979). These numbers do not account for the most recent (1979-1981) influx of Cubans to the United States. The concentration in Florida adds an important demographic factor.

Despite the federal government's effort to disperse segments of the most recent group outside of Dade County, significant numbers have established residence in Miami and the surrounding county. The Cuban elderly are concentrated in Hialeah, Miami, and Miami Beach. The five-square-mile area in central Miami known as Little Havana has confronted serious challenges over ways of absorbing the newest group while attempting to maintain its flourishing commercial, cultural, and residential characteristics. The interface among the Cuban, black, Jewish, and Anglo sectors is not necessarily one of either consistent conflict or competition.

The increasing proportion of Cubans in southern Florida is creating a need for bilingual service providers such as welfare workers and health educators. The bilingual characteristic is resented to some extent by older residents and has created some economic hardships for blacks ("It's Your Turn in the Sun," 1978). Immigration patterns of the older Cuban population include those for whom Miami is the first point of entry and those who move there after living in other areas. Factors affecting the latter group include family and friendship ties, climate, and access to services. For the older Cubans, access to health care is very important.

In the early 1960s, many middle and upper-class Cubans sought political asylum in the United States. By 1978, however, the exiles' demographic distribution reflected a socioeconomic cross-section of the island's population during the late 1950s. Approximately 17 percent of the refugee population is over 55 and 7.8 percent over 65 (Szapocznik, Santisteban, Kurtines, & Hervis, 1980).

Variations between Anglo-Americans and Cuban immigrants have been delineated by Szapocznik, Scopetta, Kurtines, & Aranalde (1978). They reported

Cubans had greater respect for a hierarchical relationship, were more likely to perceive themselves as being unable to control natural forces or to modify detrimental environmental conditions, and put greater emphasis on the immediate concerns of daily life. Hernandez (1974) reported significant differences in the Dade County Cubans, as contrasted to Mexican-Americans in San Antonio, in terms of their valuing of home ownership and their acceptance of public housing as an alternative. Of the total Hispanic population in Dade County, 88 percent lived in rental units and 66.4 percent expressed a desire to move to public housing. In contrast, in San Antonio, 60 percent of the Hispanics owned their own homes and only 15 percent wanted to move. Housing as a priority item thus varies considerably from one area of the country to another and among Hispanic subgroups. These variations reflect periods of migration and residential patterns, as well as private and public housing options.

In 1974, the Cuban National Planning Council completed a pilot study on the occupational, educational, and income characteristics of Cubans in South Florida. The findings generated a significant amount of information on the Spanish-speaking elderly in Dade County. The ethnic composition of those 55 and older included 80 percent Cuban, 6 percent Puerto Rican, and 14 percent of other Hispanic backgrounds.

Older Cubans have significantly higher education than all other Hispanic groups, and more have citizen status, especially among those who reside in Miami. But divided loyalties between their island home and the United States continue to be a dilemma. The inability to migrate back to Cuba creates a somewhat different psychological condition for Cuban elderly as compared to older Chicanos (if legal immigrants) and Puerto Ricans, who face no barriers to returning to their home areas.

The increasing political activity of the Cuban community has manifested itself in voter registration drives but it is not clear whether the older cohorts have been a target. However, the effort to elect Cubans to local government has increased the political influences that advocate for the concerns for their elderly (Hernandez, 1974).

Linn, Hunter, and Perry (1979) reported on their study of three ethnic groups of elders (whites, blacks, Cubans) who used ambulatory care in a large medical center in Miami, comparing social participation, depression, social functioning, life satisfaction, and self-esteem. The results indicated the Cuban elderly had more negative factors in adjusting. The Cuban sample consisted of 74 persons with a mean age of 73.8 years, 96 percent of whom had migrated to Miami, and whose average length of stay in the United States was 13 years. Many thus arrived after they were 60 years old. The Cubans scored lower in social participation and higher on social dysfunction than the black or Anglo groups. The Linn, Hunter, and Perry interpretation of these results provides an interesting summary of the factors that contribute to the isolation of the elderly Cubans in the Miami-Dade County area:

The results seem reasonable since acculturation is a slow process and the older Cubans would be less likely to be assimilated into the broader core culture. For example, most do not speak English; therefore, it is understandable that they watch television less and go less frequently to clubs or activities, since most of these are not conducted in Spanish. Although Miami is considered a bilingual community, it is the younger generation that has been absorbed more into the general culture. Although there is considerable visiting and socializing within the Cuban subculture, elderly Cubans may still feel uprooted from their homeland and unsettled in the new and different social milieu. The displacement may be reflected in their social behavior. (p. 280)

Data on the feelings of loneliness suggest that this feeling, when combined with other problems related to a scarcity of environmental resources, poor health, and living in exile, can create a cluster of isolators not easily removed by the individual as an autonomous entity. Perceptions of family neglect certainly can contribute to this phenomenon when individuals' most valued roles and interactions depend on contacts with relatives.

The role of the extended family in the context of the Cuban elderly population can be interpreted to reflect rapid economic and social mobility among the younger elements that provide an opportunity for an increasingly diversified range of outside social relationships and multiple social forces in the community that must be weighed against family demands. The challenge of balancing intrafamily and extrafamily connections is a pressure on the younger generations that is not present for the elders, who experience others. However, the older generation, unlike the younger ones, may be poorly equipped to generate relationships outside the family to balance their risk of isolation.

In a study in Dade County (Hernandez, 1974), Hispanic elders (Cubans for the most part) were interviewed on what they considered their most pressing needs and those of most such older ones in their area. The responses were markedly different. Individuals responded to the personal question by listing (in order of the percent of persons having the problem) housing, economics, health, family, and freeing Cuba, with loneliness being mentioned by only 2.1 percent. In contrast, on the question of major problems of Hispanic elderly they listed (in order of the number of persons including the item) language, loneliness, health, housing, economics, adapting to new environment, and children's neglecting parents.

The differences between the definition of personal problems and the perceived problems of others can be compared to those reported in the Harris survey data (National Council on Aging, 1978). That study suggested that the elderly accepted certain preset attitudes and perceptions of situations that older persons experienced and applied them to other seniors but did not regard them as problems in their own lives. It also could be said that the elderly felt uncomfortable admitting some problems, mentioned only those that were considered acceptable, and projected onto others what they knew in fact to be part of their own personal experience.

Professionals who worked with the Hispanic elderly, when questioned in the Dade County study, ranked the top four problems as housing, medical care, loneliness, and language, which is closer to what the elderly listed for others than for themselves.

The population profile and community structure of Miami-Dade County Cubans have been affected by the influx of immigrants in the early 1970s. Their impact drew national media attention at the time but that has waned in interest and now to a large extent is defined as a local and state issue.

In the initial phase of the influx, economic and social service supports poured in to help in the processing stage but the real challenge will be a long operation, requiring continuing response from all sectors of the community. It should be noted that the stability of both the Cuban and non-Cuban communities in Dade County—whites (Christians and Jews) as well as blacks—is in transition.

The shifts in resource distribution among public welfare sources and other community systems providing the bulk of public health, mental health, and social service supports and resources cannot be truly understood from afar. To appreciate the social, economic, political, and, above all, human consequences, it would be essential to understand how a new resident group with a shared cultural, familial, and political history, but largely without resources, can be absorbed into the fabric of the Cuban community and larger system.

One of the pioneering demonstration programs addressing the needs of the Cuban elderly in the Miami-Dade County area was conducted by the Spanish Family Guidance Center in the Department of Psychiatry in the University of Miami School of Medicine. The project, funded by a federal grant from the Administration on Aging, produced a procedure known as the Life Enrichment Counseling. The approach involves counselor access to the elder's environment and incorporates life review and reminiscence techniques. It encompasses two major concepts, Life Review and Ecological Assessment and Intervention, and establishes a set of assumptions that represent a model for treatment of this population (Szapocznik, Santisteban, Kurtines, & Hervis, 1980).

Of particular importance to elder Cubans is the extent to which the life review technique can help provide a vehicle for assisting them in examining the important transitions associated with exile and immigration. It also is helpful in resolving problems involving adaptation to changing cultural traditions and shifts away from the integrated family network that traditionally supported the oldest generation.

The elderly Cuban population in Dade County has important sociodemographic variations that establish unique needs (i.e., socioeconomic factors, family group structure, bilingual capacity, and familiarity with environment). The most recent older arrivals require special transition services that place a drain on the specialized programs for the senior Cubans as well as on the larger systems that serve the diversified elderly population. An analysis of the unique needs and characteristics of the elderly Cuban population cannot ignore the impact of recent historical events, largely uncontrolled by a community that is left to deal with the consequences.

The variations in value orientations of Anglo-Americans and Cuban immigrants are important in designing and providing services. Sometimes these value orientations have been held to be particularly relevant to counseling and mental health relationships. However, the theme of value differences actually is equally applicable across the spectrum of helping relationships. Value orientations of the Hispanic elderly or among their major subgroups become vital components of helping. Practitioners wishing to increase their effectiveness with Hispanic elders should assume that there are differences between Latin and Anglo cultures, as well as additional variations among the various subgroups and across component generations. Restated, elderly Hispanics as a whole have value differences that must be understood for their variations from those of Anglos, yet these systems share common elements that must be taken into consideration. Hispanics' common value systems are a backdrop for understanding the ethnic and historical factors that form the basis for uniqueness between the Chicano, Puerto Rican, and Cuban elderly and among the various generational cohorts within each of these subgroups.

Conceptually, the most important factors in understanding the variations between Hispanic and Anglo cultures can be subdivided into three primary areas: language, cultural, and community. In the language area, English vs. Spanish and Spanish variations must be considered. The cultural area consists of patterns of cooperation, temporal perspectives, family orientations, communication, and religious variations (Sue & Sue, 1977). The community factors involve the cluster of economic, geographical, political, and social components that impact on the lives of people who collectively share common environmental influences.

PUERTO RICAN ELDERS

In developing a perspective on the Puerto Rican elderly, it is important to understand that they have needs similar to those of other older Hispanic groups and that the overall goal of social policy should be to benefit all senior Hispanics while at the same time being sufficiently flexible to meet subgroups' needs in local communities and in major population centers.

Unlike the Cuban or Mexican-American elderly, Puerto Ricans have natural-born citizen status whether they reside on the mainland or the island. However, this citizenship does not preclude them from experiencing major ethnic and cultural problems associated with their minority status nor does it ensure them protection against poverty and prejudice.

Many Puerto Ricans, especially those clustered along the Eastern seaboard, came to the mainland during WW I and WW II, a movement that has continued ever since. A key factor was the availability of employment. The war period influx is one of several elements in classifying the Puerto Ricans. Sociodemographic characteristics, stress points of migration, and patterns of human service need are additional variables.

Distinctions between those who were born on the mainland and those who immigrated have relevance for identifying differences in the older population. The WW II era migration was related to the search for jobs, overcrowded population, and cheaper transportation between the island and the mainland (Fleisher, 1963). The move of the late 1940s and early 1950s was the focus of a classical sociological study by a team from the Bureau of Applied Social Research directed by C. Wright Mills. The project provided important information about the settlement patterns of the new group in New York City and examined how language and cultural differences impacted on problems they encountered on the mainland, comparing these to Cubans who had not migrated and to other immigrant groups in the United States (Mills, Senior, & Goldsen, 1950).

By that time, the Puerto Ricans were well established as a community in East Harlem. Their influx there began in WW I when that area of Harlem was largely Italian, and by 1980 contained more than 11,000 Puerto Ricans 65 years and older (Donaldson & Martinez, 1980). By 1950, Puerto Ricans on the mainland totaled 250,000 and during the next two decades increased to 1.5 million (U.S. Bureau of the Census, 1969). During the 1950s there was a marked pattern of population dispersion beyond New York City into Connecticut (Bridgeport, Hartford, New Haven, and Waterbury), Pennsylvania (Bethlehem and Philadelphia), Illinois (Chicago) and other major cities in New York and New Jersey. These areas face the impact of an aging Puerto Rican population and the need to address the health, nutrition, nursing home, home health, housing, and income supplement needs of these elderly persons to prevent the social isolation of individuals culturally distinct from senior Anglos.

Based on March 1978 data, the Bureau of Census estimated there were about 1.82 million Puerto Ricans in the United States, equalling 15.1 percent of the total Hispanic population. Of the total Puerto Rican population, 6.7 percent were 55 years and older (U.S. DHEW, 1979). As of March 1977, 38.8 percent of mainland Puerto Ricans were in the low income brackets, with families averaging only $7,669 as compared to the median income of $14,958 for all U.S. families. Nearly 30 percent were one-parent families, headed by a female, in contrast to 11 percent of the United States families (Report of the U.S. Commission on Civil Rights, 1976).

In considering how the demography of the elderly Puerto Ricans translates into service needs, it is important to recall that these persons are highly concentrated in New York City and State and that they have a pattern of migration back to the island after their productive work years have passed. This trend is reflected in the data that indicate only 2.3 percent of the mainland Puerto Ricans are 65 years and older as opposed to 3.7 percent of Mexicans and 13.3 percent of Cubans (U.S. DHHS, 1980).

The pattern of resettlement back to the island is not reserved to older age groups, and many of those who return experience problems (Maldonado, 1964), but there may be special factors involved for older Puerto Ricans. The process is stimulated by a reduction in the employment incentive to remain, the opportunity to reunite with family, and the belief that old age is better experienced in Puerto Rico. Those who make this transition in later life may base this decision on their feeling the isolation and reduction of social roles (work and family) in the midst of a predominant Anglo culture that is no less accepting of them because they are aging.

This segment in transition has potential needs of services from the mainland and in Puerto Rico, once they face the problem of reestablishment on the island. The scarcity of public and low-cost housing in the urban areas (San Juan and Santurce), the lack of health and mental health programs, the pressing demands of a large juvenile population, rising inflation rates, and complexities of political, economic, and welfare policy governance associated with the territorial status of Puerto Rico produce complex bureaucratic and community needs that impact on the older population (Metropolitan Life Insurance, 1972).

Many factors must be taken into consideration with older Puerto Ricans. The images created of the extended families from four slum areas of San Juan and their relatives in the United States in *La Vida: A Puerto Rican Family in the Culture of Poverty—San Juan and New York* (Lewis, 1966) gives a very narrow perspective of the types of poverty on the island and does not capture the variations among the elderly and their relatives. The diverse living circumstances of these older persons before their arrival on the mainland (or their return to the island in later years) is not a unicultural experience ascribable to a "Puerto Rican" culture.

Family backgrounds there vary extensively, depending upon social class and community structure. The contrasts between rural peasantry and elite landed gentry or between urban poverty and middle-class life styles provide extensive variations in family structure. No descriptions of a small sample of older Puerto Ricans can accurately reflect differences that characterize life for the landless workers as compared to the hacienda owners in the western central highland or the plantation workers on the west coast. These regional and cultural variations often are ignored by all but the most sensitive and knowledgeable professionals.

Another cultural component is the island's history. The Anglo view of contemporary Puerto Rico gives little or no recognition to the lasting impact of the Spanish colonization, including the ethnic and folk Spanish Catholic practices and traditions, nor is there an awareness of the strong influences created by centuries of African slave trade, Indian culture, or the Caribbean island culture. These influences provide a historical backdrop for contemporary racial identity and race relation factors.

The experts differ on the influences exerted by racial mixtures in the population. Donaldson and Martinez (1980) note that members of the same family may have skin colors ranging from dark to fair but that these differences usually are accepted with little tension or conflict. Mizio (1979) suggested a different set of influences. Puerto Ricans who live on the mainland are subject to racial categorization as either black or white. From a mental health perspective, being forced into a definition as either one has consequences for feelings of self-worth and poses a severe threat to ethnic identification as Puerto Rican.

The history of Puerto Rico's struggle for independence has its beloved heros who remain largely unknown to the Anglo world. Ramón Emeterio Betances, Rosendo Matienzo Centrón, and Eugene Mariáde Hostos were leaders in the struggle for political equality in the latter part of the 19th century. To some elders, these are their cultural heros, celebrated with comparable meaning as Anglo elders recall and celebrate the American Revolutionary War and founding political fathers. An elder's knowledge of history provides a dynamic addition to the cultural and ethnic movement of the national culture as it is legitimated and perpetuated in the Puerto Rican movement. The elders have much to contribute to that movement, if they could be recognized as legitimate among the younger community leaders. Their contributions serve to (a) create continuity between the island and those on the mainland, (b) provide a synthesizing focal point for cultural linking of communities in Puerto Rico and neighborhoods on the mainland, and (c) stimulate a cultural transmission function. Folklore; popular arts and crafts; individual, family, and popular customs; speech patterns; folk literature; music; religion; and superstition are the cornerstones of ethnic identity.

It is beyond the bounds of this analysis to evaluate the status of communal objectives of Puerto Ricans on the mainland. The Puerto Rican Task Force of the Council on Social Work Education established in the early 1970s gave a burning critique of social work's professional irrelevance toward the community (Miranda, 1973). The social work profession is not alone in its continued ignorance and perpetuation of the problem.

Health and social professions that assist the older Puerto Rican population may erect barriers to their own helping efforts if they (a) demand clients speak English in order to receive competent medical care and social services; (b) discourage personal connectedness; (c) challenge the right of Puerto Rican groups and organizations to control decision making for service resources for elders in their neighborhoods and communities, or (d) chastise self-help and self-determination efforts.

However, community-based organizations in areas having high concentrations of Puerto Ricans are not acting responsibly if they continue to trade off the needs of the young majority against those of elders. This only divides the community if religious and family institutions are criticized as too traditional and provincial to advance the goals of young leaders. The extended family (more correctly, the modified extended family form), which must continue to absorb the economic and geographic pressures of contemporary life, is the expected source of security for the elderly. To distort the value and appropriateness of this expectation, despite its hardships, is in the final analysis a challenge to the Puerto Rican cultural heritage.

The continued emphasis on family responsibility toward those in need is compatible with the maintenance of cultural enrichment. Social action emanating from within the community may be optimally directed if it demands reforms in welfare policy and practice that strengthen the family as a system. The Puerto Rican who grows old in an urban barrio òn the mainland, such as East Harlem, relates to an urban technological jungle (Donaldson & Martinez, 1980). The efforts of Puerto Rican community-based organizations would be directed appropriately if their social action strategies took a life cycle perspective that accounted for the special problems of both the dependent young and old.

Almost any intervention planned for providing services to the Puerto Rican elderly must consider the specific social situation, the individual, and the community. Generalizations across communities without benefit of evidence of important structural similarities may lead to inappropriate services. The efforts of the East Harlem Coalition, begun in 1973 to provide multisite coordinated services to the older Puerto Rican population, offer guidelines for a fragmented multiorganizational network.

The federal funding provided sufficient flexibility to divide Nutrition Project costs among eight centers under the Older Americans Act. This established budgetary assistance to diverse program settings to (a) provide specialized programs for small groups of Puerto Rican elders, (b) develop integrated programming to accommodate older blacks, Puerto Ricans, and whites with opportunities to work toward specialized cultural-specific needs, and (c) strengthen the common pool of resources required by all the elderly groups (e.g., home health, information and referral, escort service, and friendly visiting). The staffing patterns of these programs emphasize talent and interest in working with the elderly as more important than formal credentials so that indigenous potential is maximized. This personnel pattern is compatible with the larger movement in Puerto Rican community-based organizations to utilize every opportunity to develop new leadership capacities.

In addition to the East Harlem coalition, there are other programs designed to provide services. One of the common features of successful programs is that they are planned, managed, and monitored in the context of community realities. The long history of failures in that impoverished area of New York City may reflect an important point: the community context must be an integral part of program design and delivery. The area maintains the characteristics of other barrios in that its structure and internal governance are influenced by Puerto Rican formal and informal leadership structures and the neighborhood environment that reflects the population's cultural and familial dimensions. Zambrana, Merino, and Santana (1979) documented the process of providing home health care services to this population.

The Chelsea-Village Program, administered by St. Vincent's Hospital in New York, delivers in-home services to homebound, isolated, and aged persons through an approach that modifies traditional efforts by blending existing community resources with available professional expertise even though these practitioners may not be indigenous to the area. The team model also introduces a role for elderly persons to maintain a caregiving role that emphasizes the more informal aspects of peer helping. Older persons are trained as community health workers to perform basic monitoring, patient education, liaison, and patient advocacy. The limited number of services available to the frail homebound elderly in East Harlem does not begin to match the needs of these estimated 4,000 to 4,500 persons, of whom approximately half are black and Puerto Rican.

These programs illustrate the need to use available local resources, specific to the community, in a way that provides services that are attractive to a minority population yet still stress integration into the larger community and form linkages to programming for other elders.

MEXICAN-AMERICAN ELDERLY

The body of literature most germane to this chapter focuses more specifically and frequently on the Mexican-American elderly because they are the subgroup that dominates the geographical area where the authors' explorations were concentrated. Research among the Mexican-American elderly began in earnest in the late 1960s with the work of Margaret Clark (Clark & Mendelson, 1969; Newton, 1980). Thus the metropolitan San Francisco and Los Angeles areas and their surrounding counties have been of much interest to those concerned with this subgroup.

In California, there were Mexican-Americans, 3,335,500 or 15.5 percent of the population, according to updates completed in 1975 by the U.S. Bureau of the Census. Of these, 110,000 were over 40 and 100,000 did not live in urban areas. Poverty is pervasive; in 1975 the income for the Mexican-American family was $2,628 below the national average and per capita income was only $1,716 (Cotera, 1976). California has a relatively new Mexican-American community resulting from the pre-World War II bracero programs and the wave of immigration in the 1960s as compared to the settled older communities in Texas, New Mexico, Arizona, and Colorado. Braceros were Mexican laborers brought in under contract by local farmers and ranchers during harvest season and represented a major source of competition to Spanish-speaking residents, given the scarcity of employment opportunities. They settled mainly in clusters around industrial centers (reflected in factory labor force participation). Even the approximately 5 percent of the Mexican-American population in California that is rural has a seasonal rural-to-urban migration that generates service needs in the city centers. Many of those who are now elderly were not educated in the United States, either because they were migrants and not drawn into mainstream schools or because they started working when they were very young, which is a common expectation of a traditional village culture. Thus, they often had little education, even in Spanish. Many of the oldest of them speak an impure Spanish or regional Mexican rural lingo that varies considerably from classic Spanish.

Practitioners seeking information on the Mexican-American elderly will find help in material that summarizes and critiques the literature (Newton, 1980; Newton & Ruiz, in press). On the other hand, those wishing to learn more about specific guidelines for intervention and service planning for this population will not be comforted to discover the many important areas of controversy that exist in published sources. In addition, there are other areas, equally as important, that are relatively unexplored (Newton, 1980).

There is no agreement about the strength of the primary support system. The data focus on the extended family structure, with less attention on other aspects of the informal network. Three sources support the continued viability of the extended family (Clark & Mendelson, 1969; Sotomayer, 1973; Keefe, Padilla, & Carlos, 1979). Three others suggest that it has been eroded and continues to be reduced (Peñalosa, 1966; Maldonado, 1975; Velez, 1978). Given this conflict, several intervention issues become important. The Mexican-American elderly do not benefit from a perpetuation of the rationalization that the extended family can meet all their needs and that the capacity and willingness of the younger generation to care for them is based on many factors in the family system.

Grown children face complex factors in deciding either to return an aged parent to Mexico or to find some other feasible alternative. From the standpoint of both elders and adult children, raising grandchildren is something of value. A thin and tenuous balance may be created for the entire family if this function or others in which the younger adults may depend on the elder are broken. Failure either to belong to a supportive group or to participate in a supportive role in it could produce strains toward isolation that go unnoticed by the larger community.

Contributions from the extended family structure that promote the elders' isolation from the mainstream of formal service provision and access to the outside world are real. Older people's needs often are filtered through the family rather than through direct contact with service providers. While this often is necessary because of language barriers, is acceptable to the aged person, and is done willingly by the adult child, members of the younger generations are placed in the position of having to interpret and to try to communicate the needs of the elderly. The seniors have a strong tendency to accept the younger generation's definition of almost everything and anything around them in their external environment. To the extent that an elder is dependent upon a younger family member to assume responsibility to gauge the environment, a potential crisis exists if the latter is not around. The younger generation probably does experience stress through this form of dependency. However, the middle-aged children of Mexican-American elders still are reinforced for their socialized pattern of caring for the aged, but this pattern is shifting among younger generations.

Too little is known about the differing responses to caregiving between the Mexican-American and Anglo adult children of dependent parents. Perhaps they are more able to accept the idiosyncrasies of their elders, share the responsibilities with other family members or close friends, or place the problems in a balanced hierarchy that weighs it in relation to other competing demands. Greater precision is required in the identification of circumstances in which older Mexican-Americans do or do not receive support from their families (Newton, 1980). Furthermore, the situation facing Mexican-American elders may differ greatly from what their adult children will face when they reach a similar point of dependency on their children who are less socialized to care for the aged at all costs.

The literature is unanimous that the physical health of aged Mexican-Americans generally is poorer than that of nonminority elderly but there is a serious question whether sex differences exist (Newton, 1980). Men who were manual field and factory laborers tend to stop working at 50 or 55 because of disabilities. There are accelerated aging patterns in this population, with a differential of approximately 17 years as compared to whites. Many have no skills to acquire another job and are known to become withdrawn and therefore comparatively isolated from previous work roles at an earlier age than Anglo males.

On the other hand, women evidently begin to take over more dominant roles at this time and become more highly involved in their communities. Older men, and to a lesser extent older women, according to their position in the community hierarchy, may assume advisory roles in later life (Larrabure, 1980). From the gap in health information and data regarding the full range of possible sex differences, it is important to keep in mind that there are no ready suggestions regarding how to perform outreach, develop incentives that will encourage both older men and women to become more involved in the problems, or build better linkages between community and family resources.

The desire of the Mexican-American elderly to use formal services is unclear. The data are divided on this point, suggesting that some individuals wish to receive assistance from the family (Carp, 1969, 1970; Sotomayer, 1973; McConnell & Davis, 1977; Ragan & Simonin, 1977), and others do not want to be a burden (Bengtson, 1976; Valle & Mendoza, 1978).

Whatever the complex series of factors that contributes to the different data results, the pattern of possible nonutilization of community resources and services—mainly through inadequate knowledge compounded by language barriers—adds to this group's isolation. This could be described as an entrenched perception of nonentitlement to services. This results from the elders' not understanding what they are legally entitled to under county, state, and federal human service regulations. Cultural values also may reinforce expectations of entitlement that conflict with policies. More research is needed to clarify subjective perceptions of the influence of personal behaviors on service utilization. The lack of eligibility or the steps required of the older person to receive a service may produce a very demeaning or disheartening experience.

This combination of factors creates a vicious circle for the elderly. The "don't deserve," "won't be helped," and "can't be understood" all combine. This may approximate a type of learned helplessness that emerges in part through acculturation and in part from individual personality characteristics. The extent to which an individual personality explanation is useful is questionable because it tends to cast a sense of blame on the person without consideration of environmental influences. If large numbers of elderly Mexican-Americans do not know how to conceptualize or define their own needs so as to facilitate their access to what they are entitled to, or to advocate their rights not to be short-changed on human services, this plight cannot be rationalized away as an individual personality trait or a personal problem. They do not know how to ask for something if it is not recognized as a need that can be met (Larrabure, 1980).

A prevailing attitude that life is hard and always will be, a lack of a sense of control, and a feeling of powerlessness that afflict many of these individuals may translate into behavioral passivity and seeming indifference to their needs or conditions. They are in this sense self-isolating, but this may be the result of acculturation. Their apparently stoic and uninterested behavior (as perceived by Anglo culture) in turn discourages potential caregivers and makes complex demands on service agencies. Agencies without ample resources, including Spanish-speaking personnel, are not likely to devote time and resources to identifying and developing the utilization capacity of elderly Mexican-Americans who tend to be inconsistent and careless in their use of services designed for Anglo clients.

Self-sufficiency also is of great importance. If pride is invested in "what I can do for myself" or "what my children can do for me," much of the nonhelp-seeking behavior is understandable. Only sensitive personnel with a comprehensive understanding of Hispanic folkways, acculturation experiences, and the limitations of the existing system to meet their needs can break through these behavioral modes and extract them from self-imposed or culturally imposed isolation.

To view these problems (created by cultural differences and isolation from the service network) abstractly misses some of the hardship and suffering that they represent. Two cases illustrate how different cultural expectations, in respect to family help, and lack of connectedness to or understanding of the service system, impact on elders and their families.

Carmen Cortez

Carmen Cortez is a 58-year-old female. Although she still is relatively young, she has several chronic physical problems that include lung and cardiovascular diseases. She has extended periods of confusion, gastric distress, generalized discomfort, and considerable anxiety. For five months she alternated between stays in the hospital and in her home with an unmarried daughter. Hospitalization would be occasioned by trouble in breathing (a choking feeling), generalized fears at night, a refusal of food because of gastric distress, and refusal to walk because of dizziness and weakness.

Carmen looks much older than her 58 years; she is white-haired and toothless and her face is wrinkled. She began working in the fields at age 5, was married at 15, and had 11 children, eight of whom survived. During her married years she often worked as a field hand, as did her children. She had no education and does not speak English.

Carmen's daughter said in an interview:

> You know, I think she really likes to be in the hospital. I don't know what to do with her, I can't watch her all the time. . . . My sister has her babies, she can't run in all the time. For me to drive to the hospital every night is too much. My sister drives but is too scared to drive on the highway. . . . I'm the youngest of the children and not married, so I have all the responsibility for mother. I have no life of my own. My mother wants us to be with her and care for her. She doesn't speak anymore. She is so stubborn. . . . I know she can walk, but she says that when she stands up she feels like she is falling, and so she doesn't try anymore. When the nurses make her take some steps she cries like a child. . . . We tried to get her into a nursing home, but they keep telling us there is not room. I am so angry at that doctor, he told me there is nothing to be done, that she will never get better. He says her heart is very bad and she is too sick for an operation.

In spite of Carmen's chronic illness, her daughter is committed to helping her but is frustrated in that she does not know what to do and resentful of the burden being placed on her. She does not know, nor has she been told, how to link up with resources that would provide a home care respite. Shared responsibility for the mother is difficult because of the employment and child-rearing problems that absorb the time of other family members. They do not seem to understand the mother's real medical condition, seem to feel she could be well if she tried, and cannot locate the community resources to help them care for her.

Gabriel Homes

Gabriel Homes is 79 and of Mexican-Indian origin. He speaks no English. He understands some requests but most often fails to respond to them. Gabriel had been staying at a board and care home but now is hospitalized. While at the home he fell and broke his leg. He was hospitalized once before (briefly) because of increasingly bizarre and somewhat destructive behavior but responded quite well to chemotherapy and soon was returned to the home. Shortly afterward, his son from Colorado visited but did not maintain contact with him.

During his lifetime Gabriel worked in the fields, in a shingle factory, and for a construction company. He has the son in Colorado but doesn't know the whereabouts of his other children. His wife died quite some time ago. Gabriel yearns to see his son and doesn't understand why he cannot live with him. He often sits for hours in the sun, refusing food and drink, in a withdrawn silence. A social service worker who does not speak Spanish is his only, but infrequent, agency contact. He does not understand her when she visits his home.

Both Carmen and Gabriel expect to stay with and be cared for by family members. This traditional expectation becomes difficult with the dispersing of family in search of employment and the pressures of a modern urban existence. When their financial situation is marginal it is difficult to support another relative who does not have an adequate pension and/or may have chronic physical problems. For many there is no role or place in the family and no comfort in the unfamiliar settings provided by the community at large.

The Mexican-Americans tend to cluster in barrios and vecindades. Barrios are homogeneous Mexican-American settlements in the United States and have been one of the bulwarks against assault on the culture at large, preventing more rapid assimilation (Nava, 1973). Vecindades are smaller areas of identification, sometimes within barrios. The neighborhoods within the barrios or vecindades are the center of much daily activity for old and young. To understand how each elderly Mexican-American lives, either with or without meaningful social contacts and under what circumstances, it is essential to understand the pattern of informal relationships within the barrio and how the structure of age-specific services and problem-specific agencies relate to its internal structure.

The Mexican-American community in San Mateo County, Calif., adjoining San Francisco on the south, includes more than one barrio where the elderly are clustered. More than two decades ago, Margaret Clark, the anthropologist, completed a definitive study of Mexican-American population in neighboring San Jose (1959), with a concentration of work in the Sal si Puedes area, which was a major barrio in the 1950s that a decade later continued to be a major focal point in the life of many Mexican-Americans in San Jose. She spoke about influences over a period of 10 to 15 years because of the migrants who had entered the United States in the 50s and early 60s. Her observation, reported in the update (1970) of her original study, that these new immigrants had reinforced the Latin-American character of this one barrio seems characteristic of the development of the qualities of the others in San Mateo County. She writes:

> The past decade has seen a major change in the relationships between the Spanish-speaking community and the Anglo-American society. The social and political ferment of recent years has broken down some of the old isolation that formerly characterized the California barrios. Community leaders, social action groups, and student organizations have emerged as even stronger forces demanding attention to the social and economic evils that have beset the poor for generations. (p. vii)

The barrios in San Mateo County have their own hierarchy of community leadership. To a varying extent, these leaders resent intrusion from outside agency personnel in matters of concern to residents. Political and labor leaders tend to play an important overall function in linking the Spanish-speaking community with leadership of the various towns in the county (Daly City, South San Francisco, San Mateo, and Redwood City) and the larger county power structure. These leaders have influence on those seeking help in the barrios. They can encourage or discourage individuals from applying for outside services and can identify problems and translate barrio needs to the larger community.

In attempting to understand how the elderly residents of the San Mateo County barrios are connected into the social structure and therefore influenced by it, it is necessary to become familiar with a particular barrio. Until very recently, little or no information was available on the needs of the Mexican-American elderly in the communities where they were concentrated. To a large extent, the information that is available has neither been put to maximum utilization to resolve human service needs nor been of significant use, given the outdated and inaccurate statistics available from the previous census and its updates.

Perhaps irrespective of where and how older persons are involved with a particular barrio, many Spanish-speaking elderly do not fit into the surrounding urban community. They tend to live in the present with immediate economic and practical life matters that do not relate to contemplation of tomorrow, which to them remains vague and indefinable. Mexican-Americans, often labelled as poorly acculturated, live in the long sequence of present realities and reflect a fatalistic and accepting attitude. Since they cannot control the future, they see no point in striving to accept what essentially is unattainable (Salcedo, 1974). The dichotomy between reality as they perceive it and society's promises is sufficient to alert practitioners to the serious problems brought about by many of the same isolators that impact on other groups of impoverished urban elderly. However, those problems are made more complex by the differences in language and culture that tend to set older Mexican-Americans on ethnic islands out of sight and therefore out of mind to the Anglo navigators and captains of human services.

SAN MATEO SPANISH-SPEAKING ELDERLY

An important community survey project sponsored by the San Mateo County Area Agency on Aging documented the social and health service needs of the Spanish-speaking elderly in the county (Muller, 1978). It then delineated how they presented their perceptions of their problems when brought together in a special caucus held in conjunction with the First Annual Minority Conference in San Mateo. These information sources provide a basis for considering intervention strategies that might be initiated to meet the needs of this group.

Almost every agency faced with the problem of having to identify the special needs of a minority group within a larger population at one point will consider the value of conducting a needs assessment survey. These surveys, if ever undertaken, often must be done with limited personnel and financial resources. The original goals for such needs identification activities can be either very realistic or too grand in nature. Their results can clarify or distort actual needs, can present specific recommendations for change or conclude without offering a direction for future planning, and can become a document that is used for social intervention or filed away as evidence of the fact that at least something was done.

In the first interview, the project director explained that a little more than three years ago she had been hired by the San Mateo Area Agency on Aging to conduct a project on the service needs of the Mexican-American elderly. As with many efforts to obtain information from isolated populations, the research task in reality required far more resources than were made available to use empirical tools to gather and analyze material about complex service needs.

The original sample was much larger than the actual final 84 Spanish-speaking seniors. It was to be conducted in all four cities in San Mateo County with large concentrations of the target population, but finally was based on the two northern-most—Daly City and South San Francisco. They were selected because of their close geographical proximity, their shared service resources, and because they contained 33 percent of the Spanish-speaking elderly in the county. The sample included participants in two groups that met in the target areas. In addition to interviews conducted by the project director, herself a fluent bilingual person, Spanish-speaking seniors served as an invaluable source of outreach through their in-home interviews.

Of the 84 participants, more than half were permanent resident aliens and only 20 percent were naturalized citizens. Mexico was the country of origin for slightly less than half of the sample, with the next largest group representing countries in Central America. Thirteen had lived in the United States for nine years or less. Two-thirds were females and one-third males. They were divided into two segments with two-thirds in the young-old group (65-74) and the others 75 or older. The minority—actually 19 persons—were living alone and a majority of these reported fair to poor health.

When asked how they had learned about available social services, half said the information was common knowledge, somewhat fewer cited friends of family, and seven had no prior knowledge. A pattern of discussing personal problems with someone outside the family or friendship network was mentioned by only one person. Although the subjects consistently reported their linguistic ability in Spanish was good, the project director questioned their fluency because of low educational levels. Their adequacy in all aspects of English was rated as poor or none for more than 50 percent.

Only three were covered under private medical insurance, 28 were receiving Medicaid, and 42 MediCal, but not sure of how to distinguish between the two sources. Of 36 who reported dental problems, 21 were not receiving any form of dental care, most often because of a lack of money or access to a dentist. More than half owned their own homes and three owned mobile homes. Sixty-one of the 84 did not own cars, the majority depending on public transportation. As to employment, 68 were not working but were unable to do so anyway. Only three of those not working thought that they could, even though most expressed a desire to be able to do so. Thirteen were working part-time or full-time. Income levels were based on combined household wages. Just under two-thirds of the total sample reported incomes of less than $5,000: six had no income, three between $1,000 and $2,000, 20 between $2,001 and $3,500, and 24 between $3,501 and $5,000.

The implications of these data are analyzed in the context of an agency-consumer exchange model that delineates the functions for the two subsystems (Muller, 1978). To provide continuing delivery of services to the Spanish-speaking population, this particular agency, and foreseeably others, must be concerned about how both it and the target population function in relation to specific elements of the program.

The first function is the identification of need. To some extent, this Area Agency on Aging, through its completion of this project, has begun the difficult process of identifying the needs of the Spanish-speaking population. However, this particular survey does not specify the patterns of need throughout the entire area where the Hispanics are distributed. It points to the problems of this small sample of elders in accessing, receiving, and continuing in service after service. The responses strongly suggest that the elderly do not present their problems in a framework that fits the categories that the Area Agency on Aging is able to serve, even though it is working diligently and in many cases very successfully to provide help in a planned and coordinated manner to the majority of its Anglo target population. The seniors' tendency to identify problems and crises, rather than continuing needs, puts the agency in a position of not knowing how or what to do when its function is not crisis intervention.

The second service function involves the selection of staff members who are culturally aware and sensitive to the needs of the target population. In counties such as San Mateo, where there is significant cultural and ethnic diversity, the administrative and management functions should include a continuing personnel selection and evaluation process that identifies and eliminates behaviors that exhibit institutional or personal prejudice against the poor or minorities (Muller, 1978). Spanish-speaking elders confronted by direct or indirect prejudice from service providers tend simply not to return, to say nothing, or to give up pursuing their needs. Neither clients nor agency will benefit if the elderly do not defend their rights not to be treated as undesirables, if their informal network does not challenge practices that discriminate against them, or if the agency does not develop an effective monitoring system to avoid perpetuation of these practices. Word gets around and potential service users stay away.

The third function might be described as processing or eligibility facilitation. The organizational structure of national aging service networks produces increasing amounts of red tape. The Hispanic elderly, particularly those who are not fluent in English or well acquainted with the complexities of being processed to receive service, lack the incentive or capacity to deal with such impersonal situations. Staff members who are working to help link these people to services but who do not understand Spanish may in reality cause the elderly whose English is inadequate to miss out on assistance.

The fourth function involves making services visible in the community. If an agency issues well-prepared publicity aimed at the mainstream of elderly, it will not be recognized easily by the invisible minorities. Muller (1978) strongly suggests that in order to reach the Spanish-speaking, communication in both languages must be the rule rather than the exception. The usual modes of publicity that are more or less effective with the majority target group may not alert the informal network in the barrios to the availability of services.

If there is little publicity with the barrio leadership structure, the network upon which the Spanish-speaking elders rely may never be informed. Thus they may not know what service agencies exist and what their functions are (Muller, 1978). Failure to tap into this informal network or never realizing that efforts to do so are being misdirected can prove frustrating and costly to the agency. The result is that the agency can justifiably claim to have attempted to make its resources known in the community; on the other hand, the minority does not accept the effort as legitimate or the best that could be done. In the long run, these information distribution efforts are not always effective and keep the Spanish-speaking elderly underserved or not helped at all.

The fifth function is the attempt to establish consistency in the services and in how they are offered. Almost all of the services provided by an area agency on aging may be subject to funding reductions. Special one-time demonstration grants may be lost from one year to the next. The addition of a bilingual staff person to increase the capacity of a core service may do much to encourage its use by Spanish-speaking seniors. Individuals tend to rely on a familiar person with whom they feel they can communicate because their prior contacts have been successful.

The client thus places reliance on the individual rather than on the agency, and loss of this key contact person discourages future utilization (Muller, 1978).

The San Mateo Area Agency on Aging is an example of an entity that has Spanish-speaking elders in addition to other minority groups that experience cultural and linguistic barriers to service. One of its greatest challenges is to get its target population to fully recognize the core services it offers: Multipurpose Senior Centers, a Senior Information and Referral Office, Outreach to the Homebound, the Redi-Wheel Bus Service, Escort Service, Nutrition Centers and Meals-On-Wheels, Adult Day Health Centers, Employment Program for Seniors, Legal Services, Housing Assistance Service, In-Home Chore Services, Home Visitation, and Legislative Advocacy.

From the recommendations made at the conclusion of the demonstration project with the Spanish-speaking, it is clear that a generalized publicity approach is not effective with a community that is not seeking the offered services. Few agencies have realized that in order to help this group they must create demand for the services. To some this may appear to contradict the supposition that the Spanish-speaking elderly are at risk. To suggest that many services go by unnoticed by the Hispanic senior community would understate the problem. The general lack of understanding of the bureaucratic structure and how it operates provides a formidable obstacle for all but the most sophisticated Spanish-speaking seniors (Muller, 1978). The tasks facing the agency appear equally as formidable.

There was a period between the time the agency received the recommendations of the report and when the next significant step was taken in the county to stimulate renewed attention to the needs of this group. The action came in the form of a community forum that offered the San Mateo Area Agency an opportunity to establish dialogues with the elderly themselves and with their strong advocates in the Hispanic leadership structure of the county. This involved agency representatives who sought to gather information to provide renewed impetus to address the needs of the Hispanic elderly in the direction of their own priorities.

For the first time in the history of San Mateo County's attempt to address the issues of the minority elderly, a single meeting sought to encourage the formation of common objectives that cut across the needs of all these groups but at the same time provided an opportunity for each to explore its own individual concerns and interests. The objectives were to identify key issues in minority aging, to develop a means for including these issues in the 1981 White House Conference on Aging, and to facilitate the participation of the minority elders of San Mateo County in that conference.

The conference planners were all too familiar with the lack of cooperation that had characterized the largest minority groups of California in their efforts to gain access to human service resources in proportion to their numbers and needs and to obtain the backing of the leadership of each bloc to support a program that included several minorities. They also, most importantly, had to make everyone aware of how difficult it would be to come together to share problems and concerns.

These elderly do not often respond to the infrequent requests to voice their opinions in the planning and/or evaluation of services directed toward them. Many will not participate because they do not want to show their ignorance of the systems that are requesting their participation. To speak in public is to run the risk of making a comment that may be incorrect or inappropriate. Some of the elderly feel that since the services are ''free'' or subsidized, they should not be critical or the few to which they have access might be removed or they might be punished in some way. These attitudes were, and continue to be, what must be overcome if the Hispanic elderly are to have input into service planning.

The caucus activities confirmed the initial hesitation of the elderly to participate but also gave them a basis for greater confidence that their views were important and that their message would be heard. The following is a summary of the major dialogue of the caucus translated from Spanish.

> Today you, the Spanish-speaking elders of San Mateo County, have been brought together for the first time to talk together about the problems that you are experiencing and the needs that you have that you want to make known at the White House Conference. The responsibility that you have to try to talk about the important issues is important for you and all others like you in the United States who need to have a voice that makes it known whether or not it is difficult for you to use services; why and how the needs of Spanish-speaking elders may be different and special; and how we can make the needs of the San Mateo Hispanic elders known at the White House Conference on Aging. Some people here with us do not speak Spanish, but we will translate for them because we want them to understand. Those who are not a minority may feel like a minority and maybe this is good, even though we do not want anyone to feel like that.

The elders were then asked to speak to three questions:

1. Is it difficult for you to use the services that are available?
2. Do you as Spanish-speaking elders have special needs that are not being met and why do you think this is so?
3. How can we make your needs known at the White House Conference? (Larrabure, 1980)

The responses of a number of different participants are excerpted as follows:

> Before anything else we need people who speak Spanish to help us. . . .

We should not be called old people, you and they should call us grown-up people. . . .

More than 70 percent of us in this room own our own homes and they are putting liens on our houses. Other people put liens on our homes, then when we sell our homes we are left with having to pay an annual 7 to 10 percent. When somebody puts a lien on your house, someone from the county office must tell you. . . . I have tried to help 20 friends who have been in this situation, but I cannot do it all and there must be some better way. . . .

When I went to the Social Security office they told me that I would have to sell my own home in Mexico before I could get Social Security. . . . I do not want to have to sell the home in the town of my birth. My sister will never leave Mexico and she has a right to die in my house. I do not understand what they want me to do. . . .

I have had to go to the doctor two times a month. I have to call one week in advance in order to get the special bus. I can't use the public transportation because of my health problems. There should be better transportation for us to get to these services. . . .

The authority for housing for the elderly says to me that they will not allow people to have their family members stay with them, they won't allow my grandchild to come and stay with me so that they can help me. . . .

We have no day care centers and we and our children need respite. We will gladly take care of our sick elders but we need respite. . . .

We do not know the age limit for the services or the money we can receive. There must be some consistent age limit that applies or they must make it clear to us when we will be eligible to receive what. For many of us we will not live long enough to collect the benefits they say that we can get. . . .

Nobody is concerned that our people live alone in the hotels and that there are isolated men who know nothing about the services. . . . We have our SROs [single room occupants] too. . . .

There are fewer and fewer hospitals that accept MediCal and we don't know which ones, so people can't go to those that accept it if they don't know which ones. . . .

If a woman has worked for many years she gets Social Security and Medicare; sometimes we need these benefits before we are 60 and it isn't right that we go so long without these benefits and then have so few years to enjoy them because we don't live long enough. . . .

In the nutrition programs where many of us go there should be people to speak about the programs in Spanish. . . . The language makes it difficult for us to even get on buses and the Redi-bus does not help if you have an emergency that you can't schedule and it is terrible if you are sick and must go to the hospital. . . . We must always take somebody with us who speaks Spanish, no matter where we go . . . the services are never located where we are located. . . .

What we must do is to select a good representative to the President's Conference so that he can go to speak about our interests, one who is not a coward. We want to choose that representative and not have others do it for us. (Larrabure, 1980)

These comments by the participants at the minority elderly caucus reflected concerns faced by all seniors as well as some that are peculiar to Hispanics. Among these concerns are:

1. There was some confusion about eligibility requirements in various social programs and even between programs. This was evident in the remarks on the need to sell property to receive Social Security benefits. In reality, there is no means test for Social Security benefits but there is for other local and federal income assistance benefits available for the poor. This type of problem, as well as the one concerning property liens, suggests that the language difficulty has taken a heavy toll in communication between agency and applicant. It would seem obvious that all important legal matters should be discussed in both English and Spanish. Language problems also were a factor in the use of other services, such as the nutrition program.

2. Concern was voiced over the eligibility age for Social Security. All minority groups have a lower life expectancy than the nonminority population. (This is not true for those who do reach advanced age, at which time the death rates for minorities actually are lower than for nonminorities.) A lower age eligibility requirement for minority elders has been considered by some. However, it must be considered that shorter life expectancy is more closely related to socioeconomic class standing, directly affecting those in the lower categories. So perhaps, to be truly fair, all individuals with very low incomes should be allowed to retire early rather than to extend this privilege to some based only on minority status. It may be more beneficial, however, to concentrate energies on the unmet health and social needs that contribute to the problem of lower life expectancy among the poor. There is a need to formulate a uniform policy for age eligibility requirements across all programs to eliminate any confusion over eligibility. Among the caucus participants there did seem to be something of a contradiction: (a) a desire for uniform age requirements and (b) a desire for differential age eligibility requirements for minority individuals.

3. Concern was expressed about the inadequacy of services offered, i.e., the limitations on the use of transportation facilities that made them unavailable

for crisis situations. The inadequacy of transportation is felt by all elders who depend on public facilities. The solution to this problem, while partly dependent on better organization of fragmented programs on the local level, looks more to increased funding from all sources. The same inadequacy of services was echoed in other complaints about health services for those on public assistance, neighborhood branches of service agencies, and day care centers. It must be noted that all of these services help an elderly to remain at home and possibly prevent unnecessary use of the even more expensive total care institutions. While it is true that needed services are inadequate for all elderly, older Hispanics feel the lack even more because those that are available are geared to the need of majority group seniors.

4. The wish was expressed that older adults should be called "adult" rather than "old." This would seem to be a rejection of ageism, of being placed in a separate category. This is an issue not only with agency personnel as they relate to their clients but also in overall policy formulation. If separate programs are created with eligibility based on an identified age, the agencies then must serve a population defined by age.

5. Concern was expressed that the housing authority regulation preventing related children from staying with tenants ignored the cultural needs of Hispanic elders. There may be general reasons for this type of regulation, such as the needs of other tenants for quiet or the problems that accompany overcrowding of housing facilities, but perhaps arrangements could be worked out that would be mutually satisfactory once all parties were aware and sensitive to competing needs.

What is most important in these statements about services is the particular problems faced by Hispanic elders, e.g., confusion resulting from language difficulties, regulations that ignore cultural tradition, and differing personal life histories and experiences. Their participation in this forum gave evidence of another role: they were advocating for themselves, declaring the right to make their needs known, and wanting to help the larger society understand their isolation and entrapment. They recognized that they could not afford to lose the opportunity to have a forceful position prepared for the White House Conference on Aging.

The recommendations made by the Hispanic elderly clearly suggest issues regarding intervention and provision of services in ways that link the resources of the age-specific network with the general resources of their community, both formal and informal. However, conference recommendations, like the results of special projects, either can produce no results or lead to consequences that can have negative impact for those most in need. One of the outcomes to be avoided in this multiminority area is a misdirected sense of different needs among the minority elderly that induce competition among the black, Hispanic, Filipino, and Pacific Asian groups. At the center of all of the statements of needs and all of the urgent directives to the planners of the White House conference was a single message: give us adequate resources to ensure a quality in our lives as elders and, in the process, our dignity as people with much uniqueness but a common humanity.

WHAT ARE SOME POSSIBLE ALTERNATIVES?

It is easy to argue that coordination, advocacy, and some specialized services are needed by the Spanish-speaking elderly of San Mateo County. (The social resource system for all Hispanic elders is sketched in Figure 7-2.) To initiate and sustain efforts to bring together a better working relationship between the age-specific service network and the resources of the barrios will be far from simple. It will not be accomplished by strategies that rely on such efforts as

- the Area Agency on Aging merely developing a contract or purchase of service agreement with Catholic Charities that do not have a network of effective outreach to the Spanish-speaking elders

- establishing a token information and referral system in Spanish to take care of the problems of all the elderly

- increasing the visibility of Spanish-speaking elders on a few senior councils

- a short special demonstration project that would be unlikely to continue if federal funds or state appropriations were cut

A first step might be to develop a long-term cooperative planning relationship between the San Mateo Area Agency on Aging and the newly formed Hispanic Concilio of San Mateo County. A limited basis for a working relationship was established through the participation of some of the key leaders of the Concilio in the planning of the Hispanic caucus.

The National Concilio of America has its national headquarters in California and has been instrumental in organizing chapters in major cities throughout the United States where there are large clusters of Spanish-speaking persons. Its function is to focus on the spectrum of issues and problems related to the language and cultural differences among Hispanics and the majority citizenry that serve as barriers to the former's receipt and utilization of human services. The National Concilio was instrumental in helping form the Hispanic Concilio of San Mateo County. The local concilio has a 15-member board of directors that was installed in June 1980. It began to work to bring together, under the structure of one Hispanic advocacy organization, the key individuals in the county who could provide leadership and support to facilitate the human service provision to all barrio residents.

Figure 7-2 The Hispanic Elder and the Social Resource System

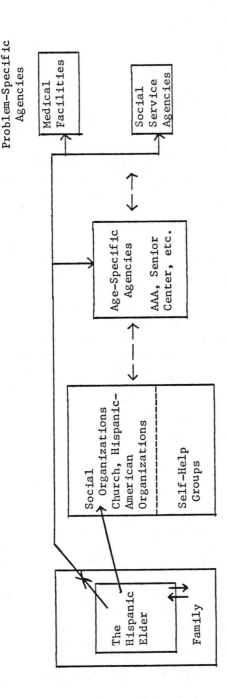

The Hispanic elder frequently has direct contact only with social organizations whose personnel are bilingual and with family members. Contact with other agencies must often be facilitated by a family intermediary. If family members are not available, contact with community organizations is hampered.

The National Concilio has taken leadership roles in many areas:

1. It has provided linkage with the United Way of America and was successful in advocating for additional funding for Hispanic agencies.
2. It has acted as liaison with key federal agencies on issues important to the Hispanic community nationwide.
3. It has helped promote the first national Hispanic Women's Conference and played a central role in the development of local concilios.

In some communities where concilios are lacking or do not focus on the elderly, assistance may be available through other local or national Hispanic-based advocacy groups. The Asociacion Nacional pro Personas Mayores (National Association for Hispanic Elderly) is unique in that it serves all segments of the Spanish-speaking elderly. The national headquarters of the nonprofit private organization is in Los Angeles, with a network of regional organizations throughout the United States (the Southeastern Regional Office in Miami, the Eastern Regional Office in New York, a liaison office in Washington, and the Midwest Liaison Office in Chicago). The association has sponsored a number of special education and research projects along with maintaining an advocating effort. Under funding from the Administration on Aging, it provided technical assistance to AoA regional offices to facilitate service delivery to the Hispanic elderly. The projects it has undertaken have helped advance the state of the art (Lacayo, 1980).

The local concilios such as the one in San Mateo County can conduct functions similar to those undertaken by the national: (a) review the demographics of the Hispanic population in relation to human service needs and resource distribution, (b) design programs that are appropriate for the Spanish-speaking community or various subgroups, (c) plan and conduct a full range of advocacy programs, and (d) identify gaps in service provision.

It is evident from the structure of the board that key people on the San Mateo Concilio also are the main links to the provision of services to the elderly. Two of the officers work directly with the Hispanic-American elderly in the county, and the executive director of the concilio is a highly respected and credentialed professional who has become well-known to the Hispanic elderly and throughout the human service network. Together, those three individuals have a wealth of knowledge about planning for the Hispanic elderly, are visible and highly political, are fluent in Spanish, are either Hispanic or have lived closely with that community, and have a track record of being highly successful advocates and organizers.

The primary thrust must be to develop: (a) a linkage between the age-specific network and the full range of other service agencies that have resources that would be valuable to the Hispanic elderly, (b) a new thrust within the barrios that involve the elderly more closely in support networks for each other and reach out to those without families or to those whose families and friends need support to continue caregiving; (c) an integrated service center that can provide a more comprehensive range of clinical assistance through the onsite availability of Spanish-speaking health professionals, and (d) draw more directly on gerontologists' increasing knowledge about the Hispanic elderly.

On these bases, a focused and formalized mechanism between the Area Agency on Aging and the concilio in the county would seem appropriate and timely. As suggested earlier, the aging service network cannot meet this group's total range of needs. The county and its resources can be coordinated because there is a mutual vested organizational interest in doing something beneficial to better serve this minority as its demands increase.

It has been mentioned repeatedly that many of these Spanish-speaking seniors remain passive and uninvolved in either generating better personal access to services or in the development of collective self-advocacy. Professionals have noted that while it is not impossible to start small groups of seniors and develop peer communication, in these groups they appear to have little self-sustaining capacity. Without constant input from a leader to provide cohesion and direction, the groups usually do not remain active and effective (Larrabure, 1980; Muller, 1978).

More efforts might be directed toward developing leadership skills among Spanish-speaking seniors in the barrio communities. The first step would involve the identification of individuals who have this potential. This would require looking beyond their membership in senior citizen programs to identify those who are vital to the barrio's social structure but are not visible to the larger community. For instance, through their parish membership, it might be possible to find some older persons who have natural leadership abilities even though neither they nor others recognize their talents to work for and with others. They may be identifiable by clergy but more often are found through lay leadership of the parish. Once identified, they could be recruited and paid to attend a Hispanic Elder Community Leadership Development Program. It could be offered by Spanish-speaking professionals from San Jose State University who have both community development and group work skills as well as knowledge of the cultural dimensions involved.

Developing the leadership skills in Spanish and having these seniors function as special advocates and organizers in the barrios could help avoid the barriers of trying to teach these other persons to work in English, which may be a major reason why some of those most able to perform these functions do not become involved. In the past there has been too little consideration of how these seniors could be mobilized for self-advocacy and outreach. The proposed program could avoid some of the pitfalls associated with superimposing ideas on this group that its members understandably reject as either inappropriate or irrelevant to their world.

As a single example, a joint project could be undertaken between the San Mateo Concilio and the Area Agency on Aging to attempt to strengthen the health and social service capacity of the Fair Oaks Senior Center in Redwood City. Its program is directed by a Hispanic administrator with great professional and personal commitment to her tasks related to the advocacy and provision of services to Spanish-speaking elders. It has operated successfully to serve numerous minorities by providing an atmosphere that allows each group the opportunity for social programming that is culturally appropriate and relevant to it. It is the appropriate site to implement a major community outreach and case management program for the isolated and impoverished elderly in that community.

Through the combined resources of the Harold D. Chope City Hospital, serving that area, and the Fair Oaks Senior Center, an adult day health center program could be developed to target its services to minority elderly. It could provide an alternative to the scarce and often unacceptable institutionalization in nursing homes, living alone without supports, or care provided by family members who themselves need support to continue to maintain caregiving to an elderly parent. This service concept could be adapted to fit the self-help mode of meeting needs. A day health care program is one way to stimulate the existing informal support network and to link its members to resources in the larger community that are essential for health and well-being. It could complement current functions and help to vitalize the Hispanic elders to redirect the trends that perpetuate their isolation.

CONCLUSION

The problems of immigrants have reached a point of heightened concern in recent years. Vietnamese, Russian Jews, Haitians, and El Salvadorans face complex political, social, and economic struggles as they adapt to the fabric of American culture. For individuals in later life, whatever their cultural and ethnic characteristics, the process of adaptation is particularly difficult. The Hispanic elderly were selected for this analysis because their numbers create serious demands for human service needs that cannot continue to be ignored.

The emphasis has been directed toward the segments of the elderly Cuban, Puerto Rican, and Mexican-American subgroups that are at greater risk of isolation because they are not as established within their communities as either those who have a family history of many generations in the United States (such as the Mexican-Americans in the Southwest), or the Cubans who arrived before the Castro revolution. Immigrants such as these brought with them different personal and financial resources or have a familial history of stabilized location in American communities.

It is crucial for practitioners to have knowledge about the Hispanic elderly, recognize the strengths within their subgroups to define and structure their destiny, and accept that they cannot and should not accept all that is Anglo without self-protective skepticism.

The neglect and disinterest among the helping professions can be reversed. Only time will tell whether the Anglo majority recognizes the Hispanic minority because of a desire for greater equality or because of political necessity. Either way, the circumstances of the Hispanic elderly must be attended to as they struggle through difficulties toward the American Dream.

REFERENCES

Bengtson, V.L. *Familiar support systems and ethnic groups: Patterns of contrast and consequence.* Paper presented at the 29th meeting of the Gerontological Society, New York, October 1976.

Carp, F.M. Housing and minority group elderly. *Gerontologist,* 1969, *9,* 20-24.

Carp, F.M. Communicating with elderly Mexican-Americans. *Gerontologist,* 1970, *10,* 126-134.

Clark, M. *Health in the Mexican-American culture* (1st ed.). Berkeley, Calif.: University of California Press, 1959.

Clark, M. *Health in the Mexican-American culture* (2nd ed.). Berkeley, Calif.: University of California Press, 1970.

Clark, M., & Mendelson, M. Mexican-American aged in San Francisco: A case description. *Gerontologist,* 1969, *9,* 90-95.

Cotera, M.P. *Profile on the Mexican-American woman.* Austin, Texas: Information Systems Development, 1976.

Donaldson, E., & Martinez, E. The Hispanic elderly of East Harlem. *Aging,* March-April 1980, pp. 6-11.

Fleisher, G.M. Some economic aspects of Puerto Rican migration to the United States. *Review of Economics and Migration,* 1963, *45,* 221-230.

Hernandez, A.R. *The Cuban minority in the U.S.: Final report on need identification and program evaluation.* Washington, D.C.: Cuban National Planning Council, 1974.

It's your turn in the sun. *Time,* October 16, 1978, pp. 48-52; 55; 58; 61.

Keefe, S.E., Padilla, A.M., & Carlos, M.L. The Mexican-American extended family as an emotional support system. *Human Organization,* 1979, *38,* 144-152.

Lacayo, C.G. The Asociacion Nacional pro Personas Mayores: Responding to the decade of the Hispanic. *Aging,* March-April 1980, pp. 12-13.

Larrabure, L.G. *The social services context of the Mexican-American elderly.* Unpublished paper, George Warren Brown School of Social Work, Washington University in St. Louis, 1980.

Lewis, O. *LaVida: A Puerto Rican family in the culture of poverty—San Juan and New York.* New York: Random House, Inc., 1966.

Linn, M.W., Hunter, K.I., & Perry, P.R. Differences by sex and ethnicity in the psychosocial adjustment of the elderly. *Journal of Health and Social Behavior,* 1979, *20,* 273-281.

Maldonado, A.W. The migration reverses. *The Nation,* March 16, 1964, *198,* 255-257.

Maldonado, B., Jr. The Chicano aged. *Social Work,* 1975, *20,* 213-216.

McConnell, S.R., & Davis, W.J. *Social and cultural contexts of aging: A decision-maker survey report.* Los Angeles: University of Southern California, Andrus Gerontology Center, 1977.

Metropolitan Life Insurance Company. *Population and health profile of Puerto Rico.* Statistical bulletin of the Metropolitan Life Insurance Company, 1972, *53,* 9-11.

Mills, C.W., Senior, C., & Goldsen, R. *The Puerto Rican journey: New York's newest migrant.* New York: Harper, 1950.

Miranda, M. *Puerto Rican task force report.* New York: Council on Social Work Education, 1973.

Mizio, E. *Puerto Rican task force report: Project on ethnicity.* New York: Family Service Association of America, 1979, p. 9.

Muller, S. *An analysis of the social service needs and social service utilization of Spanish-speaking senior citizens in northern San Mateo County.* Redwood City, Calif.: San Mateo County Area Agency on Aging, 1978.

National Council on the Aging. *Fact book on aging: A profile of America's older population.* Washington, D.C.: National Council on the Aging, Inc., Research and Evaluation Department, 1978.

Nava, J. *Viva la Raza.* New York. D. Van Nostrand Co., Inc., 1973.

Newton, F.C. Issues in research and service delivery among Mexican-American elderly: A concise statement with recommendations. *Gerontologist,* 1980, *20,* 208-213.

Newton, F.C., & Ruiz, R.A. Chicano culture and mental health among the elderly. In M. Miranda and R.A. Ruiz (Eds.), *Chicano aging and mental health.* San Francisco: Human Resources Corp. (in press).

Peñalosa, F. The changing Mexican-American in southern California. *Sociology and Social Research,* 1966, *51,* 405-417.

Ragan, P.K., & Simonin, M.S. *Social and cultural context of aging: Community survey report.* Los Angeles: University of Southern California, Andrus Gerontology Center, 1977.

Rothman, S. *The status of minority elderly.* Proceedings of a symposium/hearing on federal policy issues concerning the nation's elderly minorities convened by the National Council on the Aging, Committee of the Special Aging Populations, Jackson, Miss., 1979, pp. 99-107. (Copies available through the National Council on the Aging, Washington, D.C. 20201.)

Salcedo, C. *Mexican-American socio-cultural patterns: Implications for social casework.* San Francisco: R E Research Associates, 1974.

Sotomayer, M. *A study of Chicano grandparents in an urban barrio.* Unpublished doctoral dissertation, University of Denver, 1973.

Sue, D.W., & Sue, D. Barriers to effective cross-cultural counseling. *Journal of Counseling Psychology,* 1977, *24, 420-429.*

Szapocznik, J., Santisteban, D., Kurtines, W., & Hervis, O. Life enrichment counseling for Hispanic elderly. *Aging,* March-April 1980, pp. 20-29.

Szapocznik, J., Scopetta, M.A., Kurtines, W., & Aranalde, M.A. Cuban value structure: Treatment implications. *Journal of Consulting and Clinical Psychology,* 1978, *46,* 960-970.

U.S. Bureau of the Census. Persons of Spanish-speaking origin in the United States: November 1969, *Current Population Reports.* Washington, D.C.: U.S. Government Printing Office, p. 5 (Series P-20, No. 213).

U.S. Commission on Civil Rights. *Puerto Ricans in the continental United States: An uncertain future.* Washington, D.C.: U.S. Government Printing Office, 1976, pp. 5-9.

U.S. Department of Health and Human Services. *Health of the disadvantaged: Chart book-II.* Hyattsville, Md.: Public Health Service, Health Resources Administration, Office of Health Resources Opportunity, September 1980, pp. 6-9 (DHHS Pub. No. HRA 80-633).

U.S. Department of Health, Education, and Welfare. *Health status of minorities and low income groups.* Washington, D.C.: U.S. Government Printing Office, 1979, pp. 23-25 (DHEW Pub. No. HRA 79-627).

Valle, R., & Mendoza, L. *The elder Latino*. San Diego: Campanile Press, 1978.

Velez, C. Youth and aging in central Mexico: One day in the life of four families of migrants. In B.G. Meyerhoff & A. Simic (Eds.), *Life's career-aging cultural variations on growing old*. Beverly Hills, Calif.: SAGE Publications, 1978.

Woerner, L. The Hispanic elderly: Meeting the needs of a special population. *Civil Rights Digest*, Spring, 1979, pp. 3-11.

Zambrana, R.E., Merino, R., & Santana, S. Health services and the Puerto Rican elderly. In D.E. Gelfand & A.J. Kutzik (Eds.), *Ethnicity and aging: Theory, research and practice*. New York: Springer Publishing Co., 1979, pp. 308-319.

Chapter 8

Elder Abuse and Isolation

INTRODUCTION

Only recently has the concept of elder abuse been added to the complex range of physical and psychological ill-treatments that occur within the family context and sparked the concern of the professional community. Child and spouse abuse are so widely publicized that most every one has heard of them, although society continues to ignore the shocking prevalence rates. One estimate places the rate of child assaults at 50,000 to 75,000 a year (Lord & Weisfeld, 1974). A Law Enforcement Assistance Administration survey estimated spousal assaults numbered more than one million between 1973 and 1975 ("Spouse Abuse Cases Top One Million," 1978).

Sibling abuse is the most commonly recognized, expected, and accepted form of family conflict (Star, 1980), and has included such major acts as attempted drownings, poisonings, and setting fire to clothing (Tooley, 1977). Adolescent children also physically abuse their parents (Star, 1980). Elder abuse shares common elements with these other types of mistreatment, but also has its unique features. The differences are related to the aging process and its impact on individuals and their relationship to the environment.

Some authors have written about the problems of abuse and neglect of the elderly perpetrated by family members (Lau & Kosberg, 1979; Steinmetz, 1978; Block & Sinnot, 1979; Hickey, 1979). This includes tying senile parents to their beds so they will not wander off, overmedicating or withholding needed medications to ensure compliance, or physically striking elders who may nag, argue, or complain (Star, 1980). These studies document that the ill-treatment occurs among the noninstitutional aged who become victims of nonaccidental—probably, in an unknown numbers of cases, highly deliberate—physical abuse and endangering neglect by so-called caring persons.

The institutionalized elderly also are victims. Abuses also occur in settings designated to provide caregiving functions such as nursing homes, foster homes, and all other types of institutional and quasi-institutional facilities where people are employed and/or receive remuneration for caregiving. Like institutional-based abuse, in-community mistreatment often goes unrecognized, unreported, and unaddressed by service providers (Rathbone-McCuan, 1980).

There is much confusion about what types of caregiver actions should be categorized as abuse. A common tendency to lump together physical, psychological, and material or financial abuse is understandable. The categorization process, and attempts to define the problem, are complicated further by the probability that many forms of abuse may exist concurrently. For example, a daughter who placed her mother in a bathtub of cold water for several hours or a 19-year-old woman who confessed to torturing her father for seven days by chaining him to a toilet and hitting him with a hammer when he fell asleep are examples of physical abuse. However, practitioners would assume that some form(s) of psychological abuse also was/were present. Psychological abuse does occur frequently if there are physical acts of violence but may exist without physical mistreatment.

The severity of abuse can vary along a continuum ranging from mild to severe (Scott, 1974; Star, 1980). Efforts to conceptualize abuse in degrees of severity should be undertaken in relation to the clarification of mistreatment of the elderly. Yet this is difficult because an act of shoving, pushing, or slapping that may leave only slight skin discoloration and require no medical attention in a younger person (Star, 1980) can have more serious consequences for a frail elderly victim. Severe abuse such as burning or kicking that requires hospitalization can have very serious consequences for the aged (Rathbone-McCuan, 1980).

Some estimates of the incidence of elder abuse range from 500,000 to 2.5 million cases per year, with the highest ones including neglect in the definition. Victimization's link to the behaviors of family members as the most frequent abusers has been documented (Block & Sinnot, 1979; Douglass, 1979; Steinmetz, 1978). There is some disagreement about the characteristics of these abusers or which of the elderly are most at risk. A study commissioned by the Department of Elder Affairs in Massachusetts of more than 1,000 professionals and paraprofessionals indicated that these practitioners found physical and emotional abuses tended to be recurring, rather than isolated, incidents. Most of the victims were women who were more likely to be over 75 years of age rather than between 60 and 75. In 75 percent of those cases, the abuser resided in the same household as the victim, and 84 percent of the abuses were committed by family members (U.S. Congress Joint Hearings, 1980, p. 60).

An Ohio study in 1978 indicated that 10 percent (or a total of 39 cases of the clients 60 years and older at the Chronic Illness Center in Cleveland) suffered some type of abuse. Of these individuals, 30 were women, 21 were widowed, and 29 were white. Twelve lived alone, nine with a spouse, and the rest with children, grandchildren, or other relatives. The majority lived in private homes. Twenty-one resided in the city, twelve in boundary suburbs, and six in outlying suburbs. More than 75 percent of these abused persons had at least one physical or medical impairment. The researchers defined thirteen types of abuse, with 72 percent of the individuals suffering from two to five types and only 15 percent in just one way. The study said 74 percent were abused physically or severely neglected, 51 percent were abused psychologically, 31 percent were materially deprived, and 18 percent had their civil rights violated—a number of the elderly being victimized in more than one way. Abusers usually were the relatives upon whom the elderly depended for care and/or assistance (U.S. Congress Joint Hearings, 1980, p. 68.) The only agreed-upon common characteristic of abused elders is the degree of the dependency of the person on the family care given.

As this chapter indicates, few ironclad ideas and recommendations are put forward. The dynamics of aging as a process that impacts on the family system is well documented; the discussion of that process is brief and valuable only as a context to analyze causation and consider intervention. An attempt is made to clarify the dimensions of isolation and to suggest its multidimensional role in the lives of the aged victim and the abusing family member. The role of isolation may be central in the lives of the abuser and abused. Isolation is used repeatedly as a general description without sufficient clarification to understand its relationship to the elderly person and the caregiver.

The section on intervention is structured toward a family-based definition of the client system from the standpoint of both clinical and supportive service provision. The communitywide level of intervention focuses on outreach, crisis intervention, and human services legislation to report elderly abuse and ensure that financial and personnel resources are made available to offer qualified services. The knowledge base is growing rapidly but is not yet an adequate foundation to define appropriate interventions for the at-risk elderly. Care delivered by the family is sanctioned by society but is not widely recognized yet as a possible source of inhumane experiences and violent onslaughts.

HYPOTHESIZED REASONS FOR ABUSE

Practitioners seeking to find explanations for the conditions labeled as elder abuse will be able to identify little material that explores the reasons for such mistreatment. What material exists is based on a few studies that were conceptualized and conducted independently. Practitioners' case descriptions, taken as a group, often pinpoint the reasons individuals abuse their aged family members. Because adequate empirical and clinical data are not available to offer consistent support for one causal explanation over another, consideration should be given to the range of perspectives, which overlap to some extent.

The Revenge Framework

The revenge framework is based on the assumption that the abusers actually were, or perceived themselves to have been, mistreated in the past and thus ill-treat the parent now. For the elder abuser, the phrases "getting even for what you did to me" or "getting even for what somebody else did to me through you" are common. In the first circumstance, the elderly person is the actual target for the revenge and in the second is the substitute target. The elderly, as well as children and spouses, can be vulnerable targets who serve as symbols of those who were the actual abusers (Elbow, 1977).

The presence of a revenging behavior toward the aging parent in no way precludes the possibility that reprisal also may be taken against young children. What the framework fails to analyze, at least in this type of abuse, is why some caregivers seek revenge while others do not. A number of factors may contribute to this variation. One may be the type of earlier life victimization and its consequences. If they include a perpetuation of their victimization, the incentive for revenge may now be linked to present conditions. Another factor may be the extent to which the victimization to cause harm was intentional. If the avenger believes the actions were intentional, the motivation to take revenge can be stronger.

The Pathological Personality Framework

Various pathological personality types, developed as a typology applied to child abusers, also may be applied to those who mistreat the elderly. This typology includes individuals who are psychotic or sadistic, compulsive, have passive-aggressive or inadequate personalities, or displace aggression (Boisvert, 1972). A typology such as this is difficult to apply without empirical data on the detailed personality profiles of a large number of persons who abuse the aged members of their family.

This approach might prove fruitful if personality types were studied carefully in relation to emotional states of anger and/or rage. When the caregivers experience anger, they are dealing with an emotional reaction to the present situation in which they perceive themselves as hurt or mistreated in some way. They can easily identify the reason for anger, and their reactions are appropriate to the severity of the situation.

Rage is more complex and differs from anger. Rage involves suppressed anger and fear that have accumulated over time. After the passage of much time, the original causes are not identified easily. The rage simmers beneath the surface and is a source of terror to the individuals, who feel the pressure and fear that the dammed-up emotion may burst forth beyond their control.

Often the rage originates from the terror the individuals experienced at an earlier point in their development. If it occurred in childhood, it may have included fear and a feeling of being overwhelmed by helplessness. These individuals were not allowed to express their anger at being mistreated so they were forced to submit to the abuse and suppress their fury. As adults, they recreate the scene, only now they are in the position of power and can express or apply it (Holmes, Barnhart, Cantoni, & Reymer, 1975). By adding the distinction between rage and anger, the personality framework moves beyond merely a descriptive view of abusers to a more in-depth focus on the individuals' feelings that always will play an important role in resolving the abusive behavioral problem.

The Generational Transmission Framework

Violent behavior is assumed to be transmitted from generation to generation as a response to stress. This framework may be associated with the multiproblem family that has a history of chronic stresses and of difficulties in dealing successfully with them. There may be disproportionally more violence of all types in these families as compared to others. In many cases, inadequate financial, social, or other resources have existed over the generations. Multigenerational patterns can be identified by assessing: (a) any history of violence and chronic conditions, (b) patterns of isolation and contacts with the outer environment beyond the family unit, (c) erratic or drastic patterns of strife in family interaction, and (d) patterns of decision making and power distribution.

This framework does not offer an adequate foundation from which to generalize about how the transmitted pattern of violence is manifested in various family role relationships within, across, and between generations. Without assessment of individual families, it is impossible to determine why some direct violence toward the youngest, middle, or oldest generations, or among all of them. Furthermore, this framework has not been translated into an empirically based assessment of large family units. The framework suggests that the family system must be conceptualized as broader than the interactions between abuser and abused; however, the larger family context has yet to be applied in the multigenerational transmission research designs that have been useful in the investigation of child abuse.

A focus on only the abuser-abused subsystem seems too narrow a perspective, given the diversity of situations, personalities, overall life circumstances, and generational changes that have probable risk implications for the elderly. Efforts to better understand abusers' responses and how to meet their needs clearly are compatible with the generational transmission framework if the framework is expanded.

Absence of Community Resources Framework

The major assumption of this framework is that a lack of community resources to assist the caregiver in caring for the elderly parent leads to an expression of frustration through violent behavior. This is a widely accepted notion among the few practitioners and researchers who have considered the issues of elder abuse. However, it will remain an underdeveloped framework until there is more empirical information to document the consequences of service provision and utilization on elder abuse. It also will be necessary to explore whether providing supportive services to families can have a longer term impact on their functioning.

There should be more exploration of the emotional and behavioral consequences related to abuse (a) when resources to be made available to the caregiver and the aged do not exist, (b) how caregivers can be made aware of resources, and (c) where the help is rejected by either the elderly or the family. Practitioners' analyses consistently suggest that rejection of help by the abused person blocks further assistance and prevents the utilization of whatever may be available.

Functional Incompetency Framework

In this view of causation, the caregivers themselves are somehow functionally impaired. For example, the caregiver could be an elderly spouse suffering some level of impairment, alcoholic, mentally retarded, or psychiatrically disabled. This dysfunction, whatever its source, prevents the individual from either being aware of abusing or being able to respond nonviolently. This is a framework worth additional exploration because it provides an understanding of how functional incapacities of the caregiver may set into motion problems that also are similar to conditions of pathology, generational transmission of violence, and stress responses.

The various conditions of the caregiver combined with the demands of the elderly person translate into a type of environmental resource deficit, leaving the provider unable to perform the helping tasks. This framework also points to the need for better linkages between assessments and judgments about causation. The hidden problem of the abused elderly may be no less serious than an unrecognized dysfunction or problem in the caregiver.

Economic Exploitation Framework

This cluster of motivations involves the caregiver's misuse of economic and material resources of an elderly person in order to preserve assets or gain control over them. The actions can involve economic resource manipulation or withholding of care. The types of situations range from neglect actions by the caregiver such as failure to commit resources for expensive hospitalization that could lead to depletion of an inheritance, to death by arson or poisoning in order to collect life insurance funds available only at the death of the older person.

It may be difficult to determine how financial exploitation by the caregiver has been played out secretly over long periods, leaving the elderly person without resources and unaware that they are gone or how they were manipulated. Too little is known about how economic motives may contribute to abuse or violence. This framework cannot be compared to child abuse situations. These abused adults hold economic resources that the caregiver wants and may be able to obtain through violent, illegal, and/or inhumane actions.

The implications of these multiple theoretical frameworks for interpreting causation produce a complex, confusing, and nondirective situation for practitioners faced with intervention functions. The frameworks suggest that the following factors need to be taken into account:

1. that all that is known about the stress produced from caregiving should be screened for application to elder abuse
2. that family units may be part of both the problem and the solution but that services provided must be adapted to fit the problems in the family system
3. that three components of comprehensive services can be considered as potential requirements for intervention: clinical therapeutic counseling, supportive social services, and legal action

All of the frameworks suggest the importance of stress and isolation. Before reviewing intervention and prevention strategies, this section reviews some of the typical circumstances of caregiving that can set the stage for abuse of the elderly person and explores isolation as an emergent factor that must be included in planning interventions.

ISSUES OF STRESS AND ISOLATION IN CAREGIVING

Various sources of stress arise in late life parent-child relationships: the accumulation and expenditure of personal and environmental resources; the application of power, authority, and control in decision making; adjustment and adaptation to changes, losses, or restrictions in family roles; financial resource distribution; care and management tasks associated with chronic and/or acute medical or psychiatric illness; and behavioral consequences of substance addictions.

These stresses can be experienced in relation to activities such as helping the elderly person with daily living activities or in more complex situations demanding time and energy where adult children periodically or daily assist with needs involving decreased physical or mental functioning. Coping with the deteriorating aged parent produces a stressful situation, generally results in negative portrayals of the elderly individual's capacities, and perhaps affects the general presence of the person in the household (Robinson & Thurnher, 1979).

Responsibility to the aged member can cover a wide range of arrangements and functions. For example, the children may have to find adequate medical care, transport their parents to Medicare appointments, and make sure that prescriptions are filled and medications taken. In addition, they may have to transport physically ailing parents to social and recreational activities, find suitable living facilities for them, provide general protective services, and give them physical and emotional support (Simos, 1973).

The amount and type of support varies widely. Many levels of care are provided, and the greater the degree of dependency, the higher the level of assistance. At one level, the family does not help the aged persons. Separate households are maintained, along with regular contact and visits. The elderly maintain their independence. At the next level, they may begin to suffer some degree of impairment such as arthritis, mild confusion, or lessened ability to exert themselves. Usually, separate households still are maintained. However, the family may step in to provide help at home, run errands, and shop for and transport the older persons. At the next level, the elder may suffer a stroke and be confined to bed or a chair or become increasingly confused. Depending on how well they are managing, the family members may obtain a power of attorney and encourage the seniors to live with them. The older persons still are active. Finally, as in the case of organic brain syndrome, the family may find that it is assuming total care: the elderly need to be watched constantly, cannot be left alone, and must be helped with dressing, grooming, bathing, and feeding. At this highest level, the aged usually are in need of constant attention.

Caregivers, in assuming initial responsibility, may be ill-prepared for the great demands that may be placed upon them in the future. If at the start of caregiving the elders are at a point of high functional independence, it is neither easy nor pleasant to recognize that circumstances may change drastically. The seniors may exhaust personal and fiscal resources quickly and have to face ever-increasing activity restrictions. The heretofore unrecognized fear of personal aging may face caregivers, leading some to literally deny the aged persons' circumstances. If the problems are recognized and accepted, caregivers may or may not know where to turn for help or what steps to take.

In situations of great dependence, caregivers' functions reverse long-established behaviors. The parent who once was autonomous yet was cared for is now dependent but is not a child, despite that reliance. If positions are reversed, the adult child may have no other support to fall back on and thus becomes the supporter, helper, and troubleshooter. Usually these roles are assumed at some tangible personal costs.

Each relative interprets the experience of the aging person in a different way, yet the impact of the caregiving affects the total family system. The extent to which problems are contained or amplified seems to be related to the functioning of the whole family (Steger & Kotler, 1979). The stresses may spread to relations between adult child and other family members.

Caregiving demands can strain spousal interaction and relations with children and between siblings. The aged parent's dependencies may create forms of competition with spouse, leaving the adult child caregiver caught in the middle. The middle-aged person may have mixed feelings about the situation. An aged individual's needs can lead to confinement that can only further exacerbate the coexistence of resentment and obligations—not a comfortable situation.

Traditionally the woman in the family is expected to assume the burden of care and to conciliate the differences between her spouse's needs and those of the elderly person. This burden may become difficult to bear. If the spouse refuses to share the responsibility, and in addition expects her to provide care for his aged parents or other elderly persons for whom he is accountable, the problem is only intensified. Personal loyalties become competitive with responsibilities that others are asking or expecting the middle-aged woman to assume.

It can become a question among siblings as to the appropriate decisions concerning the elderly family member. Resentment toward siblings can occur if there is the perception that sisters or brothers (or both) are not sharing the burden (Popky-Hausman, 1979). Jealousy of a favored child also could become an issue. Power and conflict, problems of communication, and frustration can result. Any attempts at resolving the situation to the family's satisfaction can become blocked. The middle-aged person carries the responsibility of a parent's care as well as that of her family. She also faces the crises that arise from living, death, divorce, unemployment, loss, and illness. She is in a strategic yet vulnerable position because the demands placed upon her can cause role conflict and strain.

The illness of an older relative or changes in a beloved grandparent can be bewildering to young children who may feel a desire to help but not know what to do. They also may feel deprived of their parent's and the aged relative's attention and affection. They can form an alliance with the elder. Both they and the older person are dependent on the middle-aged family members. Power and control, the lack of easy access to resources, and inability to use them can be an issue for both children and the aged individual. Older children may be pressed into assisting the parents. Their reactions probably vary from rebellion to bewildered submission, which could be a strain for active children. In a sense, they can share the frustration of their elders. If they share no closeness with the elder person, friction could become open. If the young children were to become aware of a parent's abusing or conflict with the aging grandparent, internal problems can result. The young people may feel at fault or feel unable to express personal needs lest they create new abuses.

The elderly persons face a number of problems: the loss of some previous roles and resources, physical changes, and the possibility of increased dependence. Their reactions to these changes may be fear, depression, or a sense of disorientation and concern. Communication with the family may change as the older individuals age. Having little awareness of what it is to age, they find it difficult to understand their position.

Grief may express itself in the form of increased requests for attention, from which they later may withdraw. The elderly want to be supported but do not want to relinquish their independent style. Body image and physical change are sensitive areas. Disability or severe illness brings worry that a change in the balance of family resources or power will occur. Elderly parents' relationship with their adult children can influence their view about whether they could tolerate dependency. Older persons do seek contact with their families and desire their support. The loss of roles or resources involuntarily restricts their world. Loss of income also can mean that housing and transportation will be inadequate. If they live with their adult children, the elderly may not find much social opportunity unless they are fortunate. To formerly active persons, this can be a source of frustration. The loss of things once valued can be a severe blow.

Basically, older persons are faced with the challenge of relating to their adult children in the face of increasing needs and decreasing opportunities. If they suffer abuse in the home of a relative, they may have limited alternatives. To be placed in a nursing home away from family may be a worse alternative. If the abuse is severe and the elders would choose separation, they frequently are in no position to effect that change. Dependent elders essentially are cut off from others, with their only links to an outside world controlled by their abusers.

Relatives other than adult children who care for schizophrenics living at home are in comparable difficult situations. Some of the behaviors and restrictions involved in the two circumstances are similar. In both cases, the relatives must learn to live with and to deal with unpredictable, even violent behavior. The schizophrenic's lack of conversation is a particular problem for a relative such as the spouse who depends on the patient for companionship. Relatives must come to terms with difficult circumstances such as social withdrawal, underactivity, excessive sleeping, and socially embarrassing behavior. In cases of considerable disability, the relatives may not be able to leave the house even to go shopping without getting a substitute caregiver. The relatives not only may become the jailers but also, in effect, be in jail themselves (Lamb & Oliphant, 1979).

While this comparison may seem dramatic and unrepresentative of the caregiving functions and relationships between the aged and their family, it is the extremely burdensome situations that are the most difficult to transform into manageable situations. What people cope with in this aspect of family life is often very private, and it is the invisible quality of their struggle that promotes isolation.

The isolators come in many forms (Figure 8-1). Those who provide help are isolated emotionally from those they care for. In turn, caregivers and the elderly are isolated from their environment in the midst of their interpersonal separateness. After having reviewed multiple case histories, it is not possible to rank the importance of the various isolators. Usually there are multiple sources, and they interact. Once intervention is offered and services utilized, some of the isolation

Figure 8-1 Isolators in the Lives of the Abused Elderly

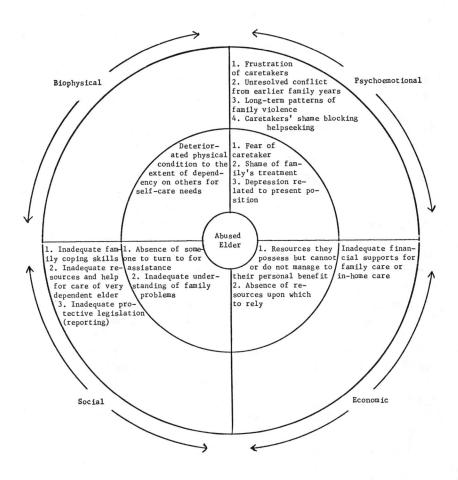

The inner circle contains isolators as they are manifested in the personal lives of abused elders, the outer circle those that abound in the environment.

problems are eliminated but others can be created. For example, the practitioner may help facilitate a decision that leads to relocation of the aged person, but that produces an institutional situation where the senior's isolation takes on other dimensions, such as separation from family. The resources commonly available to practitioners to offer to families as a means of reducing the stress of caregiving may not eliminate the isolation until the impacts of the new circumstances are handled directly through interventive efforts.

STRESS AND ISOLATION INTERACTING WITH ABUSE

Under conditions of extreme stress linked to caregivers, abusive behavior may take place. Violence and abuse are among an infinite range of possible coping behaviors that arise in such situations. In some cases, it may be an old behavior, learned from a previous situation. It may have been transmitted over generations. In still other cases, abuse may be a new behavior associated with feelings of anger and rage involving the present. Why some caregivers shift from nonabusive to abusive conduct, abandon a sense of responsibility or commitment to helping, and take up neglecting or endangering actions to others is pure speculation.

Practitioners seeking a definitive causal analysis may be disappointed by this hesitation to speculate about this problem. The state of knowledge would be increased greatly if more research studies had been completed. In any case, determining what types of families are more likely to abuse the elderly because of stress and/or isolation is a future issue; stimulating critical thinking about the potential importance of those factors is a present concern.

Any given caregiving role obviously involves helping events or actions. Some providers, by reason of personal or environmental circumstance (e.g., some type of emotional separation from the aged person or of isolation from potential supportive relationships or resources), experience stress.

Some type or degree of stress may be unavoidable but isolation need not be present. Formal and informal supportive resources and relationships can be made available to the caregiver. This is the key to intervention in cases of elder abuse. Reactions of individuals and relatives are important in considering reactions to stress since the total family has a unique responsibility for mediating this problem. Whether or not caregivers perceive/feel that circumstances associated with providing help are stressful depends in part on how the event is defined or interpreted in light of their own cultural and historical experiences. What may be stress for one family may not be for another. The following 14 conditions or factors may be related to stress and isolation in the context of elder victimization:

1. Caregivers may not have contacts with strangers, may attempt to avoid them, and may not want to make contact with a resource that involves interactions with unknown persons.
2. Caregivers are not involved in situations or have not had contacts in which to learn about supportive resources or alternatives to the current situation.
3. Caregivers react negatively to the limitations of time, money, or energy that their task places on their ability to pursue personal desires.
4. Others in the family seem unclear about what helping responsibilities translate into burdens on primary caregivers.
5. Caregivers assume that only they know what is appropriate or needed by the aged parent and reject the opinions of others.

6. Caregivers feel pushed and pulled in several directions by expectations of others regarding what assistance should involve.
7. Caregivers lack confidence in resources beyond themselves to help the elder.
8. Caregivers resent the expectations of others and consider these as additional burdens.
9. Caregivers feel they are under criticism and suspicion regarding the assistance they are providing.
10. Other family members feel that the caregivers do not have sufficient control over the behavior of the aged person.
11. Caregivers feel overqualified or underqualified to give the needed help.
12. Caregivers are frustrated by the elder's demands.
13. Caregivers feel resentment over the aged parent's very passive or very aggressive behavior.
14. Caregivers and other relatives may be in conflict over financial resources to cover the cost of care and/or the decision to make that assistance a priority economic expenditure.

These are but a sampling of the types of conditions faced by caregivers, and their feelings about them. The abusive behavior probably includes, for caregivers, some combination of symptoms involving the physiological (headaches, stomachaches, tension, backaches, stiffness in neck and shoulders, elevated blood pressure, fatigue), behavioral (crying, forgetfulness, yelling, blaming, bossiness), and emotional (depression, agitation, impatience, anger, frustration, loneliness, powerlessness, inflexibility).

Those symptoms might be a cue to pursue help if it is highly incongruent with usual behaviors and symptoms. If that pursuit leads to no source of help, or to assistance that is not appropriate to or that aggravates the situation, the isolation conditions take over. The importance they play in abuse are understood from caregivers' responses when they discuss the situation retrospectively.

Simon Sauget

Simon was a 52-year-old divorcee who lived with his mother. She had been bedridden for a year and had not been out of the house for two years. She was admitted to a local hospital dehydrated, undernourished, covered with bedsores, unable to move out of a fetal position, unable to speak, and suffering from Parkinson's disease. She had not been seen by anyone else for more than six weeks. A number of probable causal factors can be identified:

1. Simon interpreted his mother's not eating food he prepared as her spite at his efforts and an attempt to get back at him because he didn't want to cook what she wanted. His reaction was to stop making any attempt at special cooking for her.

2. Simon perceived his mother's combative behavior when he attempted to dress her bed sores as taunting him. He then in anger made the assumption that some acute pain might make her more manageable and stopped treating the sores with medication.

3. Simon's former spouse criticized his not putting his mother into a nursing home because of his financial greed. His reaction was that the mother's condition was so much like a vegetable that to do so would be a waste of financial resources he was likely to inherit. This was based on his belief that he would have to mortgage their house to be able to afford the cost of a nursing home.

In situations such as these, caregivers may think that others (including the elder) and events in their lives cause them to feel a range of emotional states and have diverse behavioral reactions that result in abuse or endangering neglect. In many cases the caregivers will blame something or someone outside themselves. The practitioner must be in a position to assess whether or not the thinking is irrational or faulty. An event or condition common to many highly demanding and difficult situations can be perceived by caregivers in many different ways.

It is not necessarily the aged person's behavior per se that prompts the caregivers to respond in destructive ways but rather what the providers think about the situation. Abusive caregivers often believe that the aged person has no right to act that way. This suggests that they feel they should have control over the situation or over the elder's behavior. The struggle to gain that control may serve to establish more stress for the caregivers and emotional isolation between them and the elderly.

Beverly Talson and Her Aunt

Beverly is 55 years old, never married, whose 85-year-old aunt has been living with her in her small apartment for several years. The elderly woman has early symptoms of senile dementia and extended periods of mental confusion. The niece made contact with the visiting nurse program asking for immediate help because her aunt was becoming unmanageable. The nurse conducting the initial in-home patient assessment observed welts and bruises on the client's cheeks, neck, and shoulders and that the niece was visibly angry, nervous, and anxious. The nurse then referred the case to a social worker to conduct a personal interview with the niece regarding her possible need to talk about the difficulty of the circumstances. The niece interpreted the interview as a supportive situation where blame and criticism were not an issue. She revealed her panic at her very rough physical treatment of her aunt during an argument over a cat that had died several years before. Because of her disorientation, the aunt had forgotten the animal had been dead for some time and had accused the niece of killing it.

The niece's abusive behavior shocked and frightened her to the point where she reached for immediate assistance. Fortunately, she made contact with an agency that had the appropriate resources to mobilize quickly. If caregivers who have demonstrated atypical abusing behaviors perceive that conduct as a cue that they need help and can make contact with a supportive resource, both the continuation of the mistreatment and its escalation may be redirected.

Here the niece recognized the danger of her psychological reaction to the aunt's behavior. She was able to assess the strain she was experiencing and, burdened by her guilt, knew she could not continue to rationalize her aunt's condition as warranting her own emotional burnout and physical depletion. Through short-term counseling she was able to work with the agency to arrange temporary placement of the aunt in a nursing home until a complete medical and psychological assessment could be made.

The cases of Simon and Beverly are examples of caregivers who were not in contact with community resources or other persons who could relieve some of their pressures. The major difference is that Simon continued to remain entrapped and isolated from resources while Beverly was able to make contact with a helping agency. Neither one was completely confined to the home because both held jobs. However, Simon had no supportive network and Beverly had felt increasing isolation from her friends because she could not maintain a balance between the role of caregiver and that of friend.

When conducting an assessment and examining the isolating factors, it is important to recognize that caregivers and abusers can experience aloneness when problems of communication aggravate stress. They feel some obligation that cannot be met, that the aged persons are too demanding and not grateful, and are overwhelmed by the elders' changing conditions. The aged may be living under circumstances of fear, experiencing profound disorientation of person and place, or responding with defensive behaviors that further provoke the situation. They may remain isolated from needed resources because of fear of reprisals by the abusers, fear of being institutionalized or losing their place in the home environment, or functionally unable to assume the tasks of seeking help. Caregivers seeking help may find that the resources of the agencies to which they turn are not appropriate or not available when they are most needed because of cutbacks in funding or failure to develop appropriate services.

There is a seemingly circular and/or mutually reinforcing relationship between isolation and stress: (a) stress produces a need for resources, (b) isolation from resources aggravates the problem, (c) the relationship between these factors is not mediated successfully by the environment, including the larger family unit, and (d) new stresses develop.

Abuse is a problem within a family that can be met by a response from without in the form of resources. Separation from information, supportive services, opportunities to discuss management of the older person, or social recognition of their responsibility can aggravate the abusers' problems. The abused elders likewise have no chance to exercise the power of choosing alternatives if they are isolated. They are entrenched in an interaction with the abusers and perhaps are not aware of alternatives at all. Isolation thus impacts on problem resolution and definition.

INTERVENTION WITH PROBLEMS OF ABUSE

For the isolated subgroup of elderly, all levels of intervention (individual, family, community, and legislative) are crucial. Implementing clinical intervention service components often is perceived as a piecemeal approach without the presence of an agency authorized to take actions beyond the scope of referral. (The social resource system for the abused elder is depicted in Figure 8-2.) The lack of legislative attention to this situation is a major problem in intervention.

If a practitioner encounters a case of adult abuse and begins to initiate the first steps of intervention, the frustration is tremendous if there is no legal authority to support the process. For example, when this chapter was being prepared, a request for case consultation was received from a former student working with a case of suspected abuse. An elderly widow, age 86, and many members of her extended family resided in a small town in central Illinois. A younger sister secretly contacted the social worker to tell her she thought the widowed sister had been a victim of beating for the second time by a male family member. The sister pleaded with the social worker to do something while at the same time indicating that she herself wanted no further involvement.

During an initial home visit to the widow, the social worker, accompanied by the younger sister, noted that while the elderly woman had sustained severe bruises for which she had been treated by a local physician, she insisted the only explanation for the injury was a bad fall in her living room while she was alone in the house. Her verbal interactions with her sister in the presence of the social worker indicated no willingness to reveal additional information and a hope that her sibling would give credence to her explanation.

Subsequently, the social worker made contact with a person at the multipurpose senior center who had worked previously with several cases of abuse. The latter carefully explained the necessary conditions for intervention and noted that they were limited, since no adult protective legislation had been passed.

Practitioners may well be acquainted with the conditions this social worker faced if she pursued this as a potential case of adult abuse. For example: (a) she lacked authority to have further contact with the elderly woman, (b) she could anticipate that no family member, including the sister who made the initial referral, would be willing to talk, (c) she faced the possibility of long and expensive legal procedures that were likely to be delayed through local courthouse politics to protect the good name of the family, and (d) she was operating under conditions

Figure 8-2 The Abused Elder and the Social Resource System

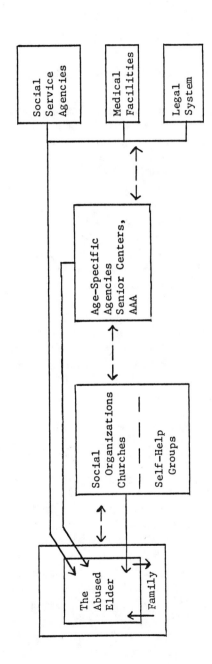

The abused elder most often is unable to seek out assistance from any organization. Many organizations are concerned with the plight of such persons but frequently can do little because: (1) they are unaware of the abuse, (2) they may lack legal support for those who would report or seek to investigate cases of suspected abuse, (3) the elder cannot or will not cooperate with outside entities against the family.

that tended to increase rather than decrease the client's potential for socialization and in-home supportive services if approached on the basis of direct intervention related to abuse.

CONGRESSIONAL HEARINGS DELINEATE PROBLEM

This discussion of intervention issues is organized to give practitioners an opportunity to note and compare the status of different adult abuse laws in the various states. This material is adapted from the published proceedings of a joint hearing before the Special Committee on Aging of the United States Senate and the Select Committee on Aging of the House of Representatives (U.S. Congress Joint Hearings, 1980). Given the rapidly changing status of adult abuse legislation among the states, readers are encouraged to obtain the latest information from officials in their own states because there obviously is a time lag in reporting and updating published information. The variations in state laws are important, especially if legislation is being proposed or an existing act is being modified. Guidelines for protecting the civil rights of these individuals have been of concern to legal specialists who have studied the problem.

Given the urgency of obtaining legislative approval of intervention, there is a need to organize groups of practitioners representing agencies with an ability to offer multiple and diverse resources to give leadership in the communication, education, and advocacy process. Such efforts are increasing. Several of those with a substantial history of community involvement are mentioned. Because of active involvement with one such well-known group in the midwest, the authors briefly analyze one program with which they have been closely connected since 1976.

It is the practitioners on the front lines who have intimate knowledge of the complex and diverse constraints that operate in the community to limit the effectiveness of intervention, if not to block it altogether. Many practitioners believe that preventive efforts must take priority—and often are too late. The view that prevention is the goal should be more than professional and political oratory, of which there has been a significant amount. To plan the direction of preventive programs should be the collective concern of the most qualified specialists in the numerous fields of family violence and intrafamily abuse.

As educators and practitioners with appreciation of and sympathetic orientation toward the need to generate knowledge based on the combined input of persons with scientific views as well as practical expertise, the authors have found the Congressional hearings on elder abuse to be one of the most valued resources for analyzing how well this problem is or is not being addressed nationwide. The hearings presented testimony from individuals from diverse sections of the country (Arkansas, California, Delaware, District of Columbia, Maryland, Massachusetts, New York, Ohio). Even more importantly, they included statements of elderly victims, some of whose testimony was shown on the television networks.

In analyzing statements by the national leaders, a certain common pattern of responses emerged. Their attitudes ranged between viewing the behavior of abusive caregivers as atrocities and deep concern over the tragedy of the victimization of the elderly.

Following are excerpts from comments by members of Congress at the hearings:

Senator Lawton Chiles, Democrat of Florida:

> Since I have been a member of the Senate I have attended many hearings that focus on unfortunate problems, but perhaps never have I attended one on a problem as regrettable as elder abuse. . . . I do know that we have shaped too many of our policies in a way that is not favorable for families that want to help themselves by taking care of their elderly and keeping them at home. Our tax policies and everything else are shaped against family care. I think we should do something about it.

Senator Pete V. Domenici, Republican of New Mexico:

> The most disturbing thing to me about the situation is the extent to which all forms of domestic violence—child, spouse, and elder abuse—mirror the deteriorating quality of family life in this country.

Senator David Pryor, Democrat of Arkansas:

> What happens if we lose our physical strength, or our money, or our ability to take care of ourselves? . . . They have to do with our basic roles in life and our well-being after a long life of working and caring for others. . . . Actually, I'm not even sure that we know what specific questions to ask . . . what can the federal government do to prevent or respond to cases of elder abuse? And, how can we do it without stepping on individual or states' rights? How can we respond in a responsible way and not be called big brother? Based on what I've learned, I can't help but wonder whether the incidence of elder abuse might be reduced if older people and those caring for them had better access to mental health services that could help them cope with stress. . . . Elder abuse is very different from child abuse in that we are dealing with competent adults. This raises some complicated questions about state protective service laws designed to help abused adults.

Representative Claude Pepper, Democrat of Florida:

Although the elderly fear crime more than any single problem, they are unlikely to report that they have been abused, even by strangers, let alone by members of their family. . . . The problem of elder abuse has no regional boundaries and occurs nationwide. Much of the elder abuse goes unreported because of the fear of reprisal and embarrassment by the elderly people affected.

Senator John Glenn, Democrat of Ohio:

We are here to try to determine what programs can be state programs and what programs can be federal programs to protect older Americans from abuse and to provide the necessary assistance that will enable families to continue caring for their elderly members.

Senator John Heinz, Republican of Pennsylvania:

I suppose that you might say that this is a terrible embarrassment to all of us to find out what other people are doing to other people. . . . We don't want to know about these things because we don't want to really believe they happen. But they do, and those are the family skeletons in the closet that must see the light of day; otherwise, we will never be able to address the problem.

Representative Mario Biaggi, Democrat of New York:

I have some recommendations, including legislative changes, that I hope this committee will consider. The first is to amend the domestic violence legislation to insure that provisions are included to help elderly victims get aid. . . . Second, early consideration of legislation to provide meaningful tax credits for individuals and families providing home care for persons over 65. Third, the early passage of legislation to expand home health care coverage under Medicare. Fourth, mandate that the White House Conference on Aging and Families place the issue on their agendas for discussion and specific policy recommendations.

Representative Mary Rose Oakar, Democrat of Ohio:

One of the things that I don't think has been mentioned is that many people who are in a position to report abuse are not protected by the law. . . . We are hopeful that the Adult Abuse Prevention and Treatment Act will provide the viable solutions to meet the critical problems of vulnerable adults who suffer abuse, neglect, and exploitations.

Representative Charles E. Grassley, Republican of Iowa:

The extent of such callous and inhumane treatment is not yet well documented, but there are indications that it may be of much broader scope than was suspected a few years ago.

Representative Marc L. Marks, Republican of New York:

If there are strong financial disincentives for an elderly person to live with their children, that adds to the tension in a family and makes it more likely that there will be some sort of abuse of the elderly person. . . . There is a large deduction in SSI benefits that an elderly person receives if he moves in with his or her children. . . . Medicare and Medicaid do not reimburse many of the medical costs incurred if an elderly person lives with his or her family that are reimbursed if he or she lives in a nursing home. . . . We give a tax credit for a working parent for child care costs, and yet we give no tax credit for working parents who want to take care of an elderly person. . . . If changes must be made in a family's home to accommodate an elderly person who wants to move in, such as adding a bathroom or a bedroom on the first floor, not only are there no tax credits to help subsidize these costs, but the family's property taxes will go up because the property has been improved.

Representative Jim Lloyd, Democrat of California:

I strongly support legislation which would provide a broad range of services—social, legal, and educational—to protect and care for victims, as well as try to relieve the problems or stresses within the family which precipitated the abuse.

Representative William R. Ratchford, Democrat of Connecticut:

The one postscript or caveat I would make is the statement of one of the professionals, and that is, if you are not going to staff systematically, you hold out false hope to the community . . . putting a law on the books in and of itself is meritorious, but it is not enough if we are not prepared to staff it.

Representative Geraldine Ferraro, Democrat of New York:

I am certainly appreciative of the fact that I am here to participate in this hearing, but I feel a great sense of frustration when you are dealing in this particular problem because if we have the people coming forward and we don't have the money to deal with the problems, it is a real concern.

Representative Dan Mica, Democrat of Florida:

It has already been stated that 15 states have elder abuse laws. You have indicated in each one of your states that the state law is adequate. Do you feel that there is need for national legislation applicable to all states? Would federal law add to the level of protection provided to the elderly by the laws of your individual states? Are there advantages to a federal law? I would like to have all of you answer.

These statements summarize some of the key issues that must be taken into account in problem analyses, documentation, and preparation of legislation. Their concerns, at least in part, echo those raised by legislators in the states where bills on abuse of the elderly have been implemented, passed, or were under review. Based on a Special Senate Committee on Aging survey conducted in March 1980 and published in the Joint Hearings report, answers to a letter sent to all governors and legislative committees on aging indicated that half (25) of the states had what the respondents considered an adult protective services law. Those responding "yes" to the question were:

State	Year Passed
Alabama	1977
Arizona	1980
Arkansas	1977
Connecticut	1978
Florida	1977
Kansas	1979
Kentucky	1976
Maine	1980
Maryland	1977
Michigan	1976
Missouri	1980
Montana	Not specified
New Hampshire	1977
New York	1979
North Carolina	Not specified

Oklahoma	1977
Oregon	Not specified
Rhode Island	Not specified
South Carolina	Not specified
South Dakota	Not specified
Tennessee	1978
Utah	1977
Vermont	1980
Virginia	1977
Wisconsin	1973

(U.S. Congress, Joint Hearings, 1980)

The analysis of findings from the responses to this question, as noted in the published appendixes of the hearing report (U.S. Congress Joint Hearings, 1980, p. 99), indicates that these state statutes protect different people. There is no common definition of who is to be protected, under what conditions protection may be offered, what protection is assured to those reporting the abuse, and the types of services to be provided and through what sources. The missing dates on passage of the laws reflects the fact that the survey did not ask that information. At least 18 were passed in the five-year span from 1976 to 80 and no fewer than eight of those in 1977.

John J. Regan, dean of the Hofstra University Law School, included in his testimony a critique of the state laws and suggestions on federal legislation. His presentation of defects, and the experiences of practitioners shared with these authors through their own exploration, suggests random development and a lack of standardization. In some cases, the laws contain mere token mentions of protective actions for the victimized elderly and lack clear reference to providing resources. Regan said the flurry of legislative activity in recent years had produced protective services laws of uneven quality:

1. Some statutes are little more than reporting laws, mandating that citizens report cases of adult abuse to a public agency.
2. Some authorize a great deal of involuntary intervention but appropriate little or no funding to provide needed services.
3. Many rely on guardianship laws derived from the 19th century to authorize intervention. These laws often are seriously defective in their worthless criteria for identifying an incompetent person, in their failure to provide even a minimum of due process for the elderly, in their overbroad delegation of power over the individual, in their blindness toward conflicts of interest between guardian and ward, and in the lack of supervision over the guardian's treatment.

4. Some fail to deal with emergency medical situations, thereby allowing hasty and often inappropriate admission into a state mental hospital or other infringements of civil rights.
5. Some permit the creation of public agency guardianships without sufficient attention to the resulting depersonalization of the guardian-ward relationship or to the inherent conflicts of interest (U.S. Congress Joint Hearings, 1980).

Regan also recommended a direction that would merit further consideration if constructive actions and initiatives are to emanate from future efforts at the federal level:

1. The welfare of the infirm elderly, institutionalized or not, is as much a federal concern as that of any other vulnerable and needy group in society.
2. Important civil and constitutional rights are at stake that often are invaded by private citizens, public agencies, and even the courts, but judicial review is unavailable because the elderly have neither the means nor the capacity to challenge the invasion.
3. Title XX of the Social Security Act and Title III of the Older Americans Act already have committed the federal government to financial support of state protective service programs without any real guidelines for protecting the interests of their clients.
4. Federal action is needed to reduce the bias toward institutionalization that permeates federal health care programs.

This brief summary of congressional concerns indicated a desire to initiate action to complement, not supersede, state intervention efforts. The next few years may see an increased trend toward state-based leadership in dealing with difficult problems such as adult abuse and other forms of intrafamily violence. Thus, it becomes important to consider how state involvement can influence the intervention process.

STATE AND LOCAL INTERVENTION EFFORTS

The passage of state measures to curb adult abuse requires much effort from dedicated persons who are willing and able to educate legislators to the realization that this problem exists, is becoming more widespread, and is sufficiently grave as to require bills to protect the elderly from victimization. Once initial steps have succeeded, additional legislative efforts will be required to strengthen laws that cannot deal adequately with the problem. In states with no legislation, the challenge is difficult.

An illustration of the issues and problems in the organizational effort needed to get protective legislation passed can be beneficial to planners in states that are in the process of, or have yet to begin, developing their legislative efforts. Therefore, this section focuses on an analysis of the law enacted in Missouri in 1980 because of the authors' detailed familiarity with the history of that five-year campaign. No evidence suggests that the effort to develop the successful legislative strategy in Missouri varied greatly from other states. This section also explores the continuing struggle in states that have passed legislation but find that broad implementation of the law faces other obstacles, such as where to place the authority for implementation. For example, if a state has divided administrative service functions for the aged among several agencies, the implementation responsibilities may not be clear. The authority may be distributed between health and aging units or placed in a special unit with linkage functions between agencies. Cost-effectiveness of various administrative structures has not yet been the focus of adult abuse research; little data is presently available.

In Missouri, community health workers and social service staff have been central to the process of identifying the problems of abuse of the elderly. Late in 1973 the director of social services at the Visiting Nurse Association in St. Louis assumed the responsibility of assembling a small group of professionals to explore how various agencies were handling cases of neglect, exploitation, and abuse. The overwhelming conclusion from these early meetings was that the effectiveness of intervention was nil if the elderly individual did not wish to accept assistance. Thereafter, about 50 social service workers decided to form a not-for-profit organization as a collective base that transcended traditional organizational boundaries from which to launch efforts to deal with this problem. The organizational base became known as the Missouri Association to Prevent Adult Abuse (MAPAA).

One of the first projects the MAPAA sponsored was a survey conducted in cooperation with the Applied Gerontology Institute at St. Louis University. The purposes of the survey were to develop a profile of the at-risk group, to explore what types of intervention were or were not available, and to discover alternative ways of dealing with the problem. Analysis of survey data indicated that the persons in need of protective services, and often not receiving them, for the most part were white, female, more than 80 years old, and suspicious of and resistant to help. In the main, they preferred to stay in their own surroundings (which often involved very poor housing conditions), had serious health problems, and often responded well to small gestures of caring and trust. Cases of self-neglect and caregiver neglect appeared to be the most prevalent problem, more so than violent forms of abuse. It should be noted, however, that physical abuse and neglect both result in endangering lives. It also was found that special skills were required to develop trusting relationships with the elderly as a first step in the intervention process.

The organization developed two major goals that were to be pursued over a five-year period: to see that (1) an adult protective service bill was developed and passed and (2) a social service delivery system was prepared to implement the legislation. To accomplish either or both goals it was important to conduct community education activities to increase the awareness of the general public and of professionals, explore a range of strategies to obtain financial resources, and build political and organizational alliances. The latter task was important because the health, mental health, social service, and aging service network resources essential for providing services were fragmented. Multiagency cooperation was facilitated by the professional associations of some of the key leaders. A central problem was that although many agencies were willing to receive information from the MAPAA, they could not find a direct channel for involvement.

Once public interest had been generated and the participation of committed volunteers was evident, the organization moved toward the legislative arena. The organization found a forceful ally in a progressive state senator who was oriented to human service and who committed herself to work with the group to develop a bill. The MAPAA was instrumental in presenting information about the problem and suggestions for specific content for the legislation, providing the resources to organize local hearings, and facilitating the preparation of testimony. The group contacted legislators and provided a liaison with other statewide organizations such as the Missouri Mental Health Association, Missouri Association of Social Welfare, and Missouri Health Care Association (the statewide scope of these organizations helped to structure broad support well beyond the St. Louis metropolitan area).

Two bills were drafted. The first one failed but a modified version of it succeeded. The first bill encompassed both protective services and more general provisions to promote independent living for the elderly. It defined a ''protective service case'' as an adult who was in need of care and resources but unable to obtain them because of functional impairment, neglect, abuse, exploitation, or wasting of personal resources. Four levels of service were proposed: case identification, investigation, assessment, and service provision. The bill provided for emergency court orders and temporary guardianship; emergency admission to a health care facility; hearings on petitions for protective services and the duties of legal counsel; and the establishment of guidelines for mandatory reporting procedures, hotlines, immunity for those reporting cases, and mandatory investigation of all cases.

This measure failed by a very small margin, significant opposition revolving around unresolved issues of civil liberty and state authority. Opponents were concerned that guardianship procedures for elders that others felt needed protective care might violate the civil rights of the aged. Some questioned the state's authority to make that decision.

The legislation was modified and presented as Senate Bill 576 during the next session, in 1980, where it passed. The strengths of S.B. 576 are that it incorporates the desired emphasis on the use of least restrictive environments; provides clear definitions of those in the various at-risk categories; mandates reporting, investigation, and court procedures; allows a peace officer to admit a needy elder for hospital care; and prohibits incompetency hearings in a mental health facility without due process of law.

However, its limitations are serious in that immunity for those reporting suspected abuses is not stated explicitly; flexibility of guardianship is lacking; and certain legal procedures are not detailed. The state agency charged with implementing the legislation faced a lack of financial resources to staff the investigative and crisis intervention phases of service adequately. MAPAA as a local organization with a statewide mobilization capacity then had to adapt its goal of increasing the capacity to provide services to the state's overall plan.

It is important to note that without expertise and resources to implement protective service features, a statute falls short. For example, the legal components of this service were expected to be costly and time consuming; once a hot-line was implemented throughout the state, the number of cases was likely to increase substantially, along with the demand for sheltered housing, health and medical services, emergency funds, longer term living arrangements, and coordination and cooperation between protective and nonprotective service providers on a statewide basis. State financial and age eligibility criteria initially were expected to preclude resources and assistance for many. This would exclude persons under the specified age, which could have serious repercussions for mentally retarded or chronically mentally ill older adults.

The MAPAA considered different service models, including a co-sponsorship role. The preferred linkage would be with an organization that had an extensive outreach component with resources that could provide emergency and crisis supportive services to assure access to the elderly. This joint programming approach would allow the MAPAA to intervene in the most difficult cases and provide counseling and clinical intervention with abusers. The limited experimental services the MAPAA funded through various small grants it had received provided an opportunity to understand major service delivery problems likely to arise if an expansive program were undertaken. It would be worthwhile for any organization to consider these questions before providing services to elderly victims:

1. With limited funding, what core services should be offered on a crisis intervention basis? A physician in-home visit, emergency transportation, homemaker services, emergency food and medical supplies, and a com-

panion to remain in the home with the elderly person up to 24 hours all seem essential.

2. What steps should be taken to develop the full range of formal and informal service referrals over time? Continuing community education will be required to ensure that work toward refining these referral functions is maintained.

3. What types of legal arrangements will be necessary to work toward maximizing the effectiveness of the different guardianship requirements and what will help to prevent the aged person from falling through the gaps between the legal, social, and health care systems? A continuum of legal arrangements, ranging from minimum to maximum authority over the affairs of an aged person, will be most effective.

4. What will be the organization's capability for ensuring access to longer term supportive services, especially if the agency itself must rely on referrals to other scarce resources such as sheltered housing or noninstitutional-based services for the chronically impaired? Careful case management and advocacy on behalf of each elderly victim can sustain continuity of long-term service use.

The MAPAA faces a series of complex questions on how to implement a viable model in view of a funding scarcity, uncoordinated service components throughout the community, and the many uncertainties created by an overall statewide program that performs many administrative and technical functions far beyond the current effort's capabilities. Those who will provide the leadership to MAPAA's effort to develop a direct service capability for the abused and neglected elderly are aware that easy solutions do not exist.

CLINICAL INTERVENTION

The parameters for clinical intervention cases of elderly abuse are ill-defined. Experimental programs with rigorous evaluation are needed. Assuming that the interactive conditions of stress and isolation are present in a significant percentage of those cases, guidelines derived from successful interventions with families under stress should be considered. Guidelines for utilizing individual, family, and group units as the forces of counseling are the following:

1. Individual-oriented counseling is most appropriate when:
   a. There is need to help family caregivers prepare for additional demands in the helping situation.
   b. There is need to help family members learn how to deal with personal stresses initiated by another relative.

   c. There is need for a role model for caregiving.

   d. There is a need to provide concrete resources and/or emotional support for the caregiver.

   e. There is a need for individuals to exercise their right to have control over personal affairs.

2. Group-oriented counseling is appropriate when:

   a. There is a need to find out how to define roles and responsibilities in the family.

   b. There is a need to gain and exchange ideas in an atmosphere of support.

   c. There is a need for information from peers dealing with a common problem or task.

3. Family-oriented counseling is appropriate when:

   a. There is a need to help the family recover the ability to provide a buffer against stress.

   b. There is a need to help balance internal family needs with environmental demands.

   c. There is a need to help the family find new ways of dealing with conflict.

Some practitioners strongly advocate family combinations where middle-aged children are provided the opportunity to participate in a group to deal with the problems of caring for elderly parents. Within such a structure family members can use others' experiences to identify a balance between themselves, their nuclear family, and their parents; to make better estimations of the extent and limits of handling duties and obligations to their elders; and to explore alternative ways of dealing with these aged individuals (Popky-Hausman, 1979).

Crisis intervention skills have much potential value for types of situations in which an immediate decision must be reached that may have long-range implications for numerous family members. Many times the need to remove the elderly person from the residence, even for a short time, creates such a crisis context for the intervention. If crisis contacts are made in the home, as often may be required, the practitioner must be particularly skillful to be able to take in stride the upheaval in the family and the extraneous interruptions that may be present.

When the crisis nature of the situation has passed and the goals of intervention are directed toward helping families deal with assistance tasks, behavioral approaches may be especially helpful for altering precipitating patterns of the elderly, reactive actions of the helping person, and the negatively reinforcing interactions between elders and caregivers.

Whether intervention is approached from an individual, family, or group orientation, there is a general caution that should be heeded. As has been mentioned, elderly victims of abuse may be impaired mentally and/or physically to the extent that institutional placement may have to be considered. This is a serious decision for both the family and the elderly. But the impairment may encourage both family and practitioner to consider such placement without including the elder in the decision-making process. It is necessary to express caution against this practice. It is inappropriate and may create an even more punitive state of isolation in the sense that the elders can be totally cut off from understanding the problems in the household situation and lose the sense of being at least partially in control of their own destinies.

Many of the public agencies likely to be contacted to handle abuse cases lack highly skilled personnel on staff and have budgetary restraints that preclude the introduction of clinical consultants. This is unfortunate since clinical consultants could (a) work with the staff through continuing review of intervention and therapeutic procedures, (b) become involved in a cocounseling capacity to strengthen the therapy from a team approach, and (c) assume a therapeutic responsibility. A qualified clinical consultant also could provide the following backup supports:

1. In-depth input into case assessment in the form of evaluating the emotional and mental status of the abused and the abuser.
2. Continued case-based educational seminars in which training materials are adapted from current situations and in which learning takes place in a manner that offers immediate feedback into the next stages of a treatment plan already in process.
3. Skills and assistance in evaluating outcomes through the preliminary, intermediate, and final stages of case assessment and, where appropriate, educating staff to use empirically oriented approaches for assessment.
4. Formal and informal resource generations that may offer some alternatives.
5. Improved recordkeeping on clinical case interventions that would facilitate future interventions if a case must be reopened or continued over a longer period.

In the final analysis, almost anything that can be suggested in regard to the possible range of clinical interventions should not be excluded categorically, given that there is almost no empirical research or even discussions of empirical case studies of intervention outcomes in cases of elder abuse. Both short-term and longer interventive approaches need to be employed and evaluated carefully. Further clarification of the dynamics of elder abuse as it varies from other types of mistreatment could provide important clues to the technologies appropriate for intervention and behavioral change.

Much research should be done on clinical intervention, ranging from the skills required to quickly identify cases of abuse to optimal approaches for termination of intervention, in order to ensure that the client will use the clinical relationship again if the need arises, and that the individual or family will be able to mobilize before a crisis. Adaptations of effective approaches in other types of intrafamily violence also should be considered but there is a lack of empirical information for treatment even in child abuse, which has been the most developed area of intervention. In all areas of abuse it is not surprising that empirical research into the relative effectiveness of interventions is almost nonexistent because most communities do not have systematic or extensive treatment programs.

CONCLUSION

An earlier section of this chapter summarized the potential causal explanations that might reasonably apply to the problem of elderly abuse. Each involved highly complex relationships and suggested possible directions for intervention. The effort to clarify and interrelate these explanations led to the development of a view of causation that interconnected isolation, stress, and resource availability.

There now is a dramatic reorientation in what is considered the best approach to deal with the increasing proportion of the older population that is frail and impaired. It reflects both a belief and a societal determination to avoid overinstitutionalizing the elderly and, therefore, assumes that noninstitutional alternative approaches are viable. The implicit and explicit message is that the family can, should, and will play an important part in the use and success of noninstitutional living for the frail elderly.

In light of what has been proposed as causal factors and the present emphasis on utilizing family caregivers, it might be expected that arrangements would break down, conflicts arise, and human beings—namely, the old—be mistreated in even greater numbers.

To prevent this possible scenerio, a number of questions must be studied in great depth. It is essential to know:

- What types of families are at highest risk for developing abusive interactions.

- What specific factors are operating in high-risk families and what is the relative significance of each factor.

- What interventions can be planned and provided to minimize the most important risk factors.

- What impact this will have on lowering the rate and severity of abuse.

- What a national prevention strategy would cost in relation to programs for other categories of abused groups, such as children.

- What solutions might imply a rethinking of individual rights and societal values toward the family and the aged.

The experiences of people as they grow older produce opportunities to provide support, reeducation, and the exploration of more or less desirable life styles for the later years. The offering of services for the elderly can produce real benefits only if they are individualized and accessible. The larger and more diversified the network of services available to the elderly, the more need there will be for a case management component available to those who must rely extensively on this increasingly complex bureaucracy.

These service bureaucracies will have to remain sufficiently flexible to offer personalized and localized outreach to the large proportion of persons who otherwise cannot take advantage of them. In all cases the desire to prevent the problem must be balanced with the need to help and protect those who already are caught in the quandary of the existence of violence toward others, especially the old.

REFERENCES

Block, M.R., & Sinnot, J.D. *The battered elder syndrome.* Unpublished manuscript, College Park, Md.: University of Maryland Center on Aging, November 1979.

Boisvert, M.J. The battered-child syndrome. *Social Casework,* 1972, *53*(8), 475-480.

Douglass, R. *A study of neglect and abuse of the elderly in Michigan.* Paper presented at the 32nd Annual Meeting of the Gerontological Society, Washington, D.C., November 1979.

Elbow, M. Theoretical considerations of violent marriages. *Social Casework,* 1977, *58*(9), 515-526.

Hickey, T. *Neglect and abuse of the elderly: Implications of a developmental model and research and intervention.* Unpublished paper, University of Michigan Gerontological Center, 1979.

Holmes, S.A., Barnhart, D., Cantoni, L., & Reymer, E. Working with parents in child abuse cases. *Social Casework,* 1975, *56*(1), 3-12.

Lamb, H.R., & Oliphant, E. Patients of schizophrenics: Advocates for the mentally ill. In L.I. Stein (Ed.), *Community support systems for the long-term patient.* San Francisco: Jossey-Bass, Inc., 1979, pp. 85-92.

Lau, E.E., & Kosberg, J.I. Abuse of the elderly by informal care providers. *Modern Maturity,* April-May 1979, pp. 10-15.

Lord, E., & Weisfeld, D. The abused child. In A. Roberts (Ed.), *Childhood deprivation.* Springfield, Ill.: Charles C Thomas, Publisher, 1974, pp. 64-83.

Popky-Hausman, C. Short-term counseling groups for people with elderly parents. *The Gerontologist,* 1979, *19,* 102-107.

Rathbone-McCuan, E. Elderly victims of family violence and neglect. *Social Casework,* 1980, *61*(5), 296-304.

Robinson, B., & Thurnher, M. Taking care of aged parents: A family cycle transition. *The Gerontologist,* 1979, *19,* 586-593.

Scott, P. Battered wives. *British Journal of Psychiatry,* 1974, *125,* 441-443.

Simos, B.G. Adult children and their aging parents. *Social Work,* 1973, *18,* 78-85.

Spouse abuse cases top one million. *Public Administration Times,* March 1978, *1,* 6.

Star, B. Patterns in family violence. *Social Casework,* 1980, *61*(6), 339-346.

Steger, C., & Kotler, T. Contrasting resources in disturbed and nondisturbed family systems. *British Journal of Medical Psychology,* 1979, *52,* 243-251.

Steinmetz, S.K. Battered parents politics on aging. *Society,* August 1978, pp. 54-55.

Tooley, K. The young child as victim of sibling attack. *Social Casework,* 1977, *58*(1), 25-28.

U.S. Congress. *Joint Hearings before the Senate Special Committee on Aging and the House Select Committee on Aging,* 96th Congress, Second Session. Washington, D.C.: U.S. Government Printing Office, June 11, 1980 (#68-4630).

Chapter 9

Elder Alcohol Abuse and Isolation

INTRODUCTION

A small number of practitioners have recognized that there is a significant problem of alcohol and other chemical abuse among the elderly. This recognition and other factors have converged to exert an influence on two major unconnected human assistance networks—those involving alcoholism and those providing service to the aging.

Both networks are increasing their attention to the alcohol-associated problems of older people. This is evidenced by (a) the National Institute on Alcohol Abuse and Alcoholism's initiatives to sponsor model treatment programs for elderly and physically and/or mentally handicapped alcoholics (National Council on Alcoholism, 1981), (b) the formation of a Blue Ribbon Commission on Alcoholism and Aging sponsored by the National Council on Alcoholism, and (c) the efforts of a few senior citizen and alcohol education programs to extend preventive and interventive information to the elderly.

In spite of these developments, however, the elderly who abuse, misuse, or are addicted to alcohol remain a forgotten, inadequately treated, or untreated group. They are isolated by life complexities and functional disabilities that prompt them to develop abusing patterns that support their drinking. The scientific, academic, and political interests in this problem will take time to transfer treatment knowledge down to local community levels where few adequate programs are available.

Older alcoholics are a hidden population who experience isolation because of their lonely life styles, who become socially disconnected because of the protectiveness of relatives avoiding the stigma of having an alcoholic aged family member, and who are rejected by peers who have strong negative biases about alcohol abuse. Unless the elderly are extremely motivated to pursue treatment, they may become captives of the conspiracy-of-denial perpetuated by significant others.

211

The proportion of elderly alcoholics is unknown and there is limited information on their treatment experiences. This chapter addresses what is known about the various isolators that prevent linking these seniors into treatment settings and suggests alternative ways of treating older alcohol abusers through the development of intervention strategies that require close integration between the alcohol and aging service networks.

THE LITERATURE AND ITS LIMITATIONS

The growing interest in the extent of alcohol problems among the elderly is evidenced by several texts that attempt to both summarize and critique the literature on substance abuse in later years (Mishara & Kastenbaum, 1980; Zimberg, 1979; Whittington & Peterson, 1979). These provide useful listings on the progression of studies that have been conducted on drug utilization, alcohol consumption, and problem drinking. The studies on drugs include investigation of a range of different types of drugs, opiates, tranquilizers, and psychotropics. They thus encompass both legal and illegal drugs.

Additional studies have been conducted on self-prescribed medications known to be serious problems for the aged (Ball & Chambers, 1970; Ball & Lau, 1966; Barton & Hurst, 1966; Capel & Stewart, 1971; Capel, Goldsmith, Waddell, & Stewart, 1972; Chambers, 1971, Kastenbaum, Slater, & Aisenberg, 1964; Learoyd, 1972; Milliren, 1977; O'Donnell, 1969; Pascarelli, 1972; Pascarelli & Fischer, 1974; Petersen & Thomas, 1975; Winick, 1961, 1962).

Most research studies on the use of alcohol are generated from samples of institutionalized elderly people. Only a few involve the aged living in the community and/or seeking treatment. Information also is available from studies with samples drawn from other countries (Baily, Haberman, & Alksne, 1965; Becker & Cesar, 1973; Cahalan, Cisin, & Crossley, 1969; Chien, Stotsky, & Cole, 1973; Chu, 1972; Epstein, Mills, & Simons, 1970; Gaillard & Perrin, 1969; Gaitz & Baer, 1973; Gillis & Keet, 1969; Gorwitz, Bahn, Warthen, & Cooper, 1970; Graux, 1969; Harrington & Price, 1962; Hoffman, 1970; Jones & Jones, 1980; Kramer, 1969; Lennon, Rekosh, Patch, & Howe, 1970; Locke, Kramer, & Pasamanick, 1960; McCucker, Cherubin, & Zimberg, 1971; Myerson & Mayer, 1966; Rathbone-McCuan, Lohn, Levenson, & Hsu, 1976; Rosin & Glatt, 1971; Schuckit & Miller, 1976; Siassi, Crocetti, & Spiro, 1973; Simon, Epstein, & Reynolds, 1968; Zimberg, 1969, 1971, 1974).

The pursuit of epidemological estimates of the numbers of problem drinkers and descriptions of drinking patterns among the elderly and other survey-based information is fraught with methodological problems. These studies give estimates of the prevalence of elderly alcohol abuse that range from 4 to 12 percent. Other professionals have suggested higher rates and suggest these are increasing rapidly.

The research methodology has not been developed to the point where either the scope of the problem or its dimensions are clearly understood and documented. Epidemiological studies rely on self-reports from interviews. The research methodologists are confronted with how to design surveys and train interviewers to ask the appropriate questions about drinking behavior and problems related to alcohol consumption. There is the tendency for many individuals, especially the elderly who were young during the Prohibition era, to be inhibited by social values and personal attitudes about drinking and thus tend to underestimate the amount of alcohol they consume and perhaps remain silent about the personal consequences of their imbibing.

Overall, the data tend to suggest that older persons drink less than the young (Mishara & Kastenbaum, 1980). This pattern of reduced heavy drinking in later years has been reported in men of 65 and women of 50 (Gomberg, 1980). Why there is a decrease is debated from many points, but eventually economic, social, and health reasons seem to converge. The health consciousness of older people also may be a factor. However, studies that merely attempt to estimate consumption patterns usually do not address the care and treatment needs of the elderly who have alcoholic problems, because the tendency for reduced consumption with age does not support the conclusion that elderly persons do not experience alcohol problems. Lowered consumption still may produce devastating physical, psychological, and social consequences.

Some of the factors likely to promote increased drinking among older people include:

- the fact that retirement may prove to be an ever more limiting and isolating experience as higher inflation provides less economic mobility and creates boredom without opportunities to seek the desired but expensive alternatives, and individuals cannot find meaningful and affordable life styles
- the awareness of death that may become an increasingly predominant preoccupation among those living alone and/or in poor health, experiencing constant pain and facing increasing chronic disability
- the loneliness that results from the loss of important social contacts and relationships.

To improve the knowledge base for intervention it is important to understand more about the late onset patterns of alcohol abuse among the elderly. Why, for instance, do some become alcohol abusers in later life and others in similar circumstances have an opposite pattern and in late life actually stop drinking? Closer investigation is needed into the risk factors of later life that could promote alcohol abuse.

The traditional approaches that provide estimates of drinking prevalence may work against detection of the problem in the elderly. Arrest statistics are not particularly useful because few law enforcement officers will charge an elderly person with drunken driving except in the most blatant of circumstances. In addition, many of the elderly no longer drive because of limited finances or physical disability.

Hospital statistics often are not helpful since health professionals either do not recognize that elderly patients have problems with alcohol or, if they do, attempt to hide the situation. There may be a greater tendency to protect older women as compared to older men during hospitalization. The private physician might prevent identification of the problem and yet be the only professional to have sufficient information about the patient's medical history to be suspicious that alcohol abuse or addiction may be a factor.

Alcoholism is a hidden problem but its nonrecognition may be greater among older women than men. Women may be more successful in their attempts to conceal their behaviors from others. Older women, like younger ones, suffer more from the stigma of being alcoholic than men do; if the community finds out about their "problem," they may pay a heavy price. Rumors about being an old sot, drunk, and with low morals develop quickly if a woman is suspected of having an alcoholic problem. These are painful burdens and may well promote additional self-imposed isolation to match the rebukes these women receive from their community.

In essence, to develop better prevalence data and to know more about the problems of elderly alcohol abusers, it will be necessary to take into more serious account the mounting experience of practitioners. They report finding more elderly alcoholics in nursing home admissions, in home health care cases, in outreach programs to the frail and homebound elderly, among tenants in senior citizen high-rise complexes and retirement communities, and among those living in isolated rural areas or inner city ghettos where they are trapped by threats of neighborhood crime.

Future research studies also will need to take into account the fact that the aged are a very diversified group. There are behavioral, health, social, and economic differences among them that place some subgroups at greater risk than others. At the very least, studies should take into account differences in gender, socioeconomic status, race, and ethnicity and their implications for treatment. Additional significant variables include the interrelationships between levels of functional disability, operative social networks, and the strength of the primary relationships to support the treatment and recovery process.

ELEMENTS OF THE ISOLATION PROCESS

Since there is little agreement about single causes of alcohol abuse in later life, it is necessary to consider a cluster of factors that may contribute to the development of this problem and possible intervention strategies. Stress, depression, and the labelling process are important in relation to the isolation experiences of older alcoholics whether they have a long or short history of abuse. (Isolators affecting alcoholic elders are detailed in Figure 9-1.)

There is no consistency in explanations of the interrelationship of stress, mental health status, and coping mechanisms among the elderly. As a causal or contributory factor, little is known about how stress and alcohol abuse operate together in late life. Some elderly persons are situational/reactive abusers and respond to crisis stress through coping approaches that involve the damaging use of alcohol. This pattern is potentially different from that of the long-term, chronic alcoholic.

Figure 9-1 Isolators Affecting the Alcoholic Elder

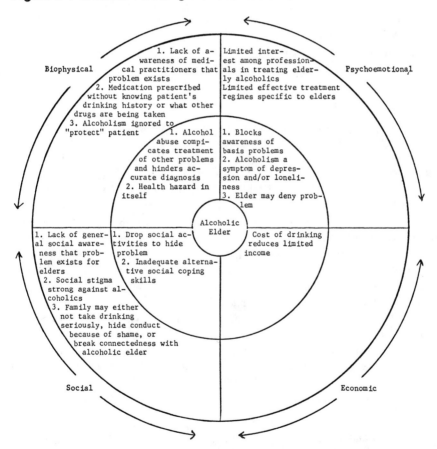

The inner circle contains isolators as they are manifested in the personal lives of alcoholic elders, the outer circle those that abound in the environment.

The typological approach (identifying and analyzing histories and patterns) to understanding the onset of alcoholism may prove a useful adjunct to the widely accepted distinction between late onset and chronic long-term abuse. The distinction is made between primary alcoholics (those with no preexisting major psychiatric disorders) and secondary ones (those with some prior pathology). The latter group is divided into two categories: affective disorder alcoholics (those with depressive symptoms) and sociopathic alcoholics (those with histories of serious antisocial life styles) (Schuckit, Pitts, Reich, King, & Winokur, 1979). This is an example of a typological approach that should be examined among the elderly, given the common problem of confusing alcoholism and psychiatric symptoms.

Research should attempt to relate life cycle stressors to an analysis of late onset alcohol abuse. Physical illness may become a more prevalent stressor among older persons, who are more prone to illness as they age and because there is a greater likelihood that the ailment will become chronic and will involve pain that cannot be eased. Accumulated stresses, such as the loss of independence and relationships, could have an effect on the late onset of abuse. The cases of two older persons who developed late-onset abuse serve as illustrations.

Garrett Reister

Garrett is 68 and was retired involuntarily five years ago. The plant where he had worked for 30 years and from which he had expected to receive an attractive financial retirement package had gone bankrupt. He therefore found himself having to rely on welfare supplements to his meager private resources. To have to turn to welfare after a lifetime of pride in his ability to support himself was more depressing than the financial deprivation. The occasional drinking that had always been a part of his social life became more extensive. While this seemed to relieve him of the pain of his reduced financial circumstances, it aggravated his diabetes.

Garrett did not seem to recognize how much more he was drinking and never mentioned it to the staff in the clinic where he was receiving treatment for the diabetes. Eventually, medical complications led to the amputation of one leg. This only intensified his depression and made him all the more unreachable to the physical therapists who tried to help him regain independence. Caregivers who by this time had become aware of Garrett's dependence on alcohol were fearful that if he were to be returned to an independent residential accommodation, he would begin drinking again. This fear led to a recommendation for nursing home placement.

Libby Patterson

Libby is 62 and in reasonably good health. Most of her adult life was spent rather unremarkably as a housewife and mother. However, about four years ago her husband, who is several years her senior, became ill with a chronic heart condition.

He is permanently unable to go out of the house without special transportation assistance or to perform self-care tasks, let alone help his wife with the many home chores he had performed in the past to maintain an old residence in manageable condition. Last year Libby's daughter's husband died in an accident. The suddenness of his death left the daughter confused and frightened and needing the support and loving care Libby had always provided in the past.

Libby's emotional and physical energy resources were being stretched to the breaking point. To continue to fulfill the needs of others, she had to ignore many of her own needs. At first her drinking relieved some of these unrelenting pressures and later helped her block out her rising resentment of the demands and needs of spouse and daughter. Recently Libby's grandson was arrested for manslaughter after an auto accident in which he was at fault. This proved to be the last straw.

Libby's drinking became so apparent that both husband and daughter began to recognize the changes in her behavior and to realize she needed immediate help. After she received alcoholism counseling she was able to focus more attention on her own limitations while her family worked to share the crises in a more constructive manner. This type of secondary gain made nonabusive alcohol consumption patterns possible again.

In both of these cases, stressful events triggered a process of isolation that led to depression, followed by drinking to relieve it. The cases differ in other respects. Garrett's situation was made more complex in that he not only concealed his drinking from health professionals but also from himself, and denial was easy to maintain. Drinking complicated his health problems, was leading to institutionalization, and therefore could be seen as an isolator. For Libby, drinking was a response to the isolation she was experiencing as she attempted to meet the support needs of those around her. Family members' awareness of her drinking did lead them to greater awareness of her needs and possibly to ending her feelings of aloneness if they could develop other patterns of communication and provide support in her care for the husband and additional therapeutic support for the daughter.

THE DEPRESSION FACTOR

Practitioners agree that depression can be a strong stimulus to the development of late alcohol abuse. The concept of depression and its numerous definitions as applied in both aged and younger alcoholics produces some confusion regarding its relation to the aging process as well as how it may serve as a causal, contributory, or associated abusing condition. The overall parameters of depression may be defined as follows:

> Since the early part of this century, mental health clinicians and investigators have grouped the depressions and other related emotional states

into the category of "affective disorders." Although a broad spectrum of symptoms, behaviors, and other states are included within this category, the person's disturbance is expressed in their mood and emotional states. As the most common conditions included among the affective disorders, the depressions are clinical states in which persistent abnormal emotional symptoms are associated with feelings of worthlessness, crying, suicidal tendencies, loss of interest in work and other activities, impaired capacity to perform everyday social functions, and hypochondriasis or bodily alterations including anorexia, weight change, constipation, psychomotor retardation, and agitation (Klerman & Weissman, 1980).

Depression often is referred to as the most common psychiatric syndrome in the aged. There is general clinical agreement that the elderly are particularly vulnerable to depression because of the numerous losses they experience and because they have less of a future in which to compensate for them. An examination of the common elements of depression reveals much overlap with the range of the symptoms experienced by the physically ill elderly patient, and with those of many aged alcohol abusers. A diagnosis of either depression or alcoholism, or a combination of both, may be hampered by the extent to which symptoms are assumed to be normative behavior and unrelated to alcohol abuse. Possible overlapping symptoms include:

1. depressed moods characterized by reports of feeling sad, low, blue, despondent, hopeless, gloomy, helpless
2. changes in posture, facial expressions, speech, dress, grooming
3. change in appetite, usually leading to weight loss
4. sleep difficulty, usually insomnia
5. thoughts of death and/or suicide attempts
6. loss of energy, fatigue, lethargy, agitation (increased motor activity experienced as restlessness)
7. retardation of speech, thought, and movement
8. decreased capacity to experience pleasure
9. feelings of worthlessness, self-reproach, guilt, shame
10. decrease in sexual interest and activity
11. loss of interest in usual social activities

A diagnosis of depression may serve to keep the alcoholism component hidden, especially if the elderly person is being evaluated in a medical setting where professionals lack geriatric alcoholism expertise and automatically associate the symptoms with a stereotypic medical condition. Failure to make a proper assessment, one which may lead to rapid identification of alcohol abuse as a primary or secondary problem, has an isolating effect. Moreover, treatment in a medical or psychiatric setting does not assure that treating medical problems will influence in any way alcohol abuse patterns during post-medical care. Analyzing the pattern of relationship between alcoholism and depression, such as that found in young adults, may be infinitely more complex when attempted with an elderly person. The evaluation activity is made more complex when the problems of alcohol abuse and depression are combined with other illness symptomology, which reinforce each other to create a complex profile of symptoms. Additional drug/medication reactions may be complicating factors, affecting the ability of the practitioner to make an accurate diagnosis of the alcohol-related problems. Among late onset alcoholics there is reason to believe that depression and alcohol abuse are inter-related in ways that resemble the depressive symptoms manifested by younger alcoholic patients (Tyndel, 1974) and clinically depressed patients that have histories of alcoholism (Reich, Davies, & Himmelhoch, 1974).

It is important to recognize that stereotypes about older alcoholics are easily generated as the results of at least two factors. First, alcoholism continues to be associated with general cultural stereotypes, as does the aging process. Alcoholism in late life may be the basis for a negative assessment of self and of others (friends or practitioners). Second, the process whereby the elderly alcoholic is so identified conforms to many of the steps in labelling. In this context, the major concern is how stereotyping and labelling may interfere with treatment.

Depending upon the pattern of onset, the life style, and the interaction between those who label and those who are labelled, the older alcoholic is likely to be described as deviant. It is assumed that personal recognition of an alcoholic-related problem does not necessarily require any individual to have to suffer the burden of a deviant label. In becoming so known, a person with an abusing or addictive condition is perceived as a problem in an all-encompassing social role (Nooe, 1980).

For example, an older man may have a period when he has a heavy drinking problem. If he goes through treatment once, he is defined as alcoholic. Because others assign that label does not ensure that the elder will define his problem in a way that is helpful. There may be a component of self-labelling behavior that is counterproductive to rehabilitation. The elderly person may accept someone's label but not have sufficient self-awareness to admit that it has therapeutic value. The labelling process may be less helpful if the connotation is negative. The elderly person, defined by others as alcoholic, may accept the label but still have no concept of what that means. Ceasing to deny alcoholism must mean more than acceptance of a condemning label.

Numerous treatment-related issues emerge from the deviance framework. Little is known about what events or conditions cue an older person's awareness of the problem. More information should be gathered to determine whether psychological, physical, environmental, or social factors are more likely to be the influential variable in an individual's identification of the problem and subsequent pursuit of treatment. Elderly persons who do label themselves as alcoholic or as alcohol abusers are the ones who will have to react to the psychological impact of the self-definition. These reactions will involve seeking external help such as by entering a treatment program, taking a self-corrective step to stop drinking without input from others in any formalized treatment sense, or deciding to take no action.

The personal reactive component of deviance theory is worthy of additional consideration in connection with many important treatment issues. First, among elderly alcoholic abusers, what factors produce strong denial patterns, and do they contribute to the hidden nature of the problem? Second, does one's personal label make any difference in the treatment approach?

If the elderly alcoholic is caught in a frequent cycle of self-criticism and self-blame and encounters practitioners who are not knowledgeable about the reactive characteristics associated with the problem, what impact will this have on the outcome of intervention? The societal response, in this case, as manifested by practitioners or other community members, also can stimulate the elderly person's experience. The fact that many of the aged person's peer group may stigmatize alcoholism may increase the isolation. Similarly, practitioners may perpetuate the cycle because they label the person as degenerate because of the alcohol-related problems, may reinforce the individual's feelings of self-worth, or merely define the elder as worthless because of the advanced chronological age.

Deviance theory as applied to alcoholism may be used to understand behaviors of the person and of the community. It is clear that isolation results when a person is consumed by both self-labelling and by the influence of the same negative cognomens from others. To understand the dynamics of isolation it may be necessary to assume that the self and community reinforcements are difficult to change unless supportive sources are available to present alternative definitions and use them to encourage continuing help seeking and thus prevent further aloneness.

A DISCUSSION OF ASSESSMENT

Treatment centers on assessment but little progress has been made toward developing an evaluation approach that fits the needs of the older alcoholic. In the last decade or so, clinicians and researchers have become increasingly aware of the need to assess the elderly person's functioning (Bernal, Guillermo, Brannon, Belar, Lavigne, & Cameron, 1977). This objective is important in the area of alcoholism-related dysfunction. It would be a valuable step forward to develop approaches that integrate the most valid and appropriate components of assessment now being used in the fields of both alcoholism and aging.

Multiple sources of measurement are necessary in evaluating the health status of any elderly person. Over time, assessment has moved from a unidimensional source (either the physician's diagnosis or the self-report of the patient) to a multifaceted approach. In the case of elderly alcoholics it is important to have an assessment completed by an interdisciplinary team, a self-report, and an evaluation based on the use of objective diagnostic tools. Taken together, measures from all of these sources provide a basis for a comprehensive evaluation.

The clinician's ratings could be made by a person familiar with alcoholism or who had expertise in gerontology, but with proper consultation from the field where the practitioner lacked expertise. A self-reported drinking history could be collaborated by an informed other. The behavioral ratings could be generated from measures of ability to perform basic actions and from indicators useful in determining cognitive functioning.

One area of potential disagreement between alcoholism specialists and gerontological practitioners is whether to include a physician in the information-gathering process. Gerontologists place great importance on a physician's input in assessment of elderly clients with chronic health problems before planning treatment. On the other hand, some alcoholism specialists would not consider this an essential component. Among the few practitioners with both gerontology and alcoholism treatment skills, there appears to be little disagreement that a medical assessment should be included in the evaluation. This would seem to be essential in modifying a younger adults' alcoholism treatment program to accommodate older alcoholics. Indeed, it is mandatory if the program is to accept elderly persons with chronic health problems and physical disabilities. In some treatments geared for younger alcoholics, the staffing patterns do not include or have the capacity to provide physician input into assessment nor is there prompt access to a doctor or to an emergency medical facility.

The issue of physician input, whether at the point of initial assessment or in later stages of treatment, illustrates one area where planning between alcoholism and gerontology experts is necessary if there are to be programs specially designed or otherwise modified to provide adequate care for the older alcoholic. Points to be considered are:

1. how to have physician input available for assessment and emergency backup during detoxification without turning an alcoholism treatment program from a social to a medical model
2. what procedures to use to continue to monitor needs and still maintain a focus on the health components of the treatment
3. how to avoid bombardment of an elderly individual who has not been involved in regular medical care with tests that might be unnecessary and inappropriate to the major focus of the treatment
4. how to define a medical consultant's functions in a treatment program and explore ways of using other health specialties such as a physician assistant or geriatric nurse practitioner that might work on the full-time team

5. how to ensure that there will be the necessary follow-up after the active phase of treatment in the inpatient program has been completed if the individual's health care needs warrant this
6. how to facilitate an understanding among community physicians who might treat the older person later in the recovery process

The assessment process also should be modified to evaluate the functional status of the elderly alcoholic. Functional status represents the level of an individual's behavioral capacities in a variety of areas including physical health, quality of self-maintenance, quality of role activity, intellectual status, social activity, attitude toward the world and toward self, and general emotional condition (Lawton, 1971). Assessing the functional status should include a determination of potential harmful consequences to self and others. Typical symptoms associated with chronic alcoholism such as falls, blackouts, delirious reactions, passing out, and trembling may have serious and complicating consequences, especially after the elderly person is discharged as an inpatient or is living at home while in treatment.

The in-home situation should be of concern while the person is in treatment not only for the influences being exerted by others to support or negate the alcoholism program goals but also to assess the adequacy of the living environment. One elderly alcoholic man who was in a very unstructured outpatient treatment program was subject to frequent passing out during drinking bouts. He had the main responsibility of caring for his bedridden wife, who received only minimal service from a home care support program. Home care staff members did not recognize the husband's behavior pattern nor its association with drinking. They did not know he was in contact with a treatment source for alcoholism. The alcoholism counselor did not know the extent of his caregiving responsibilities for his wife. One day the man passed out while cooking and gas fumes nearly killed them both. Such a common symptom may have particularly serious consequences given the living arrangement and daily routines that older people are expected to maintain in order to reside in the community. To have an accurate knowledge of the residential environment, the practitioner should visit the home before an elderly person is accepted for an outpatient program or is discharged from an inpatient unit.

There are few, if any, empirically validated social assessment protocols designed exclusively for the elderly. If the range of social history-taking approaches in younger adult and geriatric programs are examined, the variability of what is considered to be priority information becomes evident. In addition, there have been few attempts to modify drinking history protocols to account for variability in age or life stage between younger and older alcoholics. How social-psychological evaluations and alcohol consumption and utilization history-taking analyses should be modified for late life is a problem that will not be resolved quickly. A few guidelines might be helpful: (a) the older alcoholic might require different interventions, so assessment should include the type of information needed to link the older person with treatment, and (b) the degree of supportive linkages that the older alcoholic might require is much greater and not available in the traditional system, where there is little follow-up.

Where the elderly alcoholics go for treatment and how they are handled once admitted tends to depend on what facilities will accept them, given such factors as age, physical and psychological status, and/or limited or nonexistent income to cover inpatient care costs. Research on treatment is too meager to guide a rigid prescription of the optimal alternatives. However, as perspectives on treatment are being formulated, it is important to keep in mind the following types of questions:

1. Should the elderly alcoholic or problem drinker be treated in settings where younger persons also are under care?
2. Will similar treatment methods, if applied, have similar results?
3. Are there particular treatment problems that can be associated with late onset types of alcoholism?
4. Are there specific supportive resources that have special value for the elderly that are less appropriate for younger alcoholics?

TREATMENT ISSUES THAT EMERGE

The category of health and social intervention with older and elderly persons who abuse alcohol is both broad and ambiguous. The boundaries of knowledge that eventually may prove applicable in the expansion of treatment include: (a) life span developmental psychology, (b) biomedical processes and behavioral understanding, (c) studies of personality, motivation, and adjustment, and (d) socialization, attitudes, and social roles.

Despite some of the commonalities of the two fields, it has been difficult to stimulate researchers and practitioners to give priority to the dynamics of both alcoholism and aging. The problem is so basic but the knowledge so limited that the foundation for selecting what direction might be taken to plan treatment must be approached from practitioner opinion supported by a commitment for continuing empirical research into all aspects of care. (The social resource system involving the alcoholic elderly is presented in Figure 9-2.)

A framework to guide the evolution of treatment planning and delivery should explicate how alcohol abuse interferes with what older men or women are required, expected, or prefer to do in their daily lives. Environmental, physical, and social behavioral factors need to be considered carefully from both a causal and interventive point of view. To the extent that these or other factors impede performance because of or in relation to alcohol consumption, the elderly may be defined as vulnerable.

Figure 9-2 The Alcoholic Elder and the Social Resource System

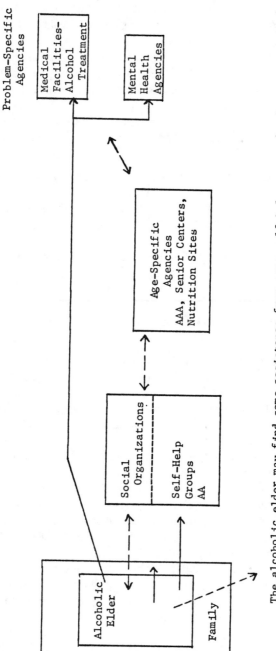

The alcoholic elder may find some assistance from some self-help groups (AAA) but for the most part they concentrate (through program focus) on young and middle-age adult problems. The same can be said for formal service agencies. Many social organizations and age-specific agencies do not want to include the alcoholic elderly. Alcoholic seniors for the most part remain outside of the social service network, which does not coordinate efforts to address these problems. Family frequently hides the elders' drinking problem and discourages or prevents contacts with social resources.

If the aged person's functional capabilities are threatened, some action may be appropriate to reduce the condition. Action may or may not require inputs from formal and/or informal helping sources. If action is taken, it may or may not produce improvement or restore the individual's performance. Ideally, treatment frameworks would address both clinical intervention and program activity. In general, clinical intervention will encompass such practitioner activities as diagnosis of alcohol-related factors, assessment of the problems of daily living resulting from the alcohol abuse or associated with it, the application of health and social technologies to treat the primary and secondary conditions, and evaluation and monitoring of outcomes. Program level intervention involves research, planning, program development, resource generation, coordination, and evaluation.

There is a range of issues that can be considered in planning an intervention program. One approach involves the modification of existing treatment that heretofore either has provided no special focus for older alcoholics or has begun to gather information about how to redesign all or part of the program to accommodate older and elderly alcoholics. A second approach involves the design of a specialized program for older and elderly alcoholics that is not necessarily based either on redesigning existing treatment or on providing services to senior as well as younger adult alcoholics.

Before considering them in detail, it is worthwhile to consider some of the broad elements required of either approach. Some treatment philosophy always is implicit, if not explicit. That philosophy is part of the framework that directs the establishment of goals and the means to meet them. The emergence of a philosophy for treating older alcohol abusers will be difficult to structure because of differences in attitudes toward such individuals.

The focus of treatment can be one variation. Some practitioners would recommend that the focus encompass both alcohol and drug abusers without differentiation as to the type of chemical involved (Community Advisory Committee, 1979). This seems to operate from the assumption that there are commonalities across the types of dependencies and that they can be handled through common treatment principles. There also is a growing pattern in substance abuse treatment programs to encompass the range of addictions in one program. This view should be examined with caution if only from the standpoint that the substances on which elderly persons usually depend are those that have been ordered by physicians and/or self-prescribed and legal. Yet a program that deals with multiple types of chemical dependency has merit and is feasible since an unknown percentage of patients will be involved in both alcohol and prescribed drugs.

From a practical standpoint, if resources are scarce, some communities may not be able to afford the most competent personnel to work with the elderly or, if affordable, such expertise may not be available. Despite limited resources, what is known about alcoholism treatment and clinical services to the elderly indicates the importance of expanding the scope of care to include involvement of family members and/or significant others. If family members can participate and are constructively supportive of the treatment goals, the effort to involve all potential significant others seems undebatable.

Another component of treatment philosophy deals with the pros and cons of developing an age-specific or age-general treatment program. The criterion of chronological age alone is not a mandatory program component. What is more important is that the elderly have a choice as to whether or not they wish to be in a setting where there are many younger persons and whether the facilities of the treatment center are appropriate for their needs. This issue is related to the all-important realization that alcohol abuse in the elderly is not usually a unitary problem and that a high proportion of those taking treatment have primary social and physical health problems that must be addressed if the alcohol dependency is to be handled adequately.

A last component, likely to be debated, is the question of goals for total abstinence or controlled drinking. These divergent objectives extend beyond the older alcoholic and are characteristic throughout the field of alcohol treatment. It would seem that there is room to redefine this issue in terms of what goals might be most appropriate and attainable for individuals, given their history, circumstances, and the behavioral dimensions of their abuse behaviors. Even those who hold that abstinence is the optimal goal will agree that chronic alcoholics who can gain more control over drinking or be less impacted upon by alcohol may have taken significant steps, even if they do not attain total abstinence.

The question of what detection/case-finding approaches to take with the older alcoholic has not been seriously considered, let alone resolved. Three suggestions have been offered as to how to establish an outreach program:

1. Develop an educational program in the outreach service of area agency on aging that is working with the frail elderly by educating them about the symptoms of alcoholism.
2. Plan and offer mass media programs that encompass both drugs and alcohol and their combined utilization as dangerous to health and likely to increase susceptibility to other disabilities.
3. Develop educational materials for health professionals, particularly home health care workers and physicians who have frequent contacts with older people thought to be very at risk of problem drinking.

Whether the older person is an alcoholic or the supportive spouse of a problem drinker, health beliefs can play an important role in the willingness of an individual to participate in the treatment process. The health belief concept has been developed into a conceptual framework for analyzing and facilitating the elderly's participation in the care system. The model is based on four generic health beliefs that may influence a range of health and health-seeking behaviors (Rakowski & Hickey, 1980):

1. A perceived susceptibility to a given illness or continued vulnerability to a current ailment would be appropriate to alcoholism if the person were to drink more frequently and/or more heavily, with notable side effects, or if the individual had been involved previously with alcohol abuse and were to realize that current behavior was promoting a recurrence of the problem that could have more serious consequences, given advanced age.
2. The perceived seriousness of the target illness would depend upon the extent to which the older person recognized some of the potential consequences if alcohol abuse became a routine behavioral pattern that could affect other existing physical health problems.
3. The benefits expected from contact with a helping source would depend on the extent to which an older person believed there was a source of help, such as Alcoholics Anonymous, that would provide nonstigmatized support.
4. The perceived cost barriers in contacting the helping source would prove to be a very tangible reason for an older person to not seek help. The cost of treatment for an individual living on a fixed income, with no knowledge of whether or not health care insurance would cover that expense or that some sources were free, would influence the pursuit of care.

Patterns of spouse behavior in relationship to the treatment of younger male and female alcoholics have not been considered carefully in older couples. One deterrent to older people seeking treatment is their belief that their spouse will leave. Limited evidence suggests that older men are more likely to leave alcoholic wives than the reverse (Rathbone-McCuan & Roberds, 1980). This pattern is supported by the caregiving roles that wives traditionally extend to ill husbands after lengthy marriages but is less common among older men when wives require care.

Knowledge about the forces that keep either older women or men as hidden victims of their alcoholism will be derived only through research. The stigma falls most heavily on the older alcohol abuser when family or close friends are rejecting. Persons who are alone, without family or friends, may find that entering treatment introduces them to a new opportunity for social participation that in itself may serve to reduce some of the isolation they had experienced previously. Perhaps the stigmatic consequences are less serious for those who are alone because they have no close intimates to label or assure them before, during, and after treatment.

Treatment involves intervention that should have clearly defined goals. Planning is at the core of any treatment program and should never be taken as less than central to all interventions. Simply stated, an interdisciplinary team or an individual practitioner formulating the treatment should initiate a plan that sets forth incremental goals, from beginning to intermediate to ultimate.

Ultimate outcomes should be framed within the context of the reasons for which treatment was undertaken in the first place. With the older alcoholic this might be initiated because somebody wants something done about the client and therefore has taken steps to get the person into treatment. However, the motives of the helping or referring person cannot be considered to be the sole or major basis for what should be happening during the course of treatment.

A second factor is what criterion was used to define the objectives toward which treatment is directed. At the very least, there should be information from the assessment that is used to establish the treatment, which should not be a standardized "come one, come all" approach.

A third factor is that when the goals are achieved, treatment can be terminated and deemed a success (Rosen & Proctor, 1978). This implies that there should be a clear differentiation between those who are in a setting for active treatment and those who are there for purposes of maintenance. The latter may be an acceptable intervention goal but should not be misrepresented or ill-defined as rehabilitation.

Intermediate goals for some elderly alcoholics may be the range of interventions undertaken during active treatment, leaving the ultimate goals to be defined when the individuals are discharged back into the community or to a more permanent living arrangement. Many times goals have to go beyond alcoholism treatment and incorporate health and social dimensions, for each of which intermediate objectives must be defined. In the long run, if the health and social problems that may have contributed to the onset of alcohol abuse or the maintenance of that pattern are not altered, those causes can resurface and initiate a cycle of "abuse into treatment and back into abuse." Most older alcoholics require a treatment plan that involves longer-range social and health care, possibly from different intervention sources over an extended period. This suggests that a case management component may be necessary.

Very few groups of practitioners have considered treatment issues seriously. Among the available materials is a proposed set of rules for conducting interventions with the elderly (Community Advisory Committee, 1979):

1. Persons important in the life of the older alcoholic should be encouraged to give facts, information, or even subjective perceptions that might be helpful in the course of treatment. It is better to obtain this information from more than one person in face-to-face communication.
2. The more specific the data to be obtained, the more useful they may prove in the treatment. The quality of this information will be important from many standpoints, including the times when supportive confrontation will be greatly needed in dealing with older persons who deny their condition. It is

important to try to obtain direct information that does not rely on hearsay or opinions about what another person thought.
3. The older persons should be given alternatives and some choices in the treatment process. Such choices should not be presented to persons who are not competent to evaluate them; on the other hand, starting to facilitate individuals' decision-making capacity during treatment can be a positive learning experience. The practitioner must be open to confronting the elderly when it is required and should be cautioned against making it easier for them just because they are old. This is a form of subtle prejudice that works against assuring that the elderly will have opportunities to deal with themselves and to make choices.

There are multiple treatment modalities that could be considered as relevant to the core program with older alcoholics. To date, nothing seems to be ruled out on the basis that it does not work. The problem is that too few modalities have been utilized in treating this group of alcoholics and systematically evaluated over time. Therefore, treatment planners should evaluate each available modality to determine whether or not it can be applied by existing highly competent treatment personnel and it is to be analyzed from the standpoint of its success with individual cases and with groups of elderly persons.

Alcoholics Anonymous, aversion therapy (hypoaversion, disulfiram/antabuse, condition reflex treatment), behavior modification, group therapy, individual counseling, family therapy, psychoanalytic therapy, and psychotherapy all are considered potentially appropriate modalities.

The limited information about the success of working with the elderly en bloc would suggest that therapeutic gains can emerge either from group involvement with alcoholics or from nonalcoholic peers. Elderly alcoholics have discontinued drinking when they were involved in group discussions and other forms of socialization therapy when the members were nonalcoholics (Zimberg, 1979). However, the seeming success of Alcoholics Anonymous in supporting older alcoholics and facilitating their recovery may be one, if not the most, viable approach for long-term maintenance of nonabusing behaviors.

The self-help AA movement is not age exclusive, does not discriminate against older people, and does not require economic resources. Groups can be formed and sustained in a number of settings, and it offers a very significant opportunity for developing new roles and forming new relationships that are more than casual senior citizen peer interactions. It also is one of the few settings or sources of treatment where remission does not necessarily have to involve institutional readmission. It places emphasis on the daily success that may have far more relevance to aged persons.

The family also can become involved in self-help. While the field of alcoholism apparently has awakened to the value of involving relatives in treatment, gerontologists only now are beginning to recognize that aging, like alcoholism, may be a family affair. The occurrence, maintenance, and remission of alcoholism may be associated with what happens within the family system. Until there is empirical documentation that families are disinterested in their elderly alcoholic members, it is better to assume that relatives must play an active role in treatment.

Among the most challenging service functions that an age-general alcoholism treatment program can undertake is the systematic effort to evaluate its capacity to serve the elderly and then to determine, within available resources, how to modify its dimensions to make them more relevant for an increased number of older patients. While each treatment involves specific issues, there may be at least a few areas that are worthy of attention by all programs because they can be anticipated as relevant, given the nature of the abuse in later life:

- Does a program have the capacity to shift its attention toward a segment of the population that may be at least two decades older than the average patient?

- Can it accommodate the likelihood that many of its older clients will have functional disabilities that will require special resources in many aspects of the treatment (physical modifications in the environment to deal with mobility problems, special nutrition needs, closer medical consultation, longer periods of detoxification, special educational materials for those with vision and hearing impairments)?

- Can it incorporate both the long-term chronic alcoholic and the late onset type and at the same time deal with a more active younger population that may be making multiple and different demands on staff?

- Can vocational rehabilitation take on a new meaning besides returning to work, given that many older alcoholics will be retired and have neither the opportunity nor the capacity to reenter the labor force?

- Can only staff specialists with knowledge in both alcoholism and aging provide adequate input to the number of elderly patients who might be admitted?

- Are other staff members willing to work with elderly as compared to younger patients for whom they may have a strong personal and professional preference?

- Is the community at large interested in supporting a program for older alcoholics and can other treatment agencies outside the service network be called upon to offer cooperation with the program?

- Can physical and occupational therapy be made available to older patients if necessary during either the inpatient or outpatient phase?

- What will the outpatient component of treatment offer the older alcoholic and if there is not such a service how will the need for it be met?

- What funding sources can be expected beyond a possible demonstration grant to ensure that there is an opportunity to provide an adequate degree of continuity—how can existing funding sources be capitalized upon and new ones found?

Clinical services must be offered in a programmatic context. How to identify resources and put them together is another aspect of intervention. The sponsorship of a treatment program may be among the most crucial factors in determining long-range effectiveness and continuation. A program model may be introduced in an institutional setting, senior center, high-rise residential program, or an alcoholism treatment effort, to name a few. However, the program must belong to the community. It must have diverse cross-sectional support and be planned and staffed by highly competent personnel.

Such issues must be considered and are equally relevant to groups that are attempting to design an innovative program without prior organizational sponsorship from an established treatment agency. Almost any type of treatment program structure could be considered relevant. One that has particular appeal is the concept of a day support center that has links to both the alcoholism and aging service networks and that can serve as a complement to existing resources in the community. The objectives of a day support treatment center would include:

- provision of direct service

- maximum utilization of all existing system resources through service linkages between primary alcoholism and the aging network service units

- incorporation of age-specific programs as well as formulation of ways to facilitate the interaction of younger persons with older alcoholics

- responsibility for helping generate knowledge and information about treating elderly alcoholics that could be disseminated to fill the major void of empirically based data

- leadership in community education and prevention efforts that may be valuable for the at-risk population

Many communities have at least some resources for alcoholism treatment and services to the elderly. Inpatient programs often are associated in some way with a medical facility and increasingly are located in acute care hospitals. The aging service networks are associated with the larger social welfare system. Together, these resources can be mobilized into a joint endeavor to plan a specialized program. As after-care services can be a weak or nonexistent component of the alcoholism continuum, and as the aging service network commits its resources to keeping the elderly outside of institutions, a day treatment program might be perceived as not duplicating existing services for alcoholics and as in line with goals for assisting the elderly.

A day treatment program could have sufficient flexibility so as to be able to help several types of older alcoholics including (a) those who had been through an inpatient treatment program and needed after-care service, (b) those who might not require inpatient care but could enter an outpatient program, (c) those who had a history of unsuccessful treatment, and (d) those for whom inpatient treatment might be financially impossible. Using a day care center to serve a highly varied population would require a trial period before the elderly person could be accepted, especially if long-term maintenance was the goal. The core interdisciplinary team consisting of a nurse practitioner, social worker, alcoholism counselor, and a recovering older alcoholic would make the final decision about admission to the program.

Admission criteria for this type of effort would require much deliberation. Those involved in planning would have to weigh the value of admitting both men and women, but perhaps having them together would be more appropriate for the elderly than for younger individuals, who may prefer same-sex therapy groups. During a trial period of perhaps a month, the staff would need to give priority to developing motivation so the alcoholics would want to join the day treatment program. However, when the team was reviewing the case after the trial, it would have to critically assess the level of demonstrated motivation.

Formal connection with a private physician or a clinic also would have to be set before admission was approved. Many persons might require active assistance from the social worker to make this linkage during the trial period. The information available from a medical examination should ensure that sufficient knowledge was available about the physical health status of the elderly individual. It should be supplemented with information about ability to function independently and to perform daily living activities.

The team also would need to assess the older person's residential resources to determine whether the helping individual they accept has an environment that can ensure adequate care and support of treatment goals.

The final criterion to be developed would be the degree of mental/cognitive functioning required before a person could be considered eligible for formal admission.

A treatment program for older alcoholics, especially one not connected with an institution, must be very clear about the types of persons who cannot be served. Establishing those guidelines should not be based merely on social class or on a poor treatment record; rather, they should be based on whether or not the program can meet the needs. If a person is too mentally and/or physically impaired, an institutional or community residential program may be the only alternative. If the person in the community taking responsibility for care does not accept the existence of the alcohol problem and does not encourage the accomplishment of treatment goals, the conflicting influences between the staff and the family or care provider will catch the elderly person in the middle.

The health care and social service components of this type of program would differ from a day care treatment component for younger alcoholics, as shown in Table 9-1. The day treatment model seems particularly valuable to older persons who are isolated and tend to be homebound. Making the program available to the more physically incapacitated would require a specialized transportation system, which would be one of the most expensive and hard-to-develop components of treatment of this type.

A benefit of the model is that it provides for the possibility of developing and maintaining social relationships that reinforce sobriety without limiting attention to other needs. With some modifications, a senior citizen day treatment program for nonalcoholic older people could be adjusted to incorporate a capacity to provide specialized services to meet the needs of the alcohol abusers within that setting.

Table 9-1 Component Activities for an Alcoholism Program

Health	Social
1. Regular health status screening opportunities would be made available and required.	1. The person would be required to become involved with AA but also would be encouraged to participate in social activities that were not focused on alcoholism recovery.
2. Physical and occupational rehabilitations would be considered a necessary counselling service.	2. More intensive case management functions would be provided to ensure that each person was receiving needed housing, legal, and transportation services.
3. Linkages would be established to a nursing home or other inpatient setting for short-term admissions in addition to readily available hospital-based services.	3. The older recovering alcoholics on the treatment team would have extensive outreach functions in the community as well as within the care program.
4. Nutrition and pharmacy input would be sought for all persons with special dietary needs and/or extensive daily medication regimens.	4. Employment and leisure/interest counseling would be equally important to ensure that those who did not or could not work would not be treated as less in need because they were retired or never had worked.

CONCLUSION

This chapter has presented the older alcoholic as a subgroup of the population at risk of isolation. The isolating process is complex and it is not clear which comes first: elderly persons become alcohol abusers because of the separateness they experience, or the reverse. In fact, both patterns probably occur and there may be a reinforcing cycle in this process. Isolation may differ between chronic alcoholics who have grown older and those whose alcoholism evolves late, but both types can and do experience isolation, with few sources of intervention to improve their circumstances. It is important for experts to integrate resources toward designing intervention programs and obtaining the necessary changes in eligibility coverage of third party payers to fully reimburse the services required to treat this group of older people.

REFERENCES

Bailey, M.B., Haberman, P.W., & Alksne, H. The epiderr⁻ ›logy of alcoholism in an urban residential area. *Quarterly Journal of Studies on Alcohol,* 1965, *26,* 19-40.

Ball, J.C., & Chambers, C.D. *The epidemiology of opiate addiction in the United States.* Springfield, Ill.: Charles C Thomas, Publisher, 1970.

Ball, J.C., & Lau, M.P. The Chinese narcotic addict in the United States. *Social Forces,* 1966, *45,* 68-72.

Barton, R., & Hurst, L. Unnecessary use of tranquilizers in elderly patients. *British Journal of Psychiatry,* 1966, *112,* 989-990.

Becker, P.W., & Cesar, J.A. Use of beer on geriatric psychiatric patient groups. *Psychological Reports,* 1973, *33,* p. 182.

Bernal, A., Guillermo, A., Brannon, L.J., Belar, C., Lavigne, J., & Cameron, R. Psychodiagnostics of the elderly. In W.D. Gentry (Ed.), *Geropsychology: A model of training and clinical service.* Cambridge, Mass.: Ballinger Publishing Co., 1977, pp. 43-78.

Cahalan, D., Cisin, I.H., & Crossley, H.M. *American drinking practices: A national study of drinking behavior and attitudes.* New Brunswick, N.J.: Rutgers Center of Alcohol Studies, 1969.

Capel, W.C., & Stewart, J.T. The management of drug abuse in aging populations: New Orleans findings. *Journal of Drug Issues,* 1971, *1,* 114-121.

Capel, W.C., Goldsmith, B.M., Waddell, K.J., & Stewart, G.T. The aging narcotic addict: An increasing problem for the next decades. *Journal of Gerontology,* 1972, *27,* 102-106.

Chambers, C.D. *An assessment of drug use in the general population.* New York: New York State Narcotic Addiction Control Commission, 1971.

Chien, C., Stotsky, B.A., & Cole, J.O. Psychiatric treatment for nursing home patients: Drug, alcohol, and milieu. *American Journal of Psychiatry,* 1973, *130,* 543-548.

Chu, G. Drinking patterns and attitudes of roominghouse Chinese in San Francisco. *Quarterly Journal of Studies on Alcohol,* 1972, *33,* pp. 58-68.

Community Advisory Committee on Aging and Addiction. *Aging and addiction in Arizona.* Unpublished report, Phoenix, Ariz., April 1979, pp. 44.

Epstein, L.J., Mills, C., & Simons, A. Antisocial behavior of the elderly. *Comparative Psychiatry*, 1970, *11*, 36-42.

Gaillard, A., & Perrin, P. L'alcoolisme des personnes agèes. *Revue d'Alcoolisme*, 1969, *15*, pp. 15-32.

Gaitz, C.M., & Baer, P.E. Characteristics of elderly patients with alcoholism. *Archives of General Psychiatry*, 1973, *24*, 372-378.

Gillis, L.S., & Keet, M. Prognostic factors and treatment results in hospitalized alcoholics. *Quarterly Journal of Studies on Alcohol*, 1969, *30*, 426-437.

Gomberg, E.L. *Drinking and problem drinking among the elderly.* Ann Arbor, Mich.: University of Michigan, Institute of Gerontology, 1980.

Gorwitz, K., Bahn, A., Warthen, F.J., & Cooper, M. Some epidemiological data on alcoholism. *Quarterly Journal of Studies on Alcohol*, 1970, *31*, 423-443.

Graux, P. L'alcoolisme des vieillards. *Revue d'Alcoolisme*, 1969, *15*, 46-48.

Harrington, L.G., & Price, A.C. Alcoholism in a geriatric setting. *Journal of the American Geriatric Society*, 1962, *10*, 197-211.

Hoffman, H. Personality characteristics of alcoholics in relation to age. *Psychological Reports*, 1970, *27*, 167-171.

Jones, M.K., & Jones, B.M. The relationship of age and drinking habits to the effects of alcohol on memory in women. *Journal of Studies on Alcohol*, 1980, *41*, 179-186.

Kastenbaum, R., Slater, P.E., & Aisenberg, R. Toward a conceptual model of geriatric psychopharmacology: An experiment with thioridazine and dextroamphetamine. *Gerontologist*, 1964, *4*, 68-71.

Klerman, G.K., & Weissman, M.N. Depressions among women: Their nature and causes. In M. Guttentag, S. Salasin, & D. Belle (Eds.), *The mental health of women.* New York: Academic Press, 1980, pp. 57-92.

Kramer, M. *Patients in state and county mental hospitals* (U.S. Public Health Service Publication No. 1921). Chevy Chase, Md.: U.S. Department of Health, Education, and Welfare, National Institute on Mental Health, 1969.

Lawton, M.P. The functional assessment of elderly people. *Journal of the American Geriatric Society*, 1971, *19*, 465-481.

Learoyd, B.M. Psychotropic drugs and the elderly patient. *Medical Journal of Australia*, 1972, *1*, 1131-1133.

Lennon, B.E., Rekosh, J.H., Patch, V.D., & Howe, L.P. Self-reports of drunkenness arrests. *Quarterly Journal of Studies on Alcohol*, 1970, *31*, 90-96.

Locke, B.Z., Kramer, M., & Pasamanick, B. Alcoholic psychoses among first admissions to public mental health hospitals in Ohio. *Quarterly Journal of Studies on Alcohol*, 1960, *21*, 437-474.

McCucker, J., Cherubin, C.E., & Zimberg, S. Prevalence of alcoholism in general municipal hospital population. *New York State Journal of Medicine*, 1971, *71*, 751-754.

Milliren, J.W. Some contingencies affecting the utilization of tranquilizers in long-term care of the elderly. *Journal of Health and Social Behavior*, 1977, *18*, 206-211.

Mishara, B.L., & Kastenbaum, R. *Alcohol and old age.* New York: Grune & Stratton, Inc., 1980.

Myerson, D.J., & Mayer, J. Origins, treatment and destiny of skid row alcoholic men. *New England Journal of Medicine*, 1966, *275*, 419-426.

National Council on Alcoholism. *A preliminary report on aging and alcoholism.* Washington, D.C.: National Council on Alcoholism, Blue Ribbon Study Commission on Alcoholism and Aging, Office of Public Policy, February 1981.

Nooe, R.M. A model for integrating theoretical approaches to deviance. *Social Work,* 1980, *25*(5), 366-370.

O'Donnell, J.A. *Narcotic addiction in Kentucky* (U.S. Public Health Service Publication No. 1881). Washington, D.C.: U.S. Government Printing Office, 1969.

Pascarelli, E.F. Alcoholism and drug addiction in the elderly. *Geriatric Focus,* 1972, *11,* 1-5.

Pascarelli, E.F., & Fischer, W. Drug dependence in the elderly. *International Journal of Aging and Human Development,* 1974, pp. 206-211.

Petersen, D.M., & Thomas, C.W. Acute drug reactions among the elderly. *Journal of Gerontology,* 1975, *30,* 552-556.

Rakowski, W., & Hickey, T. Late life health behavior: Integrating health beliefs and temporal perspectives. *Research on Aging,* 1980, *2,* 283-309.

Rathbone-McCuan, E., Lohn, H., Levenson, J., & Hsu, J. *Community survey of aged alcoholics and problem drinkers.* Unpublished monograph, Levendale Geriatric Research Center, Baltimore, 1976.

Rathbone-McCuan, E., & Roberds, L. Treatment of the older female alcoholic. *Focus on Women: Journal of Addiction and Health,* 1980, *1,* 104-129.

Reich, L.H., Davies, R.K., & Himmelhoch, J.M. Excessive alcohol use in manic-depressive illness. *American Journal of Psychiatry,* 1974, *131*(1), 83-86.

Rosen, A., & Proctor, E.K. Specifying the treatment process: The basis for effectiveness research. *Journal of Social Service Research,* 1978, *2,* 25-43.

Rosin, A.J., & Glatt, M.M. Alcohol excess in the elderly. *Quarterly Journal of Studies of Alcohol,* 1971, *32,* 52-59.

Schuckit, M.A., & Miller, P.L. Alcoholism in elderly men: A survey of a general medical ward. *Annals of the New York Academy of Sciences,* 1976, *273,* 558-571.

Schuckit, M.A., Pitts, F.N., Reich, T., King, L.J., & Winokur, G. Alcoholism I two types of alcoholism in women. *Archives of General Psychiatry,* 1979, *20,* 301-306.

Siassi, I., Crocetti, G., & Spiro, H.R. Drinking patterns and alcoholism in a blue-collar population. *Quarterly Journal of Studies on Alcohol,* 1973, *34,* 917-926.

Simon, A., Epstein, L.J., & Reynolds, L. Alcoholism in the geriatric mentally ill. *Geriatrics,* 1968, *23,* 125-131.

Tyndel, M. Psychiatric study of one thousand alcohol patients. *Canadian Psychiatric Association Journal,* 1974, *31,* 759-764.

Whittington, F.J., & Petersen, D.M. Drugs and the elderly. In D.M. Petersen, F.J. Whittington, & B.P. Payne (Eds.), *Drugs and the elderly: Social and pharmacological issues.* Springfield, Ill.: Charles C Thomas, Publisher, 1979, pp. 14-27.

Winick, C. Physician narcotic addicts. *Social Problems,* 1961, *9,* 174-186.

Winick, C. Maturing out of addiction. *Bulletin of Narcotics,* 1962, *14,* 107.

Zimberg, S. Outpatient geriatric psychiatry in an urban ghetto with nonprofessional workers. *American Journal of Psychiatry,* 1969, *125*(12), 1697-1707.

Zimberg, S. The psychiatrist and medical home care geriatric psychiatry in the Harlem community. *American Journal of Psychiatry,* 1971, *127*(9), 1062-1066.

Zimberg, S. The elderly alcoholic. *Gerontologist,* 1974, *14,* 221-244.

Zimberg, S. Alcohol and the elderly. In D.M. Petersen, F.J. Whittington, & B. P. Payne (Eds.), *Drugs and the elderly: Social and pharmacological issues.* Springfield, Ill.: Charles C Thomas, Publisher, 1979, pp. 29-40.

Chapter 10

The Chronic Mentally Disabled Grown Old

INTRODUCTION

In the process of selecting the various subgroups of elderly to be addressed as isolated populations, no preliminary attempt was made to try to rank the groups from the least to the most severely isolated. On the contrary, it was important to address the various dilemmas of each group for their unique circumstances in order to emphasize the different issues and considerations as they relate to intervention. However, it is the judgment of many experts that the life-long seriously mentally disabled individual grown old deserves to be considered as the most isolated of the isolated.

This complex chapter focuses on intervention for the chronically mentally disabled, which after all is the most important consideration. This required sifting through much material on either chronicity without specific reference to the elderly or their psychological impairment, which is a broader issue. Much of the material available to practitioners does not give operational suggestions to help provide services for this specific group.

The literature and media accounts abound with examples of cases of the chronically mentally disabled grown old and document their plight as persons in custodial institutions and other environments that neglect their human potential by reinforcing their isolation. To restate all of these studies or case descriptions would merely further legitimize these persons' extremely isolated circumstances. That seems unnecessary and almost self-defeating if the goal of problem analysis is planning better intervention.

Material from the literature describes the conditions of the population, and the somewhat questionable statistics that describe the prevalence of chronic mental disability are referenced. The best available statistics clearly underestimate the current numbers and do not give sufficiently accurate projections of the future size of this group that will be in need of treatment when life-long adult conditions

237

converge with the problems of their advancing years. The cases selected give a sense of reality to the types of situations these people face and reflect the case files of hundreds of mental institutions.

At the highest levels of public mental health service planning, several national task forces studied the complexities of this population and explored solutions to serve it better. These panels were expected to create models that would be far-reaching in nature and require the involvement of macro resources to support the continuing provision of mental health care for all mentally disabled groups. Despite the input from experts in model construction, the authors foresee some limitations.

- The larger mental health system would have to change in order to redirect more of the limited resources from acute to chronic groups or increase the resources now available to the chronic population by making new money available.

- These models would be somewhat idealistic and not immediately applicable in different states or sections of the country where the bureaucratic structure of mental health resources continued to be heavily weighted in favor of maintaining large institutionally based programs.

- The relevance of these models to communities might be merely academic since local mental health resources already were stretched to the breaking point. This stretch existed even before new service outreach to, and care of, the elderly chronic mentally disabled could be assigned by the federal government to these local and state service entities. With budget cuts being made in all service systems on the federal level, it seems unlikely that the states will receive any additional funds to implement new programs.

It may not be possible to care for this additional chronic target group. The model proposed in this chapter may provide a framework under which available local resources can be better organized to maximize the use of mental health dollars and provide a context within which a community could analyze its programs and target priorities for future development.

The recommendations posed here for developing intervention strategies are based on a single principle: the necessity of these individuals to have access to a continuum of service alternatives that meet individual needs. This principle challenges the continuation of the almost standard practice of plugging the chronically mentally disabled elderly into what is available, which usually means some form of institutional care. This is touted as an alternative to mental hospital placement. Yet whatever the deficits of the state hospital system throughout the country, such settings may offer greater protection for the chronically mentally disabled than the community facilities to which they are discharged (Subcommittee on Long-Term Care, 1976).

To the extent that any agency or community coalition makes an effort to address the needs of this group, their strategy is blatantly misdirected if it includes only the development of more nursing home beds where these elderly can be placed in order to discharge them or exit them from the mental health system. As laid out, the argument here challenges this as the only acceptable alternative to meet the needs of large numbers of these individuals, particularly if the institutional environments to which they are referred are less therapeutic and more custodial than the state hospital from which they are being discharged.

There has been frequent mention of the need to provide this group with a continuum of services. This principle has been encouraged but there has been more written about advocacy than there has been concrete action. Implementation activities are doomed to limited success unless it is possible to assure the pursuit of intervention goals that do more than dump people from one place into another. Any strategy that does not bring together the appropriate resources of the age-specific network in coordination with help from other health, social, and general welfare services cannot meet the needs of this group. Some of the attempts to do something for these elderly have resulted in little more than holding them over an abyss of continued isolation until they conveniently expire.

A SUBPOPULATION OF THE MENTALLY ILL ELDERLY

The mentally disabled elderly are a collective of diverse groups that include: (a) those who are experiencing more recent, and perhaps transient, mental dysfunctions that are a response to stressful events directly related to aging, e.g., retirement, increased physical impairment, death of spouse or friends; (b) those who are experiencing problems associated with chronic or reversible organic brain syndromes, and (c) those who have been mentally afflicted most of their lives and now are facing the combined effects of a lifetime of such disability and problems associated with the aging process. While the existence of this diversity may be recognized (Butler & Lewis, 1977), gerontologists usually have directed their attention toward late onset disorders, including those identified in the first two groups above (Butler & Lewis, 1977; Busse & Pfeiffer, 1977; Busse & Blazer, 1980). This focus on late onset disabilities leads to emphasis on stressful events that occur later in life to explain the cause of the disorders and form a basis for treatment.

There is an implicit assumption that the elderly with longstanding mental disorders are outside the province of gerontologists since their specific conditions are not related to the aging process. Whatever concern for this group does exist among gerontologists appears to revolve around deinstitutionalization and the frequent scandals associated with poor nursing home care (Donahue, 1978; Butler, 1975). Psychiatric researchers have been accused of ignoring older schizophrenics

(Bridge, Cannon, & Wyatt, 1978). Authors who discuss chronic mental disorder, while they do not exclude consideration of the elderly, focus their discussions on programs that appear more relevant for younger patients (Stein, 1979; Group for the Advancement of Psychiatry, 1978). This gap in the literature on both chronicity and mental health and the elderly leaves unexplored the process of severe disorder and the interactive influences that combine in these patients.

It has not been possible to identify accurately the numbers of elderly who are chronically mentally disabled, since there has been little consistency in the way chronic conditions are defined. The deinstitutionalization movement, stressing outpatient care, also has contributed to the difficulty in gathering accurate data (Goldman, Gattozzi, and Taube, 1981). As a further complication, the focus of this chapter, the chronically mentally disabled grown old, by definition has excluded those with organic disorders linked to the aging process. No published data attempt to estimate the total number of mentally disabled elderly throughout the nation. However, to provide a general idea of the numbers of individuals of concern in this subgroup one can look at estimates of the number of elders institutionalized with chronic mental disorder. According to the President's Commission on Mental Health (1978), in 1973 there were 70,615 patients over 65 years of age in state and county mental hospitals. There were 14,490 new admissions in 1972 and 8,222 in 1975, which indicated that the number of elders being admitted to mental hospitals was declining. As of 1973, there also were 1,534 in private mental hospitals and 5,819 in Veterans Administration hospitals.

Unfortunately, these figures do not distinguish between longstanding and recent onset mental disorders. To these numbers should be added the 193,900 patients with chronic mental disorder diagnoses residing in nursing homes, according to 1973 data. The numbers in all mental institutions represented a drop of approximately 37 percent from the 1969 total. The number of patients in nursing homes rose 100 percent during that same period. These figures illustrate the rapid shifting of elderly patients from psychiatric facilities to nursing homes in 15 years (President's Commission on Mental Health, 1978).

In viewing these statistics, it must be noted that attempting to estimate the numbers of chronic mentally disabled elderly by looking at those who are institutionalized fails to account for the many with a long history of such confinement or those discharged to the community in the 60s and 70s with no records kept on where they went (Donahue, 1978). Other factors besides the existence of mental disorder seem related to whether given individuals reach a treatment resource because of the visibility of their symptoms, their socially disruptive potential, the availability of assistance, alternative interpretations of symptoms, and symptom tolerance by significant others (Mechanic, 1969).

Some community studies have estimated the prevalence of mental disorder among the elderly. Busse and Blazer (1980) reported an estimate of 5 to 10 percent of the elderly in the community with significant or severe mental impairment.

Lowenthal and Berkman (1967) said 15 percent of a community sample of elderly had moderate or severe impairment and Abrahams and Patterson (1978-79) found 17 percent of a similar sample with psychological impairment.

These variances probably reflect differences in how disorder is defined. However, the first study mentioned did not differentiate between longstanding and recent onset of the disorder. Lowenthal (1965), in discussing a San Francisco study, stated that 65 percent of the impaired in the community reported serious psychiatric problems before age 60. Abrahams and Patterson's data divided the community elderly with psychological impairment into groups on the basis of time of onset. They divided the number of individuals who were psychologically impaired (17 percent of the total sample) into currently impaired (4 percent), currently and formerly impaired (13 percent), and formerly impaired (13 percent). Past impairment was defined as their having had problems prior to the previous three years.

These figures suggest that a majority of elders with significant psychological impairment had also had problems at an earlier age. Using these data to determine the extent to which current mental disability is linked to previous impairment may be compromised by the potential inaccuracy of recall and by defining past as prior to three years. This would mean, for example, that an individual who is now 70 and began experiencing mental problems four years ago at age 66 would be included in the chronic group even though the disorder may be linked to the aging process and of relatively recent origin.

The community studies' data also must be used with care when dealing more specifically with individuals who are experiencing severe mental disability, for some of the psychological measures used to define a case do not necessarily distinguish totally disabling chronic conditions from those of severe chronic maladjustment. What may be concluded, however, is that in reality there is no reliable count on the numbers of chronic mentally disabled elderly, as opposed to those with late onset dysfunctions. These elderly often are isolated from family, friends, community, and mental health treatment resources. They are of grave concern for caregivers in the health and welfare services who must deal with them on a daily basis without the help of community programs and services.

EXPERIENCES OF CHRONIC CASES

The experiences that the chronically mentally disabled elderly have faced can be understood by examining the history of the changing ideology of treatment. For those who came into contact with the mental health establishment many years ago and could not afford private care, the treatment consisted of placement in state mental hospitals where many stayed for the greater part of their adult years. During this extended stay the patients lost contact with and connectedness to family and community, became dependent on the institution to fulfill daily needs, and either lost or did not develop the social skills necessary to cope independently outside of an institution. Institutionalization and its consequences became a secondary condition superimposed on an original disorder.

A smaller number of the chronically mentally disabled elderly developed a similar type of dependency on their family or surrogate family group. Their adult life was spent within the family setting where they became passive and dependent. Individuals of this sort may finally come to the attention of authorities when the last family caregiver dies and some other alternative must be found.

Beginning in the 1960s, the development of the community mental health movement fostered a new view of treatment based on:

1. the evidence of unintended but powerful antitherapeutic forces inherent in large custodial institutions (Bloom, 1973; Goffman, 1961)
2. the evidence that psychotropic drugs can control psychotic behaviors to the extent that 24-hour institutionalization is not necessary (Bloom, 1973; Group for the Advancement of Psychiatry, 1978)
3. the belief that all clients, even those with severe disorders, could be treated in the community (Bloom, 1973; Group for the Advancement of Psychiatry, 1978)
4. the mushrooming costs of long-term care and the increasing numbers of patients in custodial institutions (Donahue, 1978; Group for the Advancement of Psychiatry, 1978)

This change in treatment focus was the impetus behind a two-decade deinstitutionalization thrust within the mental health establishment. At the beginning of this movement younger patients were the first target group for care in the community rather than in institutions. These cases were maintained relatively successfully in the community (Group for the Advancement of Psychiatry, 1978). This strategy then was applied to move into communities large numbers of older patients who had remained in hospitals and who continued to fill the beds of the state institutions.

The combination of heavy financial costs to state governments to maintain large hospital complexes for the care of chronic mental patients, combined with the availability of funds to finance nursing and boarding home care and the increased numbers of nursing homes available throughout the United States, all contributed to the community placement for the large numbers of these elderly persons. Indeed the need for care of discharged older mental patients developed a "veritable industry of sheltered care facilities. . . . Many attendants, nurses or aides who wanted to go into business for themselves saw an opportunity to remodel old residences into board and care homes. Others found that they could supplement their incomes by opening their homes to patients released from hospitals. . . . Many if not most of these providers . . . had neither the interest nor the capacity to provide activity and rehabilitation programs'' (Group for the Advancement of Psychiatry, 1978).

What had happened in response to the theoretical and ideological emphasis on community placement was in reality a shift in the type of custodial care setting rather than treatment and a reintegration into community life. There are a number of reasons why this outcome was inevitable:

First of all, the large numbers of patients who were moved in a very short time precluded the making of careful assessment of their needs, of local resources, and of follow-up care to ensure readjustment to community life. In retrospect, it would seem that many administrators who were in the vanguard in the decision to release so many elderly chronic cases seriously misjudged the community resources needed to provide care for these long-term patients (Bloom, 1973). An alternative interpretation was that the administrators did not bother to assess the resources and just went ahead despite the protest of a minority of professionals who anticipated the serious consequences.

The rapid discharging of many chronic patients was in fact simply a transfer of individuals from one type of institution to another. The special and extensive help these individuals needed to reenter the community and to become integrated into its fabric to the extent to which they might have been able was not seen as a priority. Discharged to the nursing home, they were being sent to a place where they could be housed, medicated, and given marginal supervision. Many of these patients never knew they had been ''liberated'' to the community.

The outcome of these inadequate procedures was the much publicized scandals of former mental patients and the inadequacy of care provided in the community (Butler, 1975; Koenig, 1978). The federal financial support policies, by providing monies for clients outside of state institutions for those without family support, encouraged discharges from hospitals and into private boarding or nursing homes. This shift could be made easily, with little attention to client preparation. For states faced with rapidly rising state hospital costs, this meant they could move large numbers of patients to other facilities and shift the financial burden to the federal government.

Secondly, the shift of patients was made with no understanding of what community resources would be needed in terms of types of residences and after-care services (Donahue, 1978). It had been anticipated that after-care could be provided by the developing community mental health centers. Unfortunately, this did not happen. The centers were not developed as rapidly as expected and those that did emerge were directed more toward outpatient services to the less severely disabled and used the more traditional approaches to therapeutic intervention. They did not have the interest, knowledge, or programs necessary to intervene with the chronically disabled (Donahue, 1978; Ford & Sbordone, 1980).

These agencies were ill-equipped to deal with the combined characteristics of a lifelong history of unbroken institutionalization or a revolving door pattern of several readmissions; a history of either many unsuccessful treatments or no treatment at all; and a continuous pattern of poverty, little education, poor occupational history, and very limited personal and financial resources.

Chronic patients are more likely to be poor, based on evidence that they are more apt to be placed in state hospitals as a treatment response to mental disorder and less likely to be considered good candidates for psychotherapy (Hollingshead & Redlich, 1958; Srole, Langner, Michael, Opler, & Rennie, 1962). In addition, of individuals who receive mental health services, many more who are of the lower socioeconomic class remain impaired than in the higher classes (Srole et al., 1962). Thus from the very beginning these clients, because of limited educational background and pressing financial and resource problems, were less likely to have the verbal skills to be successful in traditional psychotherapy, more apt to have problems associated with resource needs outside that psychotherapy's purview, and expect more concrete advice, guidance, and direct service from caregivers (Cobb, 1972; Myers & Bean, 1968).

In the absence of a meaningful response to their problems, low socioeconomic class individuals are most likely to discontinue treatment (Kline, Adrian, & Spevak, 1974). Thus, they can be viewed as continuing victims of a mental health system that has not developed the treatment approaches or given priority to their class. The elderly are among those victims (Butler, 1975; Ford & Sbordone, 1980).

Thirdly, an additional barrier to reintegration of the chronically mentally disabled into the community has been the negative attitudes against individuals so diagnosed (Donahue, 1978; Aviram & Segal, 1973). These negative attitudes have resulted in their exclusion from the community by zoning laws and neighborhood pressures to restrict development of residences, increased use of the penal code to commit individuals to mental institutions, and perhaps even an overuse of medication to leave them docile in their alternative care institutions and unlikely candidates for integration into local activities (Aviram & Segal, 1973).

Persons in this subgroup face isolators that are longstanding because their disorder has kept them apart from friends and family and those responsible for their treatment have ignored their needs. These factors are multiplied in their present circumstances since they lack personal skills and resources (as a result of past institutional care), have no social network on which to rely, and now face the additional isolators of aging, which include poverty, physical impairment, and a bias against them in the mental health establishment. (Figure 10-1 identifies isolators affecting the chronically mentally disabled.) The age-specific network does not want them, the mental health system has no room for them, and the rest of the human service agencies do not know what to do with them, so they often are ignored.

Figure 10-1 Isolators Affecting the Chronically Mentally Disabled Elder

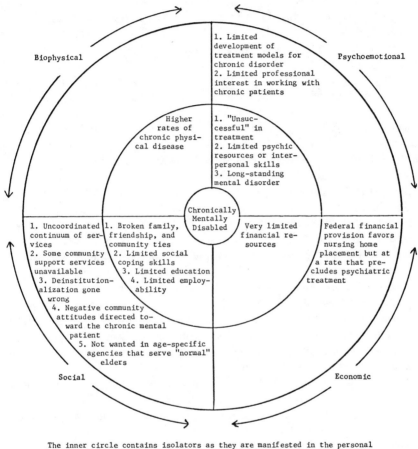

The inner circle contains isolators as they are manifested in the personal lives of the chronically mentally disabled, the outer circle those that abound in the environment.

To complete the documentation of the problems associated with intervention with the chronically mentally disabled elderly, two cases are presented. They illustrate two prevalent types of clients who come to the attention of mental health workers.

Wilbur Jones

Wilbur is 66 years old. He has never been hospitalized for mental disorder but has had significant personal and social adjustment problems throughout his life. His mental status frequently concerned medical and social service providers with whom he had contact. He never accepted nor heeded any advice to seek specific mental health treatment. Wilbur was married as a young man. His quarrelsome, suspicious behavior led to a divorce within a short time. He has lived alone since, supporting himself by a series of jobs, all of which were at a low skill level and none of which involved extensive interaction with others. This man has been unemployed for three years and is receiving a Social Security pension.

He is estranged from most family members except for one sister, Hannah, who was widowed recently and has since visited occasionally, helped him clean his small apartment, and loaned him whatever money she could afford. For some time she had been trying to interest him in attending senior center activities since he no longer was employed. She had even spoken with one of the workers at the center about Wilbur, who was alone much of the time. His only outings were riding his bicycle in the neighborhood. He never spoke to anyone.

Hannah, with the prompting of one of the center workers, did succeed in taking Wilbur to the center one day but it was hardly a successful venture. He rebuffed those who tried to be friendly and complained loudly about the food that was served. The others at the center seemed alarmed by his behavior. Later at Wilbur's apartment, he and Hannah argued because she had been quite upset with his behavior toward her friends. In the midst of this argument he threatened her with a gun he kept in his apartment and pushed her out the door.

Hannah was alarmed, and concerned that her brother might harm himself, so she called the police and told them about the gun. The police arrived in force and called to Wilbur to come out. His response was a shot from his gun. The police fired several cannisters of tear gas into the house but this did not seem to affect Wilbur. Eventually two policemen were able to enter the apartment by a rear door. They found him sitting in a chair in the living room and were able to convince him to come out of the house. Surprisingly, he seemed almost unaffected by the tear gas even though one of the policemen was overcome by it. Wilbur was taken to a psychiatric ward for treatment.

This case is an example of a lifetime of marginal adjustment, possibly exacerbated by changes associated with the aging process, that culminates in an episode of violent behavior and finally catches the attention of mental health service providers. There was need for immediate hospitalization and careful medical and psychosocial assessment to understand Wilbur's outburst more completely. The fact that he had not been in contact with mental health authorities earlier seems less related to his need than to other factors that influence whether or not an individual is brought to the attention of providers.

Wilbur is capable of meeting his own self-care needs but will require continued monitoring once his behavior is stabilized. He also may need a somewhat protective residential setting. It may be well to include Hannah in the treatment plan so she can continue support for her brother but can understand his limitations better. While Wilbur may not be able to cope with large social gatherings at the senior citizen center, he might be able to enjoy the companionship of one or two individuals, which might be arranged if he should so desire. It must be noted that a senior center or its volunteers cannot assume sole responsibility for planning Wilbur's treatment but can assist in that care by offering supportive services in consultation with mental health professionals. All of these plans depend, of course, on Wilbur's reaching stability in the hospital and whether he must face criminal charges.

Susan Este

Susan's situation is quite different from Wilbur's for she has spent a major part of her adult years in a state mental hospital. She was first admitted to the hospital at age 23 and was diagnosed as schizophrenic. She remained there for 30 years. In her last few years at the hospital she was particularly well-liked by the nursing staff. She was neat in appearance, quiet in manner, and quite helpful in ward housekeeping tasks. After her discharge she lived with her widowed mother. Her functioning after discharge was good and she was able to maintain herself and her mother's home well.

When her mother died, Susan was quite overwhelmed and distraught by the loss and by the tasks that were then pressed on her. Although she had been quite helpful with household chores, someone always had been there to tell her what had to be done. She now felt quite alone. Because of her history of hospitalization, the family doctor suggested she might need to return. She accepted his judgment and was rehospitalized briefly before being placed in the Grenor boarding home.

Susan soon fell into a routine of helping in the home and caring for some of the other residents. There were four boarders in this unlicensed boarding home, living in basement quarters. As a matter of fact, Susan soon became the sole caregiver for a rather incapacitated elderly man who was a former mental patient. This patient had been placed in the home six years earlier and because of inadequate follow-up had remained there in spite of the home's not being licensed to care for someone needing extensive nursing care. Susan developed bleeding ulcers on one leg, there appeared to be little circulation in the leg, and the danger of gangrene existed. She knew her leg needed care but didn't know how to obtain it.

The Grenors, who ran the home, were angry and insulted by accusations that they were profiteering at the expense of helpless patients. They saw themselves as offering these patients the best home that could be provided given the limited funds available. They felt that Susan's leg would be a lot better if she would stay off it, as they had told her once they saw the sores. They acknowledged the work she performed and felt that it was something she wanted to do and that it was therapeutic for her to help others. The Grenors felt harrassed by state and county officials, who frequently told them what was wrong but never offered much support or realistic advice on how to handle the situation better. Both Mr. and Mrs.

Grenor had jobs elsewhere. The money for patient care, after overhead costs, did not leave enough for either one to remain at home without income from outside employment.

The after-care worker from the state hospital seemed equally frustrated. Because of the large number of patients for whom she was responsible, she considered that the best she could do was to try to check each home once a month. The last time she was at the home, Susan had not mentioned any problems with her leg. A neighbor's complaint had led to an investigation. The subsequent revelation of Susan's need for medical treatment had surprised the caseworker, who acknowledged that the level of care and the cleanliness standards of the home were minimal, but in her opinion there were no alternatives available. She realized that the aged patient Susan was caring for needed more attention than could be provided in the boarding home, and a reconsideration of the man's status was planned. The worker was concerned, however, about the impact if he were to be moved from the familiar surroundings of the home and the personal caring extended by the others there. Reports of the situation had been on file with the department but no action had been taken that would either remove the patients or force some improvements in the home.

Susan's case points up a number of problems in the care system for the chronically mentally disabled elderly. This woman, like so many others, was removed from the state hospital system without the necessary placement planning or follow-up care. Appropriate community resources did not exist but she was placed anyway. Staff was not available to train Susan to develop the skills necessary for independent living so she was placed in a structured environment. Typical structured environments that are used out of necessity are not geared to treating clients for eventual independent living but rather to extend custodial care at minimal cost.

In addition to the systemic factors that kept Susan in this facility, personal factors were at work. She resembles many older chronic patients in that she lacks the necessary assertiveness to protect herself from exploitation. Such a lack may be a component or manifestation of a change in symptomatology called burnout. Burnout refers to a tendency, particularly during midlife, for symptoms of schizophrenia to lessen and for social adjustment and work capacity to increase (Bridge, Cannon, & Wyatt, 1978).

Even though some research has affirmed changes in symptomatology associated with aging (Sanders, Smith, & Weinman, 1967; Bridge, Cannon, & Wyatt, 1978), the dynamics behind these shifts are obscure. It may be that, like the strivings that are modified over time by all individuals, chronically mentally disabled individuals as they age give up their efforts, which may produce what others see as deviant or psychotic behavior. For the aging psychotic, burnout may well represent the acceptance of isolation from self to end isolation with others and perhaps to attain their acceptance.

Thus the transition to a quiet, cooperative passivity that gives entry to more linkages to the external environment can result in less linkage with self. Yet another interpretation that fits the aging process framework is that the intensity of the passions of seeking to work out inner feelings simply exhaust the biopsychological system. This implies that the condition is controlled biologically and not consciously by the person in a manner similar to some of the other biological aspects of aging.

Most clinicians would agree that a chronic patient with less overt symptomatology is likely to be more acceptable in the community and have more options to live outside the institutional world. However, if the elder person is to gain from these shifts in symptomatology there should be a significant other who will respond to this change with positive reinforcement. What in fact seems to have occurred is that quiet, cooperative behavior has led to exploitation by caregivers who neglect clients' needs and desires. The dependency of these clients prevents them from being able to live independently in the community without considerable support and skills training.

This is Susan's position. An entirely different outcome can be envisioned if she had been assisted to find living quarters with others who could provide her with an opportunity to develop a mutually helping relationship—one in which she could learn and increase her ability to function in the community.

These cases depict clients with different treatment histories and varied levels of symptomatology. In addition to these types, most caseloads also include clients who are markedly confused, possess few skills in self-maintenance, or are severely physically impaired. It is important to emphasize the numbers of individuals who, with less intensive skills training, could be reintegrated into the community. For clients who are more severely impaired, more extensive skills training and placement in protective settings would be necessary, at least as a first step. It should not be assumed, however, that the extra structure and care will be needed on a continuing basis nor that all chronic mentally disabled can be brought to full social functioning. What is suggested is that improvement is always a possibility and that, over time and with appropriate treatment, these clients may need less structured living arrangements and less intensive supportive care, if serious physical impairment does not occur.

INTERVENTION FOR THE DISABLED ELDERLY

Intervention with the chronically mentally disabled elderly often has been approached in a rather simplistic manner. The basic assumption seems to have been that these individuals are suffering from an irreversible chronic process for which little could be done except to put them in a structured environment to replace the custodial care offered at the state hospital. This basic assumption has led many to view the boarding or nursing home as the alternative of choice. This treatment assumption may be colored by ageism in the mental health establishment because many professionals who would advocate the placement of younger mentally or physically handicapped individuals in less structured community settings do not consider the handicapped elderly for any but the most protective setting.

Because of this bias some practitioners are less likely to perceive the possibilities of social skills learning and community care programs for the elderly. Other workers may realize that other treatment possibilities do exist but may lack the time and resources to implement plans that involve the use of these alternatives. Practitioners working in the public mental health system have been caught in the no-win situation of having to meet the cost-efficiency expectations of administrators while also making the best clinical decisions they can for their patients.

Nowhere is the double bind greater than with elderly chronic patients. There are many pressures to see the patients' potential in terms of the dollars that must be expended if they are to reach independence. This mentality and related service policies lead to a denial of the elderly persons' right to treatment and care. They also foster a trade-off of the rights of younger patients against older ones. However, the considerable expense involved in placing patients for long-term care in boarding or nursing homes, which are high in cost and absorb considerable proportions of Medicaid dollars, may reduce the expenses for mental health agencies and institutions but place a heavy burden on other budgets.

Providing treatment for elderly chronic persons would reassure recognition of the strengths and treatability of this client group. Treatment could be offered without detriment to younger patient groups if programs were to be paid for from the dollars now going to boarding and nursing home care. While good community care is not necessarily less expensive than institutional treatment, it would be cost-efficient in that hospital returns and use of costly total care community institutions will be minimized.

The ensuing discussion seeks to maintain a balance between the need to propose a system whereby adequate services to the elderly chronic patient could be provided while at the same time the reality of limited funds is recognized.

In the development of more appropriate assessment and treatment planning for the chronically mentally disabled elderly, it is essential to consider the residential need of the client, the availability of social and financial supports, and the professional supports needed to supplement family or community social supports.

The personal characteristics of the elderly that influence assessment and treatment planning include the extent to which the client is actively psychotic, in terms of acting out behavior. There appears to be some evidence that over time, particularly between 55 and 64, there is a tendency for change in the symptomatology of chronic mental disorder, more specifically in schizophrenia (Bridge, Cannon, & Wyatt, 1978). There is a tendency for many individuals to improve greatly, while for others there is a greater ability to live with psychotic phenomena.

The degree to which there are overt psychotic behaviors can be a determining factor in the acceptability of an individual in community life.

In reality many in the community already have decidedly negative attitudes toward the mentally disabled (Aviram & Segal, 1973; Donahue, 1978). The more individuals' behavior is markedly different the more likely they are to experience negative attitudes and decreased probability of access to community activities.

Other key factors include the extent of physical impairment and the degree to which clients have maintained self-care skills. Lowenthal and Berkman (1967) identified several specific self-management skills: the ability to dress themselves, to move about the neighborhood independently, to provide for personal safety, to comply with health care regimes, and to manage personal finances.

The maintenance of these skills tended to discriminate between elders with severe mental disorder who remained in the community and those who were hospitalized. This suggests that for the institutionalized elderly, treatment should emphasize the teaching of these skills or promoting a higher capacity to perform them to enable the individuals to live outside such a setting. The extent to which clients lack confidence in their ability to live in a less protective environment is a related element.

In highlighting these considerations, emphasis has been placed on current needs and level of functioning. It must be remembered that the population of concern is chronically impaired to the degree that amelioration of the primary disorder cannot be expected, nor can these persons be restored to full social functioning since their aging process is not reversible. Therefore, the treatment program should emphasize maintenance and development of the social and self-management skills that would allow the clients to live in the most nearly normal and least restrictive settings. The practitioner also must be aware that the individuals probably will continue to need support indefinitely.

Because of the extensive dependency that has developed as a byproduct of institutionalization and of the disorder, it is important that there be supportiveness and encouragement at all points during treatment. Supportiveness in this context refers to verbal and nonverbal behaviors that demonstrate the practitioner's belief that the clients are capable of learning self-management skills. Encouragement refers to positive verbal and nonverbal behaviors that encourage patients' attempts to continue to carry out self-management tasks.

The factors above are important concerns for the assessment of the elderly's whole situation, including understanding of the community where they now reside or to which they may be discharged. This assessment process begins with a chronic patient in a hospital ward after referral from a community setting or in a nonhospital placement that seems inappropriate. The assessment may occur at a mental hospital, a nursing home, or a medical facility. Regardless of the type of facility, there are standardized treatment responses that are appropriate to clients in the various situations. These responses must focus on assessment of the individuals' current functioning and of potential community resources, then making the best possible match between resources and client needs.

A carefully developed social history is the first step in the assessment process. This information includes the establishment of the existence of a longstanding disorder by means of a description of work and personal history, family relationships, current behaviors and situation, and medical and psychiatric treatment. The information should be obtained from clients and from any significant others who can be reached or from hospital records. In conducting the social history interviews, the practitioner should be particularly careful to be unhurried and allow the elderly to tell their stories without frequent interruptions for details. At the end of the statements, questions may be asked to clarify specifics.

It must be remembered that the individuals at this point are in a state of crisis superimposed on a chronic condition. Wherever they are living, the intervention may involve a change in residence. This may mean a move from one community residence or institution to another, from the community to the hospital, or from the hospital to the community. Any such change in status is likely to promote anxiety, resistance, and perhaps fearfulness or distrust. These feelings must be recognized and are best handled with patience, continued reassurance, and by involving the mentally disabled as much as possible in all decision making.

Some information on the clients' self-management capacity can be gained in the history-taking interview with both the individuals and significant others. If any observation periods are available, they can be used to support information gained in the interviews.

Those furnishing information may have many reasons for not being able to provide it accurately. It may have been assumed that the individuals were incapable of certain activities rather than really knowing whether or not they were truly incapable. The wish to have a difficult, nonproductive family member placed in an institution may lead relatives to distort the individual's capacity. That wish (or need) should be viewed with understanding. The family may face other conflicting needs and feel drained and despairing over the constancy of the burden that this one individual has imposed. Family needs must be taken into consideration in any treatment planning. As there is a beginning recognition of the problems of staff burnout for those who work with chronic patients (Mendel, 1979), that awareness should be extended to family members and their stress.

The chronically disturbed persons may distort information for a number of reasons, such as a wish to stay at or return to the hospital. Many clients are placed in more protective settings because of their fearfulness and anxiety developed through past failures at trying to manage on their own. A series of environmental stressors may prompt them to seek out the protectiveness and safety of the hospital or a sheltered setting. Thus, the more the practitioner can augment interview data with direct observation, the more reliable the information. While at first it may seem unnecessary to gather this type of history on individuals who may still reside in a state hospital system in spite of the exodus of chronic patients in the late 60s and early 70s, it may well be needed since information on self-management skills must be updated frequently.

Once relevant social history information has been gathered, it must be combined with the results of a thorough physical examination. The presence of a physical disease and/or a mobility limitation resulting from physiological factors is an important qualifier in the treatment and placement process. If the chronic mentally disabled elders' current residence is not in a hospital and there is a crisis associated with deteriorating physical condition, it may be necessary to rehospitalize them for a short time to treat the condition and/or restabilize their medications. The decision to rehospitalize must be balanced between needs created by a physical or mental crisis and the anxiety such a return may create. Depending on specific state guidelines, on the status of the chronic mental patients, or on their needs and desires, this short reinstitutionalization could be arranged at either a state hospital or a general community hospital unit.

Whether the clients must be rehospitalized or can remain in the community, social care must be instituted along with any medical treatment. This treatment should be focused on seeking the cause of the current crisis, helping the patients to understand the meaning of the event, and working with them to seek resolution. This may call for some advocacy efforts by the practitioner but this should be done only if the clients cannot handle this task themselves and always should include their participation to the greatest extent possible.

In the event that the patients are operating below their potential in self-management, every effort should be made to see to it that the hospital routine assists in the development and maintenance of those abilities. This can be done best by a teaching relationship between client and practitioner and by making the hospital stay as short as possible. For those who must remain in the hospital for a longer period, the behavioral-oriented approach introduces therapeutic intervention directed toward social learning of basic skills.

During hospitalization, the use of medication to modify behavior must be monitored very carefully so that it can aid rather than inhibit psychosocial treatment. The situation, described by Butler (1975), of "overmedicated, zombie-like persons only dimly aware of the world around them" is one where no treatment can realistically take place. Since older chronic patients often can do well with reduced dosages or elimination of psychotropic drugs (Walker & Brodie, 1980), they must be carefully monitored. Given the likelihood that the physician will not be present continuously, the observation task may fall on other staff members, particularly nursing personnel, who must translate patient response data back to the doctor.

Some of the general cautions physicians make to their medical colleagues on prescribing psychotropic medications are important: such prescriptions should be based on specific data about the patients' medical condition; a small test dosage is recommended, after which, if no major side effects emerge, the dosage may be increased until therapeutic benefits or toxicity develop; and drug-free holidays are advocated to lessen the chance of long-term side effects, especially tardive dyskinesia. If the antipsychotic medication is discontinued when early signs of this disorder appear, it usually is possible to reverse the condition completely (Walker & Brodie, 1980).

The hospital treatment also should include special attention to diet and exercise programs. Some patients, even those in institutions, may be suffering from nutritional deficiencies (Butler, 1975). For many, vitamin supplements may be quite appropriate (Walker & Brodie, 1980). An exercise program can benefit all patients regardless of their level of incapacity. Some excellent hospital unit programs involve patients, all of whom are confined to walker, wheelchair, or bed, that combine exercise with socialization and thus yield a double benefit.

For those with minimal physical impairment who might be able to function outside of a mental hospital except for limited self-management skills, this aspect of treatment is most cogent. The teaching of self-management skills begins while the individuals are still in the hospital and for maximum effectiveness should be continued during and after outside placement.

Assessment and hospital treatment should culminate in discharge planning. For many of the chronically mentally disabled, this aspect of treatment is critical since appropriate discharge planning and after-care are vital to minimize the possibility of rehospitalization. The discharge planning and implementation process is concerned primarily with making the best possible available match between client needs and resources. In reaching this goal several areas of critical concern are:

1. Determining the upper and lower levels of individuals' functional capacity and under what circumstances these are likely to be achieved. Efforts should be made to judge this through trial visits to the alternative settings being considered.
2. Evaluating the physical health problems. There is no substitute for a good medical examination before the person leaves the inpatient facility. This may be useful in determining additional medications, special dietary requirements, exercise needs, or medical problems that may require future attention.
3. Considering the range of socialization opportunities and social role possibilities to determine to what extent the elderly may be able to become more socially involved if the environment offers the proper stimulation and support. It is very easy to underestimate individuals' potential if the inpatient environment has not provided stimuli to encourage social interaction. On the other hand, some patients have been known to lose much of their socialization and capacity for social activities once they leave the hospital because

community facilities do not contain the range of program opportunities routinely available in the institution.

4. Assessing the qualities of the community alternative to consider the resources available for care as well as the potential for developing social outlets for the patients.

5. Assuring that the geographic locale of the facility meets the aged persons' needs and desires. For example, the facility should be close to family members who may wish to visit and should match the urban, small town, or rural setting from which the individuals came.

A major focus in discharge planning is the residential setting that follows hospitalization or is being considered as an alternative because the clients' current residences are unsuitable to their needs or conflict with the requirements of others (e.g., a family can no longer care for the client, or a former residence has been sold). The goal of selecting a residential placement is to seek the least restrictive setting based on, among other factors, the functional capacities of the individuals and the supports (community, professional, and family) available. The degree to which placements are successful (i.e., can be maintained) is dependent on the accurate assessment of the patients' needs and capabilities, whether appropriate locations are available, and the ability of the caseworker to marshal all potential supportive resources.

The degree to which the worker can provide for clients' needs plays an important part in the development or avoidance of potential isolation. The selection of placements often is predicated on their availability to meet the constraints of reality. On the other hand, these selections should not result in placing clients in highly restrictive settings without thoroughly investigating the community and alternative possibilities. All placements should be selected with the individuals' active participation to the extent that they are capable. If these possibilities do not exist, their development could be promoted in conjunction with other interested groups (age-specific agencies, citizen groups, mental health associations, Gray Panthers).

Placement in appropriate settings is but the first step in the continuing care needs of chronic mentally disabled older persons. It is this aspect of the service needs that is perhaps the most neglected by mental health workers. Many patients get lost in the gap between institutional caregivers and community professionals. Many of the horror stories about the fate of these elderly individuals living in substandard, if not subhuman, conditions raise questions as to whether the original problem was poor screening for the initial placement or poor monitoring of the quality of care received subsequently. It is clear that many of these abuses arise because there is no long-term monitoring of these patients. Without proper monitoring it is difficult to know:

- whether the patients are adapting successfully and if not, why not

- whether the facility is staffed and has adequate resources to care for the patients' range of needs

- whether there are abuses and neglect

- whether the individuals are satisfied

Many of those who are most critical of the use of these community facilities for the chronic mentally disabled aged do not give enough attention to different approaches that could be used to monitor patients and how resources could be introduced to support the facility's efforts to care for these individuals.

The range of settings recommended for the chronically disabled usually includes facilities that cover a continuum based on the degree to which the residence is protective and restrictive and the extent to which the elderly require medical services (Group for the Advancement of Psychiatry, 1978; Doherty, Segal, & Hicks, 1978). An overview of the continuum of residences needed is presented in Table 10-1. This listing also links the residences to staff needs, treatment requirements, and type of client they can serve.

In this model, in moving from Level 1 to Level 5, the residence aspect becomes less restrictive. Levels 1 and 2 essentially are closed systems. Residence and treatment are provided in one location by a full team of treatment specialists. Treatment is directed toward rehabilitation. It would be anticipated that both of these could be temporary alternatives. Clients who improved either physically or mentally would have the choice, in consultation with a social worker, to move to a less structured residence (Levels 3, 4, or 5). While Levels 1 and 2 are envisioned as potentially temporary it also must be stated that some whose condition does not yield to treatment would stay there indefinitely. The nursing home should be envisioned as a treatment, rather than a custodial, setting and as being most appropriate for those with significant physical impairment in addition to functional disabilities. As a treatment setting, the home should include diet and exercise regimens that encourage the maintenance or improvement of physical functioning (Whanger, 1980).

The chronically mentally disabled elderly are likely to have ignored proper health care regimens in the past and now probably need remedial attention. The nursing home program also should be directed toward psychosocial treatment. A major problem in providing such services is that staff members have little or no time for continuing one-to-one or group treatment. The budget is too small to ensure that the nursing home is provided with special consultants to meet these patients' socialization needs or to design reality orientation programs or therapeutic environments. Neither can these facilities count on the community to show concern about the elderly. Even family involvement is not certain.

The presence of clinically trained staff could help families develop positive and supportive, rather than isolating, relationships. For example, some placement units have helped community groups set up special friendly visiting programs by student volunteers who are interested in working with the elderly. They also have assisted in coordinating the planning and implementation of training programs for the recreational staff to upgrade knowledge about the special needs of the mentally disabled elderly.

Levels 3, 4, and 5 are residences of varying types of structure and protectiveness. Level 5 is, of course, unstructured and a totally independent living arrangement. While these levels are a continuum directed toward less restrictiveness, there would be no imperative for any patients to move from Levels 3 or 4 to Level 5. This is because it would seem unwise to keep changing the individuals' residences to meet program objectives unless they request it. A client in a Level 3 facility who improves to the extent that less supervision is necessary would require less staff intervention and could assume some therapeutic, yet nonexploitive, helping functions with other patients.

Treatment variability is achievable by having that aspect of the residential programs linked to a central unit, perhaps designated as the coordinating transition center, where support can be mobilized to help individuals move from one care level to another. It is important that support always be available and that all treatment be directed toward developing independence (to the extent that this is possible) as well as self-care and daily living task management skills appropriate to the residence where the persons are to be transferred. The residential aspect of the program focuses on small group living, in a therapeutic milieu, to provide the needed social participation opportunities and the stability of the few persons with whom close interdependent relationships can develop.

In the treatment programs for Levels 3, 4, and 5, the focus is on developing better health and appearance and modifying overt symptomatology (e.g., not talking with or referring to "voices" but understanding them as a private phenomenon). Many chronic mentally ill individuals learn to avoid discussion of such events in public. This is a relevant example because this type of behavior is a major barrier to such persons' acceptance in the community. While this may be the emphasis of the program, it may well be rejected as an emphasis by the client. To a certain extent some accepted level of socialized behavior is important in group residences. If the elderly cannot conform to house rules, they would be free to choose an independent living situation. This availability of choice is dependent, of course, on the availability of other alternatives and the clients' ability to maintain themselves.

The treatment center for Levels 3, 4, and 5 is envisioned as including structured care programs and recreational and social events for all residential facilities. The center is seen as problem-specific rather than age-specific in that its services would be provided for chronically mentally disabled individuals of all ages. For the

Table 10-1 Program Model for Residence Placement

Levels of Care	Residential and Staff Needs	Treatment Needs	Type of Patient
1.	Hospital: This could be a unit in a general hospital or a mental institution. Staff would include a full complement of mental health workers, psychiatrists, psychologists, social workers, nurses, occupational therapists, etc.	Complete medical and social diagnostic workup. Treatment of acute conditions (frequently more related to organic syndromes). This facility also would handle involuntary placements where danger to self or others is involved.	Individuals with extensive psychiatric impairment.
2.	Nursing home care: Staff would include psychiatric and medical consultation, physician's assistants and/or nurse practitioners, nurses, aides, social workers, recreation therapists, etc.	Rehabilitative treatment including socialization groups, physical therapy to maximize mobility, exercise, toilet retraining. For severely physically impaired patients, this most likely would be a permanent placement.	Individuals with extensive physical impairment.
3.	Protected group residence: This facility should contain no more than 10 to 15 individuals. It might include the foster family plan for one or more clients. Staff would include live-in house parents who could be unimpaired elderly paraprofessionals. Other services would be available at the center that the residents attend daily.	Behavioral treatments to improve physical condition and appearance, e.g., exercise, diet information and planning, daily self-care habits such as bathing and hair care, control over overt symptoms, care of personal property. There also would be small group excursions into the community to attend cultural, social, and recreational events and to learn how to perform daily living tasks.	Individuals with no more than limited mental or physical impairment, including those who are quite dependent and fearful of independent living. This would include the young old who have been institutionalized and do not know how to manage daily living tasks.

4. Group living residence: No staff would be present but 24-hour assistance for crisis situations would be available. The residence could take the form of shared apartments or publicly subsidized rooming houses, to replace the squalor found in the SRO's [single room occupancy], for those who wish to live alone. The unit would be visited regularly to make sure there were no violations of health or safety regulations.

Periodic review of cases to see whether all individuals can continue to manage this level of independence. Activity center would be open to residents primarily to provide crisis assistance and as a social and recreational outlet.

Individuals with no significant physical or outwardly manifested psychotic behaviors.

5. Independent living: This would include residence with family members or an apartment or room quite independent from a subsidized residence. Services would be available on call from client or family in case of a crisis.

Center open for help when needed.

Individuals with no significant physical or outwardly manifested psychotic behaviors.

elderly who participate and are more capable, the center staff would attempt to provide linkage to the age-specific network. Consultants from this unit could maintain a continuing effort to assist in program development in nursing homes. It would be imperative to have outreach staff because chronically mentally disabled clients in crises may cease visiting the center at the very time they need services and support the most.

This general description of levels of residential and treatment needs is a preliminary framework for evaluating the resources of any community and is intended to broaden the practitioners' search for resources and conceptualization of the range of needs for clients that have been grouped as the chronically mentally disabled elderly (Figure 10-2). The framework assumes that each community must view its resources in the light of what should be available, plan future programs that can be linked together in a service continuum, and better organize resources to maximize their usefulness. Practitioners must utilize community resources creatively, help the aged plan the best possible residential and treatment program, and serve as organizers of fragmented services to the best advantage of the clients.

An example of this process is the services available in St. Louis and how they could fit into the framework of the care and residential programs. Among services available for the chronically mentally disabled elderly are:

The St. Louis State Hospital, which contains a geriatric unit and a Community Placement Unit; Places for People, Inc., a community activity and residential program for chronically mentally disabled clients; the Community Mental Health Clinic; a number of boarding and nursing homes; two Area Agencies on Aging (city and county) with their network of age-specific services but with no formal working agreement for programming for elderly chronic patients; a geropsychiatrist, available for consultation and based at a local university medical center; various public and private social welfare services that could be utilized by these clients; and facilities to meet a range of medical care needs.

One unique feature of the Missouri State Mental Health system is the statutory requirement that patients be followed up by the Missouri Department of Mental Health after they leave a state institution. Placement and follow-up care are provided by several community placement units throughout the state that assume responsibility for interdisciplinary mental health care.

One of these units is located in St. Louis and is attached to the St. Louis State Hospital. Its function in the process begins when a patient has been assessed as ready for discharge. The patient's planning then becomes the responsibility of the Community Placement Unit (CPU), which finds an appropriate placement, helps the person make the transition, then continues to monitor the care provided in the community setting. The unit also has the continuing responsibility to see that psychological, social, and health care needs are met for as long as that person is placed, to the extent that these services are available.

Figure 10-2 The Chronically Mentally Disabled Elder and the Social Resource System

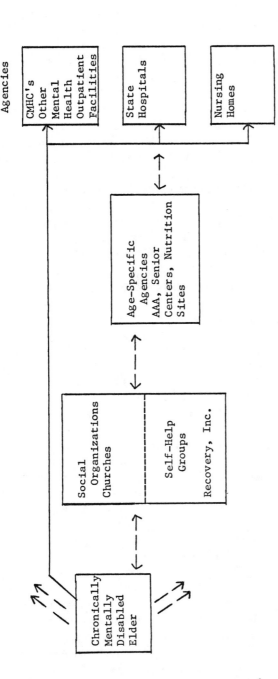

The chronically mentally disabled elder is not welcome in most social organizations, self-help groups, or age-specific agencies. Those who do apply are referred quickly to problem-specific agencies or are discouraged from attendance. Few problem-specific agencies are prepared to handle chronic disorder or elders so treatment is reduced to maintenance medication and/or nursing home placement. Little interaction or communication exists between the problem-specific agencies and the aging service network. Few or no family resources are available.

The problems facing the CPU are similar to those of discharge planning workers in other areas. One serious problem is the limited availability of good residential facilities. The shortage is particularly acute for low-income clients, who constitute a majority of the chronically mentally disabled elderly. Many of the nursing homes have limited social and recreational programs. However, the most serious deficit is in protected group residences.

Another problem is that sufficient staff time is not available to develop linkages to other systems such as the age-specific service network on a regularized basis and to give more extensive attention to upgrading the clients' self-management skills or confidence about task performance. The caseworker often is limited to taking advantage of growth skills or increased confidence in capacity, should it occur, to move the elderly toward more independent living. The clients do have the benefit of a backup team that is directly orchestrated by a mental health professional (usually either a social worker or psychiatric nurse) who is part of that team.

The clinical intervention possibilities, the monitoring of the direct care provided, and the opportunity for integrating the mental health support services with the long-term care setting probably are greater in this system as compared to community placement programs in other states where patients are given a hospital discharge and then are no longer considered state responsibility. Since most of the chronically mentally disabled elderly will require long-range care and treatment (as is true of all such individuals regardless of age) this is an important provision.

The disadvantage of this program is that it tends to become encapsulated and isolated from other community systems. In an urban center such as St. Louis, where hospital and after-care residences are in the same geographic area, this problem can be minimized. However, in rural areas the hospital after-care worker may have minimal knowledge of the communities in which clients may reside and limited opportunity for case management and location of local support systems. Community workers from other agencies may ignore these clients since they consider the elderly as still part of the state mental health system. Some of these problems could be minimized if CPU worker caseloads were controlled to allow the necessary time for community work in after-care.

There are numerous examples of how this structural approach may benefit elderly chronic mental patients who are likely to require quasi-institutional or nursing home placement. For instance, the responsibility for evaluation of assessment made by inpatient staff members often can occur in a vacuum unless they have some knowledge of the setting where the persons are to be discharged (placement after leaving the hospital). Frequently, the in-hospital treatment team is not involved in the after-care function unless the discharge plan involves returning to a home with which the staff is familiar because of interaction with family or other persons residing there during the hospital phase.

The community placement unit can be contacted in advance of the discharge review to provide suggestions about local settings. While it might be argued that where patients go once they have attained the maximum benefit from inpatient treatment is of no concern to the hospital, such a position seems to be quite inappropriate for this population in that the chronically disabled need continuing care to maintain maximal social functioning.

Once the team makes the decision about destination, the case is formally referred to the Community Placement Unit. The patient remains on a to-be-discharged status in the hospital until an alternative can be identified. A number of patients may be backlogged—that is, they remain on the inpatient unit until the new residence has been obtained. This waiting problem usually occurs because the CPU cannot identify an appropriate facility, because the funding arrangements get caught up in bureaucratic red tape, or because the patient does not agree to accept the alternative. On the other hand, this period may have some obvious benefits to the elderly, including the likelihood that they will not be rushed through the process and into the community irrespective of whether or not the setting is at all appropriate or is agreeable to the client.

A very important CPU function is to facilitate the exploration of possible alternatives with the elderly. Some patients, particularly those who have been on the inpatient units for a considerable time, may have grown accustomed to the hospital environment, finding in it much security and a sense of belonging, to the point where they will resist leaving to go to an environment they regard as threatening. For some, departing from an environment into which they have become integrated is a severe loss, similar to any elderly person who is being relocated involuntarily.

The CPU staff members can help introduce the patients to alternatives in the community and work with them to decide whether what is available is acceptable. Having the opportunity to visit a setting does not ensure that the patients' decision will be the correct one, that no pressure will be exerted on them if the staff feels that the clients can make a satisfactory adjustment to the setting, or that the elderly will or can control that decision.

A visit does afford some opportunity to explore what is or is not acceptable and to explain the process to patients. The limits of their understanding and ability to assess what is satisfactory obviously will depend on the degree of their functional capacity. Rarely, if ever, is it a practice to not take patients to a potential community setting simply because they appear too disoriented to comprehend the environment. Unfortunately, some patients really can comprehend very little but they should retain the right and opportunity to make that initial visit.

Once a site is selected, the CPU takes responsibility for processing the final application. If this responsibility were not assigned to the unit, patients without family members or other legal guardians would be left to the charge of persons unfamiliar with their particular circumstances. Throughout this process the facility also has the opportunity to become familiar with the CPU's expectations regarding the patients' individual treatment. Members of the CPU staff make initial as well as continuing evaluations of the elderly persons' adjustment to the facility as well as monitoring of their care. The potential for a significant authority and advocacy function is placed in the hands of these staff members.

The continuing monitoring process can identify problems in adaptation, shifts in functional status, and the extent to which the facility is attempting to meet the care plan, and can provide crisis intervention that may involve getting patients to a medical facility or returning them to the psychiatric unit. Whether or not this potential can be developed depends greatly on the time allotted for these functions and the talents and interests of individual workers in carrying them out.

A significant asset for placement planning in St. Louis is the availability of a program designed specifically for the chronically mentally disabled patient, Places for People, Inc. This program is linked to the CPU in that it shares responsibility for some patients who are placed in independent living residences. It provides services to these clients but leaves the monitoring of the residences to the CPU worker. Treatment programs and recreational and social events are offered. It is unfortunate that more centers scattered throughout the metropolitan area to serve larger numbers of clients are not yet available. For the benefit of elderly clients, better linkage to the age-specific network also would be beneficial.

The example of the St. Louis programming for the chronically mentally disabled elderly was presented because it provided many of the basic elements of the recommended framework of service needs. While much has been done, it is clear that much is left to be done. There is a need to broaden residential resources, provide more time for placement staff to become involved in developing such assistance, and expand community treatment services for chronic clients.

The development of programs to reintegrate the chronically mentally disabled into community life is still in a fledgling state, yet if real meaning is to be given to local placement, this is the area in which energy must be concentrated. To do otherwise would be to leave chronically mentally disabled elders in a continuing state of isolation whether they are placed in a hospital or in a community residence.

CONCLUSION

This chapter has described the chronically disabled elderly and their needs and presented an overview of treatment programming to meet those requirements. The proposed programming reflects the planning that is being developed for all chronic mentally disabled individuals regardless of age. Some modifications have been made to take into account the added problems that occur when the factor of age is added to chronicity.

The elderly chronic is less likely to be actively involved with immediate family members, so working with relatives has not been stressed. In cases where family members are involved, it is essential that they participate in the planning process so that their needs and views can be considered. Planning for the chronically mentally disabled also emphasizes their involvement in some type of work, whether competitive or protected (Test, 1979). This aspect is less relevant for the elderly because work is a real possibility for only a small minority. Sheltered workshops are a more realistic alternative.

The programming discussed reflects the more recent awareness of the services and needs of the chronically mentally disabled and the problems created by their discharge into a community that is ill-prepared to address those demands. Existing complex and entrenched problems can impede the establishment of adequate programs. Public funding for continuing care of the severely mentally disabled often is so little that it prevents the implementation of programs proved to be effective, such as those described by Fairweather, Sanders, Cressler, and Maynard (1969) and Test and Stein (1977). For programs that are established, funding limitations frequently prevent their instituting all the services that the staff realizes are needed.

Implementation of more innovative models of service delivery frequently has been blocked by an entrenched bureaucracy that is linked to continuation of the traditional mental hospital system (Turner & Shifren, 1979). Some professional disciplines are reluctant to come to grips with the fact that their treatment orientation has little or no relevance for chronic patients.

Treatment approaches that are beneficial only to members of the young, middle, and upper socioeconomic classes who have less severe dysfunctions must be augmented by newer methodologies that can ameliorate as much as possible the more disabling manifestations of severe disorder (Group for the Advancement of Psychiatry, 1978). These clients will not be "cured," given the state of knowledge of the more severe and persistent disorders, but they can be helped to function at higher levels (Anthony, 1979).

While community-based treatment may be more desirable for the mentally disabled, residents often are concerned about having chronic mental patients in their neighborhood. Public attitudes toward mental disorder generally are negative. Little distinction is made between individuals who are actively psychotic and untreated and those who are frightened and withdrawn and of little danger to anyone.

This community bias against chronic mental patients must be added to that against even the healthy elderly. A church in Rhode Island that was planning to use its facilities to provide day care activities for the elderly ran into opposition from its neighbors in its upper-middle-class section. They instituted various legal actions to stop the development of such activities because they felt the center was a business that would depress area real estate values ("Eldergarten More Costly," 1980).

In a preliminary report on a project directed toward the resocialization of chronically disabled elders in the community, Kultgen, Habenstein, and Green (1980) report limited success at reintegration but were able to achieve a neutral response from the community, which at least accepted the presence of the group with beginning signs of accommodation. Test (1979) stresses the effort that must be made to work with landlords, volunteers, neighbors, etc., to enlist their understanding and support of these elderly. Cutler (1979) reports on several isolated programs to reinstitute community responsibility for chronically mentally disabled individuals (not necessarily elderly). He suggests that these programs could function well if attention were directed to these issues:

- Mental health services should be available. Any volunteer social network needs the encouragement and support, in cases of crisis, of a mental health worker.

- Mental health workers and local community groups should collaborate in their efforts.

- Individuals in the community who become involved with the chronically mentally disabled elderly should not be expected to be junior therapists.

- The mental health workers should be trained in consultation skills to help community groups continue their efforts.

It would seem quite appropriate to enlist the energies of senior citizen groups to campaign for greater community acceptance and understanding of the chronically disabled.

More attention must be given to the professional staff phenomenon referred to as burnout. This term has been used in this chapter to refer to a client condition that results in reduced active psychiatric symptomatology, but it also can involve changes in the behaviors of their professional helpers (Mendel, 1979). In this sense, burnout refers to the failure, wearing out, and exhaustion of professionals and paraprofessionals who provide health care. This is most likely to occur in professionals who deal with the neediest and most resourceless. The chronically mentally disabled elderly obviously constitute such a client group.

Helping professionals often view themselves as able to cure a client or eliminate an emergency according to the ideals of the medical model of treatment. Supportive care without end for chronic conditions with a group of clients who are not accepted in the community and who cannot excite public concern because they function only marginally at best does not lead to the professional satisfactions that can result from treatment with other types of caseloads. Staff burnout takes the form of detachment, intellectualization, departmentalization, and withdrawal. Anger may be directed toward the patients for their inability to improve; they may be labelled as inadequate; or the therapist may become bored. When this condition affects a number of staff members in an organization, the antitherapeutic potential for clients becomes obvious.

Blame for failures often is directed toward the organization, the community, or other agencies. The organization can initiate a number of measures to prevent burnout: (a) recognize and discuss the problem, (b) provide a mix of clients so that any one worker would not have a total caseload of chronic patients, (c) have team responsibility for a client to ensure any one worker a rest from a particularly difficult situation, (d) provide research and educational programs that add refresher activities, and (e) change to a mental health rehabilitation model of care that stresses supportive care for chronic patients (Mendel, 1979).

This listing of problems associated with the development and delivery of services to the chronically mentally disabled elderly is broad and extensive enough to make it understandable that so little has been done to help this group of clients. Some of the recommendations for service delivery can help reduce the problem. These emphasize a broader range of problem-specific services and residences; an acceptance of the chronicity of the disorder; integration of resource development and consultation with patient care; and the development of newer, more appropriate models of treatment.

It must be recognized, however, that the development of services and community acceptance of these dysfunctional individuals is not an easy task nor will it be accomplished overnight. However, if practitioners accept the social responsibility of providing appropriate care for all members of society, it is a task too long ignored. The potential of this segment of the elderly population will not be understood until such services are offered and client outcomes are evaluated thoroughly.

REFERENCES

Abrahams, R.B., & Patterson, R.D. Psychological distress among the community elderly: Prevalence characteristics and implications for service. *International Journal of Aging and Human Development,* 1978-1979, *9*(1), 1-17.

Anthony, W.A. The rehabilitation approach to diagnosis. In L.I. Stein (Ed.), *Community support systems for the long-term patient.* San Francisco: Jossey-Bass, Inc., 1979.

Aviram, U., & Segal, S.P. Exclusion of the mentally ill. *Archives of General Psychiatry,* 1973, *29*, 126-131.

Bloom, B.L. *Community mental health: A historical and critical analysis.* Morristown, N.J.: General Learning Press, 1973.

Bridge, T.P., Cannon, H.E., & Wyatt, R.J. Burned-out schizophrenia: Evidence for age effects on schizophrenic symptomatology. *Journal of Gerontology,* 1978, *33*(6), 835-839.

Busse, E.W., & Blazer, D.G. (Eds.). *Handbook of geriatric psychiatry.* New York: Van Nostrand Reinhold Company, 1980.

Busse, E.W., & Pfeiffer, E. (Eds.). *Behavior and adaptation in late life* (2nd ed.). Boston: Little, Brown and Co., 1977.

Butler, R.N. *Why survive? Being old in America.* New York: Harper & Row Publishers, Inc., 1975.

Butler, R.N., & Lewis, M.I. *Aging and mental health: Positive psychosocial approaches*. St. Louis: The C.V. Mosby Company, 1977.

Cobb, C. Community mental health services and the lower socioeconomic classes: A summary of research literature on outpatient treatment. *American Journal of Orthopsychiatry,* 1972, *42*(3), 404-412.

Cutler, D.I. Volunteer support networks for chronic patients. In L.I. Stein (Ed.), *Community support systems for the long-term patient*. San Francisco: Jossey-Bass, Inc., 1979.

Doherty, N., Segal, J., & Hicks, B. Alternatives to institutionalization for the aged: Viability and cost effectiveness. *Aged Care and Service Review,* 1978, *1*(1), 1-16.

Donahue, W.T. What about our responsibility toward the abandoned elderly. *The Gerontologist,* 1978, *18*(2), 102-111.

Eldergarten more costly than expected. *Unitarian Universalist World* (11)12, August 15, 1980.

Fairweather, G., Sanders, D., Cressler, D., & Maynard, H. *Community life for the mentally ill*. Chicago: Aldine Publishing Co., 1969.

Ford, C.V., & Sbordone, R.J. Attitudes of psychiatrists toward elderly patients. *American Journal of Psychiatry,* 1980, *137*(5), 571-575.

Goffman, E. *Asylums*. New York: Doubleday and Company, 1961.

Goldman, H.H., Gattozzi, A.A., & Taube, C.A. Defining and counting the chronically mentally ill. *Hospital and Community Psychiatry,* 1981, *32,* 21-27.

Group for the Advancement of Psychiatry. *The chronic mental patient in the community* (Vol. X, Publication No. 102). New York: Mental Health Materials Center, 1978.

Hollingshead, A.B., & Redlich, F.C. *Social class and mental illness: A community study*. New York: John Wiley & Sons, Inc., 1958.

Kline, F., Adrian, A., & Spevak, M. Patients evaluate therapists. *Archives of General Psychiatry,* 1974, *31,* 113-116.

Koenig, P. The problem that can't be tranquilized. *The New York Times Magazine,* May 21, 1978, pp. 14-17; 44; 46; 48; 50; 52; 58.

Kultgen, P., Habenstein, R., & Green, P. *Modes and dynamics of support for deinstitutionalized elderly mental patients: A case study in therapeutic intervention*. Unpublished paper presented at MCSRA Training Seminar, Denver, 1980.

Lowenthal, M.F. Antecedents of isolation and mental illness in old age. *Archives of General Psychiatry,* 1965, *12,* 245-54.

Lowenthal, M.F., & Berkman, P.L. *Aging and mental disorder in San Francisco: A social psychiatric study*. San Francisco: Jossey-Bass, Inc., 1967.

Mechanic, D. Sociological issues in mental health. In L. Bellak & H.H. Barten (Eds.), *Progress in community mental health* (Vol. 1). New York: Grune & Stratton, Inc., 1969.

Mendel, W.M. Staff burnout: Diagnosis, treatment, and prevention. In L.I. Stein (Ed.), *Community support systems for the long-term patient*. San Francisco: Jossey-Bass, Inc., 1979.

Myers, J.K., & Bean, L.L. *A decade later: A follow-up of social class and mental illness*. New York: John Wiley & Sons, Inc., 1968.

President's Commission on Mental Health. *Task Panel Reports* (Vol. 2). Washington, D.C.: U.S. Government Printing Office, 1978 (Stock No. 040-000-00391-6).

Sanders, R., Smith, R.S., & Weinman, B. *Chronic psychosis and recovery: An experiment in socioenvironmental treatment*. San Francisco: Jossey-Bass Inc., 1967.

Srole, L., Langner, T.S., Michael, S.T., Opler, M.H., & Rennie, T.A.C. *Mental health in the metropolis: The midtown Manhattan study* (Vol. 1). New York: McGraw Hill Book Company, 1962.

Stein, L.I. (Ed.). *Community support systems for the long-term patient.* San Francisco: Jossey-Bass Inc., 1979.

Subcommittee on Long-Term Care of the Special Committee on Aging. *The role of nursing homes in caring for discharged mental patients,* U.S. Senate Supporting Paper #7, Senate Subcommittee Report. Washington, D.C.: U.S. Government Printing Office, 1976.

Test, M.A. Continuity of care in community treatment. In L.I. Stein (Ed.), *Community support systems for the long-term patient.* San Francisco: Jossey-Bass Inc., 1979.

Test, M.A., & Stein, L.I. A community approach to the chronically disabled patient. *Social Policy,* 1977, *8*(1), 8-16.

Turner, J., & Shifren, I. Community support systems: How comprehensive? In L.I. Stein (Ed.), *Community support systems for the long-term patient.* San Francisco: Jossey-Bass, Inc., 1979.

Walker, J.I., & Brodie, K.H. Neuropharmacology of aging. In E.W. Busse & D.G. Blazer (Eds.), *Handbook of geriatric psychiatry.* New York: Van Nostrand Reinhold Company, 1980.

Whanger, A.D. Treatment within the institution. In E.W. Busse & D.G. Blazer (Eds.), *Handbook of geriatric psychiatry.* New York: Van Nostrand Reinhold Company, 1980.

Chapter 11

Alzheimer's Disease and Isolation

INTRODUCTION

Alzheimer's disease has a major isolating influence for both the affected individual and the family. The elder person can experience isolation because of the fear connected to the realization of cognitive decline. That fear may far exceed the dread of death. Alzheimer's disease leaves in its wake a residue of continuing disability, degeneration, and dehumanization. The person's life style is affected because of mental and physical decline so pervasive that even the simplest aspects of the daily routine change. These changes lead to ever greater dependency on the environment and preclude the individual's ability to maintain a diverse and satisfying social existence.

The etiology of Alzheimer's disease is little understood. Frequent treatment procedures can only moderate associated symptoms rather than affect the disease directly. This leaves the patient and the family to struggle with a dysfunction that has no cure and to live with myths and labels of senility and brain syndromes that are perpetuated by uninformed medical practice.

This chapter meets four objectives:

1. It illustrates how a chronic disease can produce major problems of isolation for the elder and the caregiving family.
2. It illustrates the complexity of intervention for a multisymptomed degenerative condition that produces cognitive deterioration.
3. It explores some of the aspects of Alzheimer's disease as a chronic condition prevalent among the aged that produces profound isolation and complex caregiving problems.
4. It outlines treatment strategies that merit developmental and clinical practice research.

The first section gives an overview of Alzheimer's disease, including a definition of the condition, its parameters, and some aspects of diagnosis. Part of understanding the disease is the ability to distinguish it from other conditions in the older population and recognize its probable distribution among that group and its cluster of symptoms.

The next section analyzes the disease from a family context, mentions its various phases, and emphasizes the diagnostic phase. A multiphased family caregiving illustration is presented. A framework of multiple phases of progressive impairment approaches the disease from the standpoint of stages of caregiving. The starting point is the prediagnosis phase when the individual and significant others live with the fear and confusion of early cognitive losses. A range of isolators is suggested that may come into play before the search for a "why" ends in a diagnosis of such dire consequences as to impact forever on the family group. In many situations, proper diagnoses never are completed so that intervention technologies are not applied.

The third section describes various intervention approaches. A focal point for intervention should be on community-based caregiving, usually performed by the family. The burden of care, with limited support from formal resources, isolates the family group. Several directions are proposed to help families provide care under conditions that are potentially less stressful and isolating than is characteristic of situations without supportive intervention. Practitioner intervention is a potential complementary adjunct to the help that family members can derive from participating in Alzheimer's disease support groups. But the types of approaches clinicians can apply are not well formulated nor have interventions been the focus of developmental research.

The authors' clinical practice experiences and those of others who specialize in work with Alzheimer's cases suggest that treatment should be directed toward patient management to extend the length of time a person can live outside of an institution and reduce the likelihood of burnout in the family. The intervention phase when family caregiving becomes impossible and institutional alternatives must be sought is very important. The care of severely regressed Alzheimer's patients may be an opportunity for active treatment if nursing homes become something more than custodial environments.

The conclusions indicate strong support for the burgeoning efforts of national organizations and societies for education, research, and improved quality of caregiving. These entities, in conjunction with other interest groups providing quality care for chronically dependent people, may find a common challenge to radically reform the health and social care policies that control what options are available. The Alzheimer's groups may be able to develop strong coalitions for advocacy and change to establish some greater equality both for those who become dependent and for those who carry the burden of that dependency through care given to victims they love.

OVERVIEW OF ALZHEIMER'S DISEASE

The lack of information about the disease and the difficulty in making an accurate diagnosis complicate practitioner understanding. Only very recently have medical researchers directed their investigative efforts toward Alzheimer's disease to: (a) conduct studies to test various causal hypotheses, (b) evaluate the capabilities of existing medical technology as useful in the diagnostic process, (c) assess the effectiveness of various treatments, and (d) determine how medical care can be linked with other health and social service supports.

However, the current status of knowledge about all aspects of the condition can be defined as unknown. Gruenberg (p. 103, 1980b) said of the disease:

> You can have it. You can have genes; you can have slow viruses, you can have social stress; or you can have survival of the unfittest because of the lowering of the mortality rate. There are a number of hypotheses that are perfectly credible. That is why I did not pick any, because they are all equally credible to me.

Ambiguity and differences of opinion obviously characterize the knowledge base surrounding the cause and treatment of Alzheimer's disease.

This section introduces very selective information in order to provide an overview of the parameters of the disease. It explores how terminology has served to confuse rather than clarify Alzheimer's disease as a separate condition. An effort is made to give information regarding the incidence and prevalence of the condition but existing statistical data were expected to become outdated as new and more refined epidemiological surveys were conducted. The final part of the section describes some of the procedures used to diagnose the disease and determine the level of cognitive dysfunction.

Definition and Parameters of the Disease

The name Alzheimer's disease formerly was used to denote a condition of progressive idiopathic dementia that began before the age of 65, thus leading to the label of presenile dementia. It now is generally accepted that this is quite similar to idiopathic dementia that occurs later in life, in that post-mortem examinations of after-65 persons also have revealed similar brain changes (Raskind & Storrie, 1980). Because of these similarities, the name now is used to denote progressive idiopathic dementia regardless of age of onset. In the American Psychiatric Association's DSM-III, *Diagnostic and Statistical Manual of Mental Health Disorders* (1980), Alzheimer's disease is included in the disorder labeled primary degenerative dementia. This broader category is further subdivided by age at onset (before and after 65) and by the additional presence of delirium, delusions, or depression.

Primary degenerative dementia is typified by an insidious onset of dementia with a gradual downward progressive course for which all other possible specific causes have been eliminated. The essential features of dementia include memory loss; impairment of abstract thinking, language, and judgment; and impulse control. Degenerative dementia is characterized by cerebral changes, i.e., cortical atrophy, neuritic or senile plaques, and neurofibrillary tangles. Kahn and Miller (1978) point out that there is some controversy over the relationship between cerebral change and intellectual impairment. It appears that many individuals, who were found at autopsy to have a marked degree of brain change, evidenced no dementing process before death. Kahn and Miller (1978) also note that individual behavioral differences as responses to brain damage may be related to nonphysiological factors such as occupation and education, personality, physical mobility, etc.

Alzheimer victims also may have related behavioral and emotional changes. An individual with an organic mental disorder may manifest behavioral and emotional symptoms as a result of brain damage or as an indirect reaction to cognitive loss. In DSM-III (1980) it is suggested that for individuals who view cognitive impairment as a loss and/or serious threat to self-esteem, severe emotional disturbance may occur. The forms of this disturbance are somewhat linked to premorbid personality traits. Thus the compulsive individual may be particularly intolerant of reduced intellectual capacity and react with fear of loss of control. "There may also be severe depression leading to suicidal attempts" (DSM-III, 1980, p. 102). Other responses to cognitive loss include excessive orderliness, confabulation, paranoid ideation, irritability, temper outbursts, physical aggression, and decreased impulse control and social judgment.

These associated features are related to the affected individual's personality and education and the severity of cognitive impairment. The severity of the associated behavioral manifestations is not necessarily correlated with the degree of cognitive impairment, so an individual with rather mild impairment still may manifest significant disturbance (DSM-III, 1980). This point may be most significant in treatment planning for if, indeed, some of these related features are a reaction to loss and the affected individual's response to the symptoms of the underlying organic mental disorder can be modified, management of patient care in the home may be possible and/or simplified.

The course of primary degenerative dementia is one of gradual decline (DSM-III, 1980), although Raskind and Storrie (1980) suggest that some patients will have "plateaus of cognitive dysfunction which can last from months to years." Life expectancy from onset of the disease is about five years but is difficult to document because the time of the initial manifestation is difficult to pinpoint. Gilmore (1977) conducted a three-year follow-up study of individuals with dementia who were living at home. His sample included 12 mildly demented subjects (some intellectual deficits but still well integrated into society and able to care for themselves), 13 moderately impaired (more severe cognitive impairment and needing some supervision in self-care), and three severely demented subjects (incapable of self-care and totally dependent). Of the 12 mildly demented subjects, nine were dead at the time of the follow-up, one was hospitalized, and two were unchanged. Of the 13 moderately demented subjects, five were dead, five hospitalized, and three unchanged at follow-up. Two of the three severely demented subjects were dead at follow-up and the remaining one was unchanged. It appears that the degree to which the patient is demented is not the critical factor in predicting life expectancy. Though life expectancy is shortened by Alzheimer's disease, its progression is by no means rapid. This means that there can be a period of years for which care must be provided.

The conditions/symptoms of Alzheimer's disease of direct relevance to isolation (Figure 11-1) are those involving intellectual impairment and its infinite implications for both the individual and the caregivers (and others closely connected to the person). A brief description of the symptoms of intellectual impairment prepared by the National Institutes of Health to educate the general public about the behavior manifestation of the disease emphasizes that forgetfulness of recent events begins so gradually and is so minor that the individual or family may not be alerted. Raskind and Storrie (1980) concur in mentioning memory loss as the first sign of Alzheimer's. The earlier symptoms of mild forgetfulness may lead to no particular crisis point in living arrangements but over time suggest to the family that more checking must be done to protect the elder and those in the immediate environment from harm. Thus, the victim's forgetting to turn off a stove or failing to lock a door requires that someone else check to make sure this has been done.

As the disease progresses, impairment of abstract thinking and judgment along with personality changes and loss of impulse control may occur. Impairment of judgment and, particularly, lessened control over aggressive and sexual impulses, are difficult for the family. If there has not been a definitive diagnosis, the family may fail to understand the cause for these changes, much less form any plans for dealing with the symptoms.

It is in the emergence of these other symptoms that real family crises may occur in the caregiving process. Impaired judgment may lead an elder to enter into financial deals that result in loss of assets. Hostile, irritable behavior may alienate family members who have been assisting in meeting everyday needs. Impairment in abstract thinking may mean that the individual no longer can maintain employment.

It is at this point that the disease generates isolation for both patient and family. They are alienated from each other by symptoms neither understands. The individual may realize that something is wrong but not know how to evaluate the changes. Perhaps the patient will keep this awareness fearfully bottled up inside, reaching out for any possible external explanation, including blaming others. Family members are confused and may be unable to discuss problems with the

Figure 11-1 Isolators Affecting Those with Alzheimer's Disease

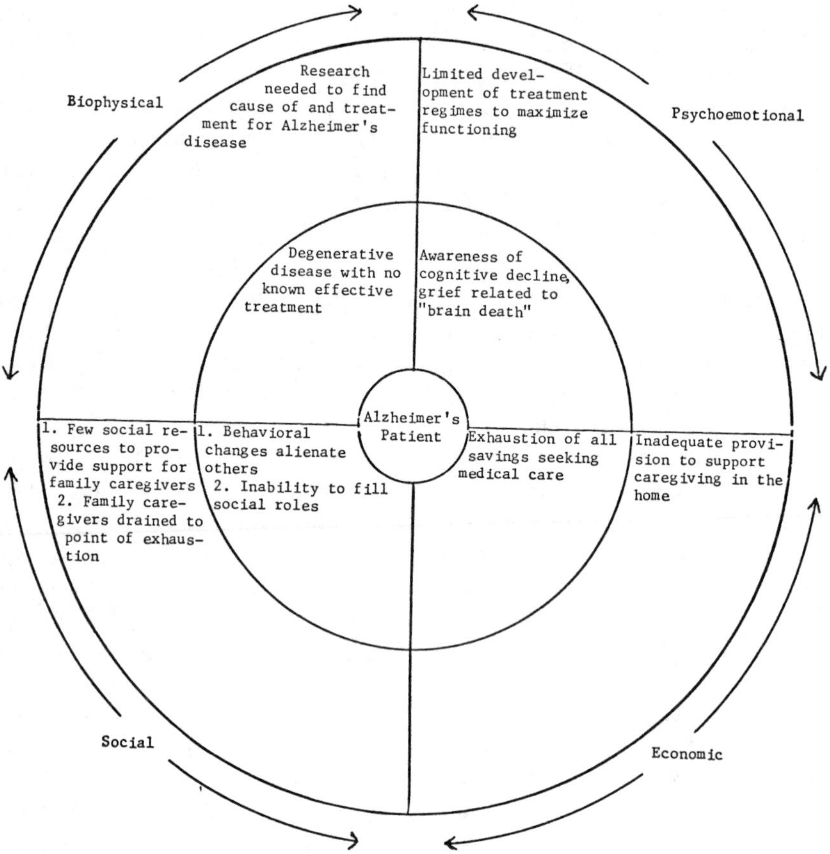

Research needed to find cause of and treatment for Alzheimer's disease

Limited development of treatment regimes to maximize functioning

Biophysical

Psychoemotional

Degenerative disease with no known effective treatment

Awareness of cognitive decline, grief related to "brain death"

Alzheimer's Patient

1. Few social resources to provide support for family caregivers
2. Family caregivers drained to point of exhaustion

1. Behavioral changes alienate others
2. Inability to fill social roles

Exhaustion of all savings seeking medical care

Inadequate provision to support caregiving in the home

Social

Economic

The inner circle contains isolators as they are manifested in the personal lives of Alzheimer's patients, the outer circle those that abound in the environment.

patient. The person's behavior may cause such embarrassment that social events are avoided and ensuing family resentment toward the victim may increase barriers that block understanding and deepen the isolation for both.

Incidence and Prevalence of Alzheimer's

The prevalence rates for primary degenerative dementia are reported (DSM-III, 1980) as ranging between 2 and 4 percent in those who are 65 years of age and older. Rates for those over 75 are higher, but no specific data are supplied. Because of the recent change (DSM-III, 1980) in the classification of Alzheimer's disease, which now includes dementia (in addition to presenile dementia) of a similar type in older age subjects, incidence rates of the disorder as now defined would not be reported in earlier epidemiological studies. However, it is possible to get a general understanding and overview from these studies.

A major contribution to the understanding of the epidemiology of Alzheimer's disease, or rather the broader category of senile dementia, is to be found in a 1947 study by Essen-Möller in Lundby, Sweden, and in a 1957 follow-up by Hagnell. The 1947 study showed a point prevalence rate (counting all the cases at a given point in time) for senile dementia in those over 60 years old to be 2.3 percent for men and 3.2 percent for women. By 1957, the point prevalence had increased to 4.9 percent for men and 5.7 percent for women (Gruenberg, 1980a; Gruenberg & Hagnell, in press). The apparent increase was thought to result from a gain in the effectiveness of treatment for pneumonia that appears more frequently in patients with dementia and in the past was a cause of death early in the course of the disease, thus extending these victims' longevity (Gruenberg, 1980b).

This would suggest that increasingly effective treatment for potentially fatal physical diseases common to individuals with senile dementia, with more patients living to advanced ages, coupled with limited progress in preventing or curing the dementia itself, will result in expanding prevalence of those with senile dementia. This longer life expectancy may mean a larger number of patients will reach the advanced stages of this disorder and require extensive physical care. This possibility suggests that efforts must be increased to treat the dementia itself and/or face tremendous demands on long-term care facilities.

Wang (1977) in a comparative analysis of 17 reports on senile dementia describes prevalence rates ranging from 1.6 percent to 9.1 percent for severe dementia (for studies that differentiated between severe and mild cases) and 2.6 percent to 24.7 percent for mild dementia. For a total rate, the reports ranged from .5 percent to 31.8 percent (the study that reported a .5 rate did not provide a breakdown between mild and severe dementia). The span of results may be accounted for by methodological differences that included varying ages ranging from over 60 in one study to another restricted to those 74 to 76, and populations in different countries and from various areas (urban, rural, etc.), with quite different backgrounds. There also may be significant differences in the way the disorder was defined, particularly since the studies were conducted in many countries (Wang, 1977).

The comparison among countries, however, did provide information that suggests potential increases in the prevalence rates of dementia over time. For example, in China, where only 5 percent of the population survive to age 65, the prevalence rate is reported at .5 percent in those who are 60 or older. By comparison, the U.S. rate in those 65 and older is 31.8 percent. From such a comparison, it could be concluded that selected survivorship in the aged population contributes to a healthier group of elders. Less selective survivorship means higher dementia rates among the larger numbers of aged who survive.

Using this information, it might be predicted that as the aged population in the U.S. continues to increase, so will the prevalence of this disorder (Wang, 1977). Eisdorfer (1981) suggested a doubling of the rate of dementia every five years after the age of 65. Thus, since the fastest growing segment of the population includes those over 75, a growing prevalence of those with senile dementia should be anticipated. Based on what is known of incidence and prevalence rates for Alzheimer's, it could be assumed that there are 1 million severely demented and 3 million mildly to moderately demented persons in the U.S. today. Tower (1978) stated that two-thirds of the cases of severe dementia had classic Alzheimer's disease. Considering all these studies, the potential increase in prevalence in the older American population is alarming and the demands for future care will be staggering.

Components of Diagnosis

Unfortunately there are no simple laboratory diagnostic tests or effective psychometric examinations to determine the presence of Alzheimer's disease (Butler, 1978); there is considerable difficulty in evaluating altered brain function in the aged (Zarit, Miller, & Kahn, 1978); and evaluating change in intellectual functioning is particularly difficult since the decline in abilities is neither abrupt nor focal (Fuld, 1978).

The advent of computerized axial tomography (CAT scanning), an x-ray technique that visualizes intracranial contents, heralded a new era of diagnosis of the disease (Butler, 1978). It is becoming increasingly available as part of the comprehensive diagnostic package. Gruenberg (1980b) feels that this technique holds promise for picking up plaque formation and slight degrees of atrophy. However, even if this could be done, there is not always a definitive link between the formation of plaques and diagnosis of Alzheimer's disease.

Zarit, Miller, and Kahn (1978) note the longstanding lack of agreement among psychologists concerning which test to use in the assessment of a patient with suspected brain damage. Those used include vocabulary tests, the Halstead-Reitan Neuropsychological Battery (which includes the Halstead Category Test, the Halstead Tactual Performance Test, the Digit Symbol and Black Design Tests from the Wechsler-Bellevue Form I, and the Trail Making Test, Part B), the Wechsler-Bellevue Scales, and many others. Psychometric tests, while extensive, have proved inadequate in that they are difficult to administer to elderly populations and often do not differentiate between psychopathological conditions (Kahn & Miller, 1978).

The inadequacy of psychometric tests has led to the adaption of clinical scales such as the Mental Status Checklist, Dementia Rating Scale, Psychogeriatric

Assessment Schedule, the Mental Status Questionnaire, or the Face Hand Test (Kahn & Miller, 1978). These clinical scales are most useful in that they can be administered to patients of varying condition, have diagnostic cutoff points, provide a quantifiable index of severity, and permit differentiation between impairment resulting from depression and from organic damage (Kahn & Miller, 1978). In practice, Alzheimer's disease is best diagnosed after thorough medical and psychological testing that eliminates other possible explanations for the clinical presence of dementia (Butler, 1978). However inexact the diagnostic process, it is important to pinpoint irreversible dementia in its earlier stages so that treatment plans can be instituted that will help the individual maintain maximal functioning as long as possible.

It is clear that some Alzheimer's patients have other people in their environment to thank (or hate) for noticing changes in intellectual functioning. That is not to say that individuals are not aware of these changes but their recognition by others tends to reinforce self-recognition or challenge self-denial. In the case presented later in this chapter, it is noted that the observations of others led to an eventual diagnosis. Information provided by caregivers describes the long and frustrating processes of seeking an explanation of why and what is occurring to account for intellectual and behavioral change.

The neurological evaluation, psychometric tests, and clinical scales are one aspect of diagnosis. The other aspect is the conveying of this diagnosis and its implications to patient and family. Brief guidelines for conveying the diagnosis are important because family members have told repeatedly of horrifying and devastating encounters with practitioners who give the final and accurate diagnosis of Alzheimer's (U.S. Congress Joint Hearings, 1980). In addition, the extent to which practitioners may have assistive guidelines available at this point may improve communication with both family and patient when providing the diagnostic results.

The practitioner who diagnoses Alzheimer's disease probably cringes at questions from individuals and their family members such as "why me," "why us," "what can you do to help," "where do we go from here." On the one hand, information that there is no known cure for the disease and/or few interventive treatments that have a consistent positive effect is devastating to those who ultimately must struggle with the consequences of a no-guarantee treatment. On the other hand, the practitioner must not give information that contradicts the scientific and medical practice knowledge about the course of the dysfunction— that it is largely nonreversible through medical intervention.

A FAMILY PERSPECTIVE ON ALZHEIMER'S DISEASE

Isolators associated with Alzheimer's disease have a profound impact on the family system. The focus in recent years has been on understanding the family and its relationship to its members as well as on the community and helping professions outside its boundaries (Robin-Skynner, 1981). Alzheimer's disease is a nonnormative event (Bourque & Back, 1977) that has similarities to other chronic diseases to which families must adjust. However, the cognitive degeneration experienced by the individual has special consequences for relatives that are not understood well by those in family practice (Lezak, 1978; Morycz, 1980; Farkas, 1980; NIA Task Force, 1980). The initial phase of the illness may not bring about major changes in the family nor may its members perceive the situation as distressing. However, over time the family unit does become disorganized. Perhaps as many as 2 million families are impacted by this disease in various ways.

Phases of the Illness

Eisdorfer (1981) suggests that the phases of response in the family follow what appears to be a pattern that begins when the person is first afflicted by symptoms up through the final stages of the disease. Phase 1 of Alzheimer's may be described as a time when there is questioning and suspicion that something is wrong with the family member. During this period, the observations that some things are different are not yet confirmed by a formal diagnosis.

Sometimes crisis events become the transition into Phase 2 that involves a search for medical information. A medical diagnosis is obtained but it may involve a long and expensive series of medical and psychiatric contacts. These prediagnostic or postdiagnostic contacts may have provided inaccurate information or may be denied and therefore rejected by the family one or more times before there is a form of initial acceptance. The end of this phase may involve acceptance of the irreversibility of the condition and the requirement of having to live with a disease whose course varies significantly from individual to individual and for which all treatments are experimental.

Phase 3 may cover an extended period of caregiving while the individual lives in the community with increasing dependency on environmental resources. The caregiver's efforts usually increase to the point where patient management demands overwhelming time and energy (sometimes leading to the provider's illness or alienation from others) and alternatives are seriously considered.

Phase 4 is a period of transition from living in the community to institutional placement. A variety of community resources may be explored but few are found adequate for any period of time so institutionalization occurs, sometimes involving several placements.

Phase 5 involves the patient's shift from having marginal functional capacities to a vegetative condition that may continue for a long time.

The time before formal diagnosis of Alzheimer's disease is a period of questioning. Usually persons with the disease and those closest to them know something is wrong but the problem cannot be identified. Sometimes a major communication problem emerges between the affected individual and family members, close friends, or associates at work. People look for explanations about what is occurring. Sometimes when the affected person is near retirement, an adjustment-to-retirement problem is cited to explain signs of confusion and mood shifts. As retirement may be perceived as a less traumatic and less common event for women, their symptomatology may be excused by others as depression or as a postmenopausal reaction.

Two spouses described how these explanations were offered as justification for problems that had not yet been diagnosed. George Booker had retired early from his job at an auto assembly plant. Just before his departure, his wife had noticed that he was showing signs of animosity toward those on his shift, many of whom he had worked with for a number of years. Mrs. Booker attempted to talk about his anger toward them, believing that his coworkers were giving him a hard time because they were jealous of his early retirement.

Several months later, after George had retired, the couple took a brief trip to Iowa for a family reunion. While there, George became very argumentative with several cousins about trivial topics related to duck hunting (a sport they often had shared). Other relatives commented about how strangely George was behaving but everybody seemed willing to accept that he was just having a bad time with retirement and really should not have left his job so early.

Finally, when George was to meet his oldest cousin for a hunting trip and ended up not being able to find the cabin where they had been meeting for 15 years, the retirement readjustment rationale was dropped. In this situation, an explanation was evolved from mutually reinforcing perceptions of various close family members. It continued to be an acceptable and comfortable definition of the situation until George's behavior proved so startling and incongruent that other explanations had to be sought.

In the case of Flora Stefler, her symptoms extended throughout the time she was going through a late menopausal transition. Unlike George, Flora encountered the additional problem of an angry spouse who constantly threatened to leave her if she did not stop "acting crazy" because she was going through the change of life. Mrs. Stifler lived through a difficult period of separation from her second husband, whom she had married shortly after the death of her first.

Mr. Stifler remained estranged from Flora until there was some medical evidence to suggest that her symptoms were related to a physical and not a psychiatric condition. He later returned to live with her throughout the period when she was undergoing the hit-or-miss series of medical diagnoses before the final and accurate pinpointing of Alzheimer's disease. The guilt her husband had experienced from misjudging Flora was a sufficient motivator for him to not proceed with the divorce he had planned. Another factor was that he wanted to ensure that she would receive the medical testings and hospitalization under his medical plan.

Diagnostic Event as a Peak Period of Isolation

Eisdorfer (1981) suggests that the response of the patient and family upon hearing the diagnosis of Alzheimer's disease is comparable to those who receive a terminal diagnosis. Simply stated, they are responding to information that equates to "your brain is dying and there is nothing that we can do." A diagnosis of terminal cancer is a relatively familiar concept, if for no other reason than the attention given through dramas, documentaries, and soap operas; however, the diagnosis of Alzheimer's may be poorly understood. For the majority of patients the information required to interpret the diagnosis may take time, but at some point irreversibility may become translated into terminality.

If the patient's cognitive losses are sufficient to influence the ability to process abstract information, the capacity to cope with diagnostic results also may be reduced. Distortions may occur as anxiety is mobilized and concern about death may be transformed into terrifying ideas or delusions (Spikes, 1980). A patient with severe cognitive impairment may never associate losses with the symbolic meaning or context of death; the implied losses of irreversible Alzheimer's disease already are a reality into which the patient has cognitively faded, preventing the illness itself from having psychological meaning. This point suggests that the disease, which can follow widely different courses, is a variable that will interact with the response to its presence and probable consequences. There is no way of estimating the proportion of patients who, at the time they receive this diagnosis, are beyond having the cognitive ability to understand vs. the proportion who experience a depressive response, concomitantly influenced by cognitive interpretations and personality factors.

The meaning of a diagnosis of Alzheimer's disease for individual and family will vary according to the impact that loss has on relationships and daily activities. However, their responses form but a brief moment in a long and complex series of crisis events to be dealt with in the future. A neurological consultant brought in to conduct the testing procedures to determine the diagnosis probably is involved in only a single event that in itself will not influence the longer-term adaptive responses. However, for the family, this moment is a crisis. Even though they may have no further role to play, practitioners with the power to define the unknowns through diagnosis need to be aware of and concerned about what will happen in the future lives of the individual and family. The health professionals who will continue to be involved in the case are key sources of positive or negative influences on subsequent adaptation and decision making.

A variety of factors can contribute to feelings of isolation during the diagnostic phase. Some of the more common are:

- Family members are given information too technical for them to understand so they remain confused and too frightened to seek clarification.

- Younger family members may be panic-stricken by a potential genetic predisposition to Alzheimer's and a common genetic defect between it, Down's syndrome, and certain hematological malignancies (Cohen, 1979).

- Families are not given information about community resources that might be helpful.

Isolation as Reflected in a Case Illustration

The purpose of this case illustration is to help the understanding of the various phases that families experience in the progression of the illness. Throughout, this chapter has presented the perspectives of the individual who is victimized by the illness and of the family that provides care. Both are appropriate areas for further research because it is important to plan intervention according to documented perceptions of problems that extend over time.

The Rocklers are a typical case of a family impacted by the disease and the caregiving process. Several families were interviewed to determine some of the important variations in such situations. Several of these variations seem important to point out before the dimensions of the Rocklers' experience are summarized. For example:

- The importance of having economic resources to cover the cost of the diagnosis and of acute and long-term care cannot be underestimated. It is the exceptional family that does not encounter serious financial hardships because of the illness. Some are significantly benefited by either comprehensive insurance policies, continuing incomes, or extensive savings, but many are left impoverished and then must turn to third party reimbursement sources, which often are inadequate. At the onset of diagnosis, it is possible to inform families about some of the predictable caregiving requirements so they can estimate the costs and their own resources. However, some families are not able to initiate early financial planning because they cannot or will not face the prognosis once a diagnosis has been made. Even when such planning is taken seriously, many families find they cannot predict what could happen (e.g., unemployment or the consequences of rapidly rising inflation). The original financial plan may have to be modified many times to adjust to alternative expenditures, depending on the services required for the patient.

- The availability of adequate medical services and resources from social and mental health agencies also varies from community to community. Having access to a university teaching hospital where there is an Alzheimer's research program and clinical treatment program is the exception rather than the rule. Many families must rely on general acute care hospital settings and nonspecialist medical help, leading to diagnosis and treatment of a lower quality.

- The community may lack supportive resources (Figure 11-2) for the families of Alzheimer's patients and other diseases so the relatives will not have this network to help lessen the burden. This may mean that the family will not have access to updated information on the disease or to informally organized services to help out and provide respite care.

The Rockler family consists of Alex, who at age 57 first gave indications of the disease; his wife Sherry, who was 50 when his illness was diagnosed; and their three daughters. Vicki, the eldest, was 27 at the onset and was living away from home, pursuing a career and caring for two young children after a recent divorce. Heather and Holly were 19, living at home, and going to a local university. The twins were moderately dependent on their parents' dual incomes to help them with college expenses. Alex worked as a data tax process analyst for a major local industry and his wife was a secretary in a small private law firm. The illness was diagnosed in January 1978. The period before the diagnosis involved the initial phase when the family had no idea that Alex was experiencing changes in his cognitive functioning. After symptoms were apparent, the family devoted much effort to obtaining a thorough and accurate diagnosis of his condition.

Sherry was alerted to serious functional problems through people who worked with Alex. For several months before she was called into the office to discuss Alex's performance problems, he had been making serious processing errors that coworkers had been covering without confronting him or reporting them to the supervisor. The consistency of his errors and his seeming increased inwardness alerted his supervisor that there was a problem of some significance. His initial discussions proved unhelpful because Alex denied he was having any difficulties. The supervisor believed that Alex was not aware of the extent of his inability to handle basic information.

The supervisor then called Sherry. She described her sense of panic during the meeting:

> I couldn't bring myself to believe what Mr. Knowles was saying about Alex and its implications for him. I didn't even think about myself or my daughters, just Alex. His work was always something he enjoyed and the source through which he had made very good friends. Several times he had been honored by his company when he headed up the United Way contribution for his section. I was told that Alex would have as much sick leave as necessary but that I had to try to get him to a psychiatrist or a doctor because the situation was getting to the point where they did not want him at the office.

The first professional contact was with a private psychiatrist who admitted Alex to the hospital for tests. The consulting neurologist then confronted Sherry alone, without Alex present, with the diagnosis that "his brain was shrinking." This

Figure 11-2 The Social Resource System for Those with Alzheimer's Disease

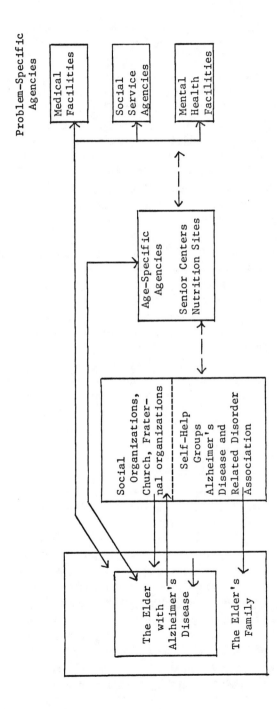

The elder in the early stages of Alzheimer's disease may be active in social organizations and age-specific agencies. As the disease progresses, these agencies are at a loss as to how to handle its behavioral manifestations. At that point, most agency contact is with problem-specific organizations and caretaking family members.

terrorized Sherry, who had to respond to both the psychiatrist and the neurologist. She could not believe what they were telling her. After this preliminary diagnosis Alex went on disability leave from the company for six weeks.

The insurance covered another diagnostic workup that lead to a referral to a psychiatrist affiliated with a research project. This psychiatrist played an important role in the diagnostic process. Sherry did not want to believe that there were no drugs that could help Alex and did not understand where to turn for help. She recalls that the psychiatrist was able to talk to Alex about the necessity of taking the option for early retirement that the company was willing to arrange and helped Sherry to cope with a very strong depressive reaction that almost brought Alex to the point of psychiatric hospitalization. The psychiatrist also was very firm with Sherry about the importance of continuing to keep her job. "When he said that I might need that job, I didn't believe him, but I never had better advice in the long run," she said.

During the next phase of Alex's illness he remained fairly active in the simple daily routine of picking his wife up from work, making daily visits to his father at a local nursing home, and completing some tasks in the home. Holly, one of the twins, became so upset at her father that she moved out of the house and spent several months having no contact with him. The other daughter, Heather, took on two part-time jobs to be able to continue in college without the financial support from her parents. Sherry remarked that Alex's major symptoms seemed related to poor timing. She said: "He was driving daily out to the nursing home to visit with his father. He seemed to be preoccupied with keeping a very tight schedule for the visits and while he was vague when asked about the visits each day, he said that Pop was becoming more feeble yet not describing any details. He would always call me to tell me that he had come back from the nursing home, which I thought was strange."

In reality, he was going to the nursing home every day but often simply walked into his father's room, sat for a few minutes, then left. Over time, he stopped having any real communication with the staff and sometimes had a hard time finding his way around the nursing home, with which he was very familiar. At one point a new orderly mistook Alex for a patient.

Sherry recalled other incidents that indicated ever greater confusion on Alex's part. About a year after the diagnosis, the police called her office to explain that they had traced a prank caller to her telephone number. An elderly woman had complained of constantly getting calls from someone who never said anything, just breathed into the phone. It turned out that Alex had been trying to dial Sherry's number but consistently had mixed up one digit. She was able to obtain a special phone hookup whereby Alex could call her by pressing only one digit.

Sherry could see that Alex was deteriorating rapidly in what he could do, including no longer being able to drive to familiar places. However, she also resented how all of the doctors kept telling her that he could only get worse. Alex's symptoms also included a slow but consistent decline in his ability to comprehend what he read. This had been one of his most important activities just after he retired. He also no longer could sign checks properly. He lost his ability to perform sexually, which was one of the most upsetting of his symptoms. Several times he became so enraged at himself that he would throw himself against the wall.

Later in the course of his illness, this behavior was described as the catastrophic reaction in which the Alzheimer's patient has a very strong and sometimes violent reaction to a personal limitation. Yet at that point his wife did not understand what he was experiencing. Sherry lamented that she wished she had been able to respond better and consistently tell him how much she loved him and that she was perfectly content just to hold him at night.

The approach she took was to say nothing for fear she might make the situation worse. Throughout this period Sherry continued at the law office. She noted that she was blessed by the fact that Alex maintained a regular nightly sleep pattern that allowed her to get her rest when she needed it. Her job provided her with an alternative to the constant caregiving that she might otherwise have encountered had she not been a working woman.

By the early part of 1980, it had become impossible to keep him at home and she was beginning to become desperate as to what do do next. She said:

> Alex simply could not remain at home and I could not ask my daughters to disrupt their lives by becoming a regular sitter for their father. I was torn between giving up the job and keeping it. I was fortunate that I could take a short leave from the job as one of the partners in the firm had retired and I wasn't needed until the new partner came. But I knew that after that either I had to find some arrangement to keep Alex during the day or else give it up. . . . Because of the money, I felt panic and terror greater than I can describe.

Sherry was fortunate to have been able to have Alex referred to a new clinical evaluation center directed by the geropsychiatrist who previously had been helpful. That referral provided an opportunity for Alex to be hospitalized for a complete physical workup and several other diagnostic tests. The clinic had social work staff members who were in a position to provide her with counseling about future caregiving alternatives.

The social work staff began intervention with a session at which the worker provided Sherry with information about caregiving options that would be safe for Alex and allow her to continue to work. The types of programs available in senior citizen centers, day care centers, and in-home care services were explained. As Alex had not been involved with any type of socialization since he retired that required him either to be out of the house in a supervised situation or to face the demands of a new social situation, it was felt that a senior citizen program should be tried. If that could not be managed, Sherry would want to consider a day care center with more structure.

Alex briefly attended a senior center program near their home. With the help of her daughters, Sherry was able to work out his transportation to and from the center. Its environment was relatively unstructured, with meal programs that were designed for a lot of socialization and recreation but without supervision. Most of the recreational activities required cognitive abilities that were beyond Alex, so he could not participate. On three occasions, he became very upset and had to leave.

Subsequent to that, placement in a moderately structured day care program was sought. This program was just getting started and had hired the full complement of staff. The day care center wanted to try to serve Alex, so in consultation with the geropsychiatric clinic, the social work staff worked on a program plan. For a while, the program was able to serve Alex but he could not maintain his daily attendance to ensure that his wife could return to her job.

The day care staff recommended that Sherry explore an institutionally based day care program that offered a more protected environment where he might be able to rest more and have more opportunity to be quiet during periods of the day. The only program available in the community with a highly structured day hospital setting was explored as a possibility. The staff informed the family that it could serve the highly physically impaired but could not deal with senile persons who were ambulatory or were management problems. The staff did suggest that Sherry try to get him into a private sitting service in a retired person's residence. The woman recommended was contacted and arrangements were made to take Alex to her home on a trial basis to see how he adapted.

The social worker went with the Rocklers the first day and provided what information he felt might help regarding Alex's management. They left Alex there and in less than four hours the sitter called Sherry to report that he was violent and she could not accept him under those conditions. During the next several days, the clinic staff met with Sherry several times. A decision was made to try to admit Alex to the inpatient part of the clinic in order to provide Sherry with a brief respite and an opportunity to explore what to do next. The clinic defined the admission of Alex as a crisis intervention situation and hoped he would be there no longer than three days.

The social worker arranged to visit Sherry and her three daughters in their home to discuss the next steps. Before the meeting he had prepared a list of several nursing homes that had beds available if the family were to decide to initiate placement. Recognizing that Sherry was very sad at the possibility of having to institutionalize Alex, the social worker hoped the immediate family could support her in making the difficult decision. At the session the family reviewed what had been done over the last 16 months while Alex had been cared for at home. Each of the daughters felt that Sherry's well-being had to take priority over Alex's.

It was one of the twins who recommended the idea that finally brought the family together on the placement decision. After Alex no longer had been able to visit his father at the nursing home, Holly had begun visiting Pop on a regular basis. She liked the staff people and felt they would be able to provide care for her father in a way that Sherry would find acceptable. An interim nursing home arrangement was set until the family could make the placement in the home they desired. During that time some consultation was given to the family about how to help the staff learn patient management techniques to avoid unnecessary medication for behavioral control. Within a month the final nursing home placement was made and the family had received a commitment from the administrator that everything possible would be done to make the setting a permanent home for Alex as the staff had tried to do for his father.

There are other potential isolators not reflected in the Rockler case. For example:

- The affected patient can develop other physiological illnesses that make deterioration more rapid and/or caregiving more complex and expensive.

- The primary caregiver can develop stress-related conditions that endanger that person's physical health and mobility (e.g., cardiovascular problems).

- The family can experience disappointment when an experimental treatment produces only short-term improvements and the patient returns to the same or a worse state.

- The family loses its laughter and joy because guilt and fear can be oppressive for all its members.

During most of the phases of the disease, family members provide important supportive functions such as patient care (feeding and emotional support that becomes more extensive in later phases), economic functions involving the material base of the family that may become depleted over time, labor that cannot be distributed equally, residential functions that place limitations on where and how the family lives, and legal and decision-making functions that are complex.

These basic family functions are influenced by the presence of Alzheimer's disease, which is a nonnormative event. It leaves the family impacted by the care of an older person who is not following the normal aging process. The disease creates abnormal cognitive deterioration that differs from cognitive changes associated with normal aging. A practitioner working with older relatives not impacted by Alzheimer's disease can apply a normative aging cycle framework to understand family organization and structure. However, this is inappropriate for Alzheimer's disease families because they perform basic functions in a situation of sustained disruption.

Other chronic illnesses that do not have the characteristics associated with Alzheimer's disease are normative in the later stages of the family aging cycle because the presence of chronic impairments is so common among the elderly. In other types of dementias, however, most chronic impairments do not destroy the cognitive capacity in a manner similar to Alzheimer's disease. The experience of the older Alzheimer's victim is not normal and the family group is encountering atypical adaptations. Many of these adaptations foster isolation within and beyond the boundary of the family system.

INTERVENTION APPROACHES

Many practitioners are unfamiliar with the issues involved in caring for the Alzheimer's patient even though cases may be referred to them for services. Their lack of information and practice skills is understandable because of the limited availability of knowledge on the potential for treatment of these patients. The notion that dementia is a result of the aging process that needs only custodial care would certainly discourage attempts to investigate the disease more closely. In many communities there is little or no organized effort to deal with the treatment of Alzheimer's as a special illness and as a problem of families requiring special assistance from health and social service agencies.

Notable exceptions to this are two national organizations devoted to community education advocacy, family support, and self-help effort. One group, the Alzheimer's Disease and Related Disorder Association, has developed a number of local chapters (among the first to be established are those in Seattle, San Francisco, Minneapolis, Pittsburgh, Boston, New York, Chicago, Baltimore, Boulder, Denver, Washington, and Westchester County, N.Y.) and several state associations. The other major group is the National Alzheimer's Disease and Related Disorders Association. These two can play important roles, especially with family members who are involved in caregiving and decision making (Barnes, Raskind, Scott, & Murphy, 1981).

This section acquaints practitioners with several intervention approaches that may be appropriate for helping the family and the affected individual. The goal is to suggest directions for future treatment and to advocate for a commitment to undertake developmental research. As more research is undertaken on the treatment of Alzheimer's disease, new approaches will emerge.

Behavioral Caregiver Training for Family Members

The family does not stand outside of this disease, but rather in its midst. Those affected include members who are involved routinely in caregiving and those less frequently and less directly involved. The affected person is central to the dynamics of daily family functioning so all members may need assistance to deal with the isolators mentioned previously in every phase of the illness because crises and stressors are emerging continually. However, a majority of families do not receive regular professional intervention oriented to their needs. The reasons help is not available are complex and include such factors as:

- the lack of linkages between acute and long-term medical care organizations and family therapists, which increases the likelihood that no referrals for family-oriented intervention will be available

- the problem that few can afford continuing family therapy in addition to the expenses involved in other aspects of treatment and management

- the situation involving diagnosis of the disease, including the lack of referral of the family to nonmedical sources of help

- the extent to which this type of intervention has been bound to the psycho-analytic modes of practice oriented toward conceptualizations not easily adapted to the circumstances of the family struggling with Alzheimer's disease

Some of the approaches in family-oriented intervention may be more useful than others. However, there has been little systematic investigation into the various methodological approaches that might be more or less beneficial to family units facing these circumstances. The approach applied should be compatible with any individual intervention being provided to the patient and be directed toward issues that family members consider important.

Before considering one approach to family intervention, it should be noted how important it is for practitioners to know their limitations. The problems associated with Alzheimer's disease are multifaceted and complex. Counseling about treatment issues and patient management techniques should not be offered unless the practitioner has expertise and other practice competencies. In these areas, it may be necessary to seek consultation and make referrals.

The potential value of providing behavioral training to the caregiving relatives is explored as a form of intervention that makes this function less burdensome and may increase the effectiveness of home care of the patient during the phase in which it is feasible and is desired by the family. Caregiving relatives definitely need support and social relationships outside the family group to reduce the isolation they encounter. They also need concrete help for dealing with the day-to-day aspects of caregiving. For that reason, clinicians, as counselors to the family group or the single caregiver, would be wise to avoid ethereal intervention approaches. Getting down to basic problems is important; the sometimes expensive and drawn-out aspects of a clinician's supportive intervention simply may not be appropriate, let alone effective, to handle the problems.

In the practitioner-family relationship envisioned, the therapist's role is that of an active trainer and consultant. The general model would focus on the family as the major connector to the patient while the practitioner would be centering on ways to help caregivers manage the patient. Caregiver training with parents of young children has been determined to be valuable for several reasons (Gordon & Davidson, 1981) that potentially are applicable to family members in Alzheimer's cases. Given the large numbers of Alzheimer's patients being cared for in the community, there probably never will be an adequate supply of clinicians to provide continuing therapy to family members, many of whom may find the idea of receiving therapy too costly and/or stigmatic. The structural arrangement of in-office therapy does not bring the clinician into the home environment.

In working with caregivers, assessment is an important step. Even if providers participate in group training sessions with other families, each group must be assessed individually. There are many different models of behavioral assessment that could be applied but as a general guideline the step-by-step outline by Gambrill (1977) and the practice guide developed by Keefe, Kopel, and Gordon (1978) may be instructive for the practitioner not familiar with the subject.

The initial interview(s) with the caregiver(s) (family members dealing with in-home supportive functions on a regular basis) should be directed toward:

- the major problems being encountered that are the focus of caregiver concerns

- the way the patient and the providers are responding in specific situations thought to reflect the problem(s)

- the background of the problem(s) such as onset, frequency, and other characteristics

- other information about the environment

An interview suggestion from the Behavioral Parent Training Model (Gordon & Davidson, 1981) that seems directly transferable is to ask caregivers to describe a typical day. This can provide them with a structure for discussing their daily routines as well as patient management. If the intervention is to proceed within a behavioral framework, the clinician must apply a systematic approach to understanding the patient's conduct.

An important facet of research into this approach would be to identify the types of measurement procedures that are useful. As caregiver training is the intervention, an assessment of how it fits the situation must be completed. Like any other intervention, caregiver training should not be undertaken just because "it's a good idea."

Certain conditions might lead a clinician not to suggest training the providers. For example, many caregivers and patients live in circumstances where resources already are so stretched that introducing special devices for ease of management such as specific bathing chairs or automatic door control devices might be impossible to obtain because of costs. Interpersonal relationships within the family system, especially between those who share the care functions, may be so riddled with conflict that cooperative management approaches could not work until, or if, these were eliminated. The anxiety, stress, and physical health problems of the caregiver might be too serious—even of a crisis nature—to allow that family member to take on more demands in the midst of dealing with these problems. Assuming that training is provided, continual monitoring of progress is essential.

The types of behavioral strategies that could be applied to training caregivers have not been tested empirically so the selection of techniques to help families deal with care and management problems remains open-ended. Based on information by Eisdorfer (1981), a technique similar to a behavioral procedure known as stress-inoculation appears to be compatible for helping families prepare for increasingly demanding caregiving tasks. If made available to families at an early phase, shortly after diagnosis and/or before the emergence of disturbing behaviors, it might well prevent some disruptions.

Stress-inoculation training as developed by Meichenbaum and his associates (Meichenbaum, 1975; Meichenbaum, 1977; Meichenbaum & Novaco, 1978) is a multiphased procedure applied to diverse clinical populations, and to a lesser extent on a preventive basis with a nonclinical group, to handle one aspect of interpersonal conflict—the experience and control of anger (Novaco, 1975, 1977). As a general model, it involves three stages. As adapted for helping caregivers deal with anger arousal in daily management, the focus would include:

- a conceptual framework for understanding how caregivers come to experience stress from that relationship, how their anger responses may trigger catastrophic reactions from the patient (Mace, Robins, Abrams, Ehrlich, Floyd, & Lucas, 1980), and the personal consequences of stress for them over time

- the presentation of alternative responses that involve behavioral and cognitive coping skills rehearsal such as role playing and guided practices

- the opportunity to use/receive continuing consultation from the trainer/consultant

Given the analysis of the reports from family members, groups are helpful for several reasons, including the support provided among members and the opportunity to learn from others. By assigning a format for primary caregivers from various families using a combined educational and support group approach, the behavioral training program also could introduce important opportunities to build relationships among a diverse array of relatives. This format might be especially valuable in situations where Alzheimer's family support groups had not been developed in the community.

Another format might be to apply training to numerous members in the family who are proposing to share caregiving functions. This procedure offers the possibility of cognitive preparation for either ever more difficult and demanding caregiving situations or patient behavioral patterns that repeatedly provoke anger.

Behavioral Interventions with the Affected Individual

Alzheimer's disease is a condition that usually affects developmentally mature older people. At the onset of the cognitive dysfunction, a variety of behaviors are manifested that have not been the focus of systematic assessment (no information has been found upon which to generalize a sufficiently concise description). Over time, progressive deterioration of cognitive functions makes basic self-care behaviors impossible for the patients. They move to increasingly fewer behaviors over which they have control; in order to continue to be maintained day to day, that control must come from the environment. The societal expectations of elderly persons is that they gradually will become less independent and require support, but it is that process of becoming dependent, through cognitive losses, that places individuals with Alzheimer's disease in a unique situation.

It can be hypothesized that in the absence of some type of planned intervention to facilitate the individual's performance required to meet daily exigencies, it is impossible to determine whether the rate at which a patient loses performance capacities can be reduced and whether losses of some capacities, however minimal, can be prevented. In the context of current clinical intervention with Alzheimer's disease, there appear to be few guidelines for introducing individually oriented treatment focused on the patient's performance capacities.

If the goal of intervention is to help the person maintain as high a level of performance as is feasible given the level of cognitive capacity, it will be necessary to identify what in the patient's environment will maintain that ability. It becomes essential to utilize environmental events in a way that is supportive, not negative, of performance ability while at the same time assuring that they are not introducing more stress into the life of an individual who is struggling to cope with losses. A primary condition of Alzheimer's disease is the loss, or reduction in frequency, of appropriate social and self-management behaviors.

The focus of a behaviorally oriented intervention plan would be to maintain certain activities that were within the capacity of the individual, teach new behaviors, and decrease or eliminate others. Two areas where behavioral intervention could be applied are self-care and social interaction skills. The self-care area is important because of the powerful significance that independence in daily living activities has for most older people. The social skills area is important to maintain contact and minimize isolation. These performance areas also may be of major importance in relation to the patient within the context of the family group.

To determine whether or not behavioral intervention principles could provide a useful framework for working with the Alzheimer's patient, it will be necessary to pursue developmental research. Several obvious steps to launch such a research effort would be to systematically inventory the behavioral deficits/performance skills capacities of Alzheimer's patients, explore these in relation to cognitive function capacity, and review the potential applicability of various behavioral intervention technologies/procedures that have been applied successfully in other areas of behavioral change.

The Baltes and Barton (1977) statement about the probable value of behavioral intervention with the elderly and Edwards' (1980) review of behavioral modification strategies with the elderly are beginning points to explore future strategies. Based on their critiques, the application of selected behavioral modification approaches to self-care tasks, social skills, and some of the behaviors associated with Alzheimer's disease (temper, physical aggression, impulse behavior) is recommended.

A limited number of technologies that have been applied to geriatric patients (primarily in institutional environments) to modify behaviors that are characteristic of some Alzheimer victims include changing feeding behaviors by using foods as reinforcers (Baltes & Zerbe, 1976), increasing verbalization among isolated elders by providing prompt social reinforcements (MacDonald, 1978), and altering daytime sleep patterns through the addition of a roommate (Will & Cone, 1976). Expert clinicians wanting to facilitate family management of problems in the home of an Alzheimer's patient (Mace, et al., 1980) suggest points relevant to evaluating future exploration of behavioral intervention. For example:

- Can the home environment be utilized as the setting where intervention is applied, given the amount of control and structure in the daily routine that would be necessary?

- Can family members be taught to appropriately apply the approaches to patients, given the demands of routine caregiving?

A significant amount of developmental research will be required to determine what techniques would be effective and for which patients, as well as under what conditions they would not work.

Raskind and Storrie (1980) report several other therapeutic approaches for working with demented patients. The first is reality orientation therapy. Unfortunately, many patients are isolated in their homes. If they are in a day care center or a group home, this approach utilizes a small group format with frequent meetings. The focus is on using visual and auditory cues to reinforce awareness of time, person, and place orientation. The exact form of the group activities would depend on the level of impairment of the patients and would range from keeping diaries and discussing daily activities to the use of visual and auditory aids to reinforce basic time and place awareness.

Reports from various studies of reality orientation groups show mixed results. When used with less than severely demented patients, this approach may have a negative effect in that the sessions are seen as boring and useless. Milieu therapy, as modified for demented patients, emphasizes individualized programming for each client and the use of the total environment to offer opportunities available in the outside community. Since the opportunities that are offered should depend on patients' capacity, homogeneous grouping of these persons would be important to take maximum advantage of this program.

As the situation now stands, a large proportion of the older population with Alzheimer's disease is in a position of not being properly diagnosed or, if diagnosed, of not receiving any active treatment beyond drugs. While medications for managing some of the endangering and/or intolerable symptoms associated with dysfunctions may be of considerable value, they are not doing much to remediate Alzheimer's disease. Raskind and Storrie (1980), in a review of pharmacological treatment of dementia, noted that it was more effective for the associated behaviors (paranoid states, nocturnal delirium, agitation, hostility, impulsivity, depression) than the dementia itself.

The choice of antipsychotic medication would depend on the patient's condition and on possible side effects that any one drug might cause. Possible side effects, e.g., tardive dyskensias, lethargy, increased confusion, disturbance in cardiac rhythm, and conduction, are associated with specific pharmacological agents and should be prescribed with the patient's total physical condition guiding the choice. The pharmacological agents used to treat cognitive losses appear to produce only mild improvement so much research is needed to explore the potential of such treatment for dementia.

To assume that older persons suffering from Alzheimer's disease cannot benefit from intensive clinical intervention is to thwart any effort to help them maximize their potential. The exploration of behavior intervention in the context of daily life routines for in-home or institutional care would seem to be a fruitful direction in a relatively uncharted therapeutic area.

Optimizing Care during Nursing Home Placement

The placement of Alzheimer's patients in a long-term care institution because they no longer can be maintained at home marks another phase of the illness. Finding the best institutional situation is difficult. Given the limitations of Medicare and Medicaid and the expensive costs of this illness in earlier stages, money usually is an object. The availability of institutions where a therapeutic environment is maintained with room to admit these patients also can be a problem. It becomes even more difficult if the patient has aggressive behaviors or is highly disruptive. Practitioners can facilitate the family's selection of an institution if they are familiar with the types of environmental factors that are conducive to optimizing the patient's capacity. They also can provide guidance as to what to request from the staff or in some cases even provide consultation to the nursing home regarding how to structure the environment for the patient.

The type of care to be provided will depend on the level of incapacity; however, assuming even marginal capacities, some types of environments clearly are preferable to others. The ideal situation for caring for these patients would involve a specialized intervention plan for each individual to help that person cope more effectively as well as environmental modification to meet the individual's needs (Miller, 1977). In fact, many nursing homes may approach these patients from a perspective of overcare, which can lead to retarding the capabilities they have.

Too much assistance in performing everyday activities can prevent the patient from realizing functional potential. Social learning theory indicates that loss of opportunity to perform activities reduces skill capacity (Edwards, 1980). For examples, minimal feeding capacity can be lost if a patient is not allowed to feed himself or herself; behaviors appropriate for social interactions will be stifled if there is no opportunity to communicate.

Before a patient is placed in a nursing home, attention should be given to many environmental aspects that can make a facility more or less appropriate. Instructional guidelines about facility selection, available to the families of Alzheimer's patients through the Department of Psychiatry and Behavioral Sciences at the Johns Hopkins University, suggest that it is important to make person-to-person contact with the administrator or director of nursing (both, if possible, as well as any therapeutic consultants who might be on staff). At that time it is possible to receive information and to give a detailed but honest description of the patient.

Obtaining information about the financial procedures and accreditation standing is important (Mace, et al., 1980) and relatively straightforward; however, evaluating the quality of the care in a particular facility may be more difficult. In communities where there are groups of people concerned about the care of Alzheimer's patients, it may be possible to make contacts with other families who have had experience in selecting a facility. If this input is sought, it becomes important to recall that patients are different, no matter how similar their level of disability. It is important to explore both the positive and negative features of a facility, because all institutional settings have both. There is no substitute for spending time in a facility. A family should be concerned if the facility does not invite a member to visit or seems to stall at the request for a visit. Practitioners can help facilitate inquiries if the family has no contacts with others who have gone through the process.

The environments of nursing homes differ. There are many settings that lack the simple features needed to introduce environmental restructuring efforts to make changes beneficial to the care of Alzheimer patients. Factors involved include physical barriers, staff characteristics, equipment and materials, staff-resident relationships, dimensions of resident participation and staff performance, training and supervision of paraprofessional staff, and program packaging and dissemination (Edwards, 1980). Assessing these aspects of a facility requires more knowledge than most family members have. If practitioners feel uncomfortable as to their ability to make these estimations, contact can be made with the local Area Agency on Aging, which may have extensive information about the local facilities through the nursing home ombudsman program.

Through whatever combination of sources the information can be gathered, the following points are relevant to the institutional care and living environment of Alzheimer's patients:

1. Dietary resources and dining conditions: will patients be able to make choices in the food; will they be isolated if their eating behaviors are not acceptably neat; will their eating be viewed as a problem if staff time is required to help them feed themselves or keep them company while they eat; are there possibilities to meet changing dietary demands with medication changes and/or new nutritional requirements?

2. Orientation and stimulation programs: is there a continuing program of activities to help residents maintain identification with their community as well as the immediate environment; are individual programs developed for more disoriented patients or groups of patients; is therapeutic work with impaired patients considered a priority; are staff members trained to develop these special programs and/or are consultants regularly available to them?

3. Basic supportive therapies: are occupational therapy, speech therapy, and physical rehabilitation available for individual patients; are patients evaluated systematically to determine whether there is need for additional therapies or modifications in the programs developed at the time of admission; are disoriented patients eligible to participate in therapies?

4. Bladder and bowel training: what are the activity limitations placed on incontinent patients; are special training programs available; what are the attitudes of staff members toward patients who have offensive excremental behaviors?

5. Leisure and recreation programs: are these available on a daily basis for all residents; are the types of programs offered designed to meet different needs among the resident population; are there opportunities for personal choice regarding participation?

6. Special physical exercise programs: what priority is given to physical exercise; do physically immobile residents have some continuing opportunity for

exercise; is there proper supervision of disoriented patients during exercise periods?

7. Homelike qualities of the environment: are patients wearing their own clothes; do they have access to personal possessions and adequate privacy; are the furnishings pleasant and comfortable?

The list of items to be evaluated before the nursing home placement is very long. While many features are general and equally important to all older persons, others may be very important to the Alzheimer's patient. A general rule of thumb for making a decision of where to place these patients is to select a facility that has more of the elements of the type of care the person requires and is accustomed to receiving at home. When practitioners are working with families to make decisions on placement, they should be prepared to help them cope with what they perceive as a crisis transition point. Even if caregivers are burned out from the unrelenting demands of home care, there still may be much ambivalence and anger over the situation.

Depending upon the level of cognitive functioning, patients probably will react differently to changes in environment that also separate them from what is both familiar and beloved. Realizing that it may be difficult to know the experiences of the patient in the nursing home placement, it is appropriate to encourage family members to prepare the individual as best as they can and then provide strong support during the placement and shortly thereafter until some positive adaptation has been made by the family as a whole.

CONCLUSION

These devastating and dehumanizing diseases [organic brain diseases] are feared by all and, tragically, are considered synonymous with old age by many. The fears surrounding the organic brain diseases are not surprising. It is hard to imagine what might be more frightening than the prospect of "losing our minds and being put away" (Butler, 1978, p. 5).

This chapter has been the most painful part of the book to write because it represents a disease of isolating desperation that impacts so extensively on the lives of older Americans and their families. The authors could not help but think that death comes as a blessing to many of those affected and to their families. Any practitioner who becomes acquainted with dynamic individuals and their loved ones who have had their lives turned inside out will understand the importance of national advocacy for catastrophic health insurance coverage.

The description of the disease is brief and tentative because there are few facts about it that are free of clinical and empirical debate. Several perspectives on intervention that reflect the thinking of some of the most knowledgeable clinicians have been explored but these are little more than a best effort to apply the authors' practice insights to a highly complex illness. Our support of continuing research to determine effective clinical intervention is an important personal and professional priority.

REFERENCES

American Psychiatric Association. *Diagnostic and statistical manual of mental disorders* (3d ed.) (DSM-III). Washington, D.C.: Author, 1980.

Baltes, M.M., & Barton, E.M. New approaches toward aging: A case for the operant model. *Educational Gerontology*, 1977, *2*, 383-405.

Baltes, N.M., & Zerbe, M. Behavior management and self-maintenance in nursing homes. *Nursing Research*, 1976, *25*, 24-26.

Barnes, R.F., Raskind, M.A., Scott, M., & Murphy, C. Problems of families caring for Alzheimer's patients: Use of a support group. *Journal of the American Geriatrics Society*, 1981, *29*, 80-85.

Bourque, L., & Back, K. Lifegraphs and life events. *Journal of Gerontology*, 1977, *32*, 669-674.

Butler, R.N. Alzheimer's disease—senile dementia and related disorders: The role of N.I.A. In R. Katzman, R.D. Terry, & K.L. Bick (Eds.), *Alzheimer's disease: Senile dementia and related disorders* (Aging, Vol. 7). New York: Raven Press, 1978, pp. 5-9.

Cohen, G.D. Research on aging: A piece of the puzzle. *The Gerontologist*, 1979, *19*(5), 503-508.

Edwards, A.K. Restoring functional behavior of senile elderly. In J.M. Ferguson & C.B. Taylor (Eds.), *The comprehensive handbook of behavioral medicine* (Vol. 3), *Extended applications and issues*. New York: S.P. Medical and Scientific Books, 1980, pp. 45-63.

Eisdorfer, C. Lecture presented April 6, 1981 as visiting professor, the Jewish Center for Aged Associates, St. Louis.

Farkas, S.W. Impact of chronic illness on the patient's spouse. *Health and Social Work*, 1980, *5*, 39-46.

Fuld, P.A. Psychological testing in the differential diagnosis of the dementias. In R. Katzman, R.D. Terry, & K.L. Bick (Eds.), *Alzheimer's disease: Senile dementia and related disorders* (Aging, Vol. 7). New York: Raven Press, 1978, pp. 185-193.

Gambrill, E.D. *Behavior modification handbook of assessment, intervention, and evaluation*. San Francisco: Jossey-Bass, Inc., 1977.

Gilmore, A. Brain failure at home. *Age and Aging*, 1977, *6*, 56-60.

Gordon, S.B., & Davidson, N. Behavioral parent training. In A.S. Gurman & D.P. Kniskern (Eds.), *Handbook of family therapy*. New York: Brunner/Mazel, Inc., 1981, pp. 517-555.

Gruenberg, E.M. Epidemiology of senile dementia. In S.G. Haynes & M. Feinleib (Eds.), *Proceedings of the second conference on the epidemiology of aging*. Washington, D.C.: U.S. Department of Health and Human Services, 1980a, pp. 91-97.

Gruenberg, E.M. Epidemiology of senile dementia (conference discussion). In S.G. Haynes & M. Feinleib (Eds.), *Proceedings of the second conference on the epidemiology of aging*. Washington, D.C.: U.S. Department of Health and Human Services, 1980b, p. 104.

Gruenberg, E.M., & Hagnell, O. The rising prevalence of chronic brain syndrome in the elderly. In L. Levi, & A.R. Kagan (Eds.), *Society, stress and disease: Aging and old age*. London: Oxford University Press, in press.

Kahn, R.L., & Miller, N.E. Assessment of altered brain function in the aged. In I. Stiegler, M. Storandt, & M. Elias (Eds.), *Clinical psychology in gerontology*. New York: Plenum Press, 1978, pp. 43-69.

Keefe, F.J., Kopel, S.A., & Gordon, S.B. *A practical guide to behavioral assessment*. New York: Springer Publishing Co., 1978.

Lezak, M.D. Living with the characterologically altered brain injured patient. *Journal of Clinical Psychology*, 1978, *39,* 592-598.

MacDonald, M.L. Environmental programming for the socially isolated aged. *Gerontologist*, 1978, *18,* 350-354.

Mace, N.L., Robins, P.V., Abrams, J., Erlich, P.J., Floyd, J.M., & Lucas, M.J. *Family handbook: A guide for the families of persons with declining intellectual function, Alzheimer's disease, and other dementias.* Baltimore: The Johns Hopkins University Press, 1980.

Meichenbaum, D. A self-instructional approach to stress management: A proposal for stress inoculation training. In C.D. Spielberger & I.G. Sarason (Eds.), *Stress and anxiety* (Vol. 1). Washington: Hemisphere Publishing Corporation, 1975.

Meichanbaum, D. *Cognitive behavior modification*. New York: Plenum, 1977.

Meichenbaum, D., & Novaco, R. Stress inoculation: A preventive approach. In C.D. Spielberger & I.G. Sarason (Eds.), *Stress and anxiety* (Vol. 5). Washington: Hemisphere Publishing Corporation, 1978, pp. 317-330.

Miller, E. The management of dementia: A review of some possibilities. *British Journal of Social and Clinical Psychology*, 1977, *16,* 77-83.

Morycz, R.K. An exploration of senile dementia and family burden. *Clinical Social Work Journal*, 1980, *8,* 16-27.

NIA Task Force. Senility reconsidered. *Journal of the American Medical Association*, 1980, *2٤٠,* 259-263.

Novaco, R. *Anger control: The development and evaluation of an experimental treatment*. Lexington, Mass.: Lexington Books, 1975.

Novaco, R. Stress-inoculation approach to anger management in the training of law enforcement officers. *American Journal of Community Psychology*, 1977, *5,* 327-346.

Raskind, M.A., & Storrie, M.C. The organic mental disorders. In E.W. Busse & D.G. Blazer (Eds.,), *Handbook of geriatric psychiatry*. New York: Van Nostrand Reinhold Company, 1980, pp. 305-328.

Robin-Skynner, A.C. An open-systems, group analytic approach to family therapy. In A.S. Gurman & D.P. Kniskern (Eds.), *Handbook of family therapy*. New York: Brunner/Mazel, Inc., 1981, pp. 39-84.

Spikes, J. Grief, death, and dying. In E.W. Busse & D.G. Blazer (Eds.), *Handbook of geriatric psychiatry*. New York: Van Nostrand Reinhold Company, 1980, pp. 415-426.

Tower, D.B. Alzheimer's disease: senile dementia and related disorders: Neurobiological status. In R. Katzman, R.D. Terry, & K.L. Bick (Eds.), *Alzheimer's disease: Senile dementia and related disorders* (Aging, Vol. 7). New York: Raven Press, 1978, pp. 1-4.

U.S. Congress Joint Hearings. Testimony before the Subcommittee on Aging of the Committee on Labor, Health, Education, and Welfare, and the Committee on Appropriations, House of Representatives, 96th Congress. *Impact of Alzheimer's disease and the nation's elderly*. Washington, D.C.: U.S. Government Printing Office, 1980.

Wang, H.S. Dementia of old age. In W.L. Smith & M. Kinsbourne (Eds.), *Aging and dementia*. New York: Spectrum Publications, Inc., 1977, pp. 1-22.

Will, J.A., & Cone, J.D. *Reducing daylight sleeping in an elderly man.* Paper delivered at the meeting of the Midwestern Association of Behavioral Analysis, Chicago, May 1976.

Zarit, S.H., Miller, N.E., & Kahn, R.L. Brain function, intellectual impairment and education in the aged. *Journal of the American Geriatrics Society,* 1978, *26*(2), 58-67.

Chapter 12

Conclusion

The original purpose of this final chapter was to point out a number of important research and training issues involving problems of isolation among the elderly. During the last stages of information gathering, it became obvious that the political tides were turning from moderately liberal to very conservative toward human welfare programs and entitlements. More importantly, the attitudes of the general public seemed clear—booms rather than butter—which provide little impetus to the search for new solutions for social problems.

Many of the issues discussed here lack an adequate empirical knowledge base, and little intervention outcome research is available to substantiate the effectiveness of the services being offered to the various subgroups. The need for research is obvious. However, at a time when the programs and entitlements upon which people depend were being threatened, it was hard to justify research as a greater priority than the provision of basic services. Just that type of resource trade-off may confront the entire field of gerontology.

From the standpoint of determining what practitioners lack to service the isolated elderly adequately, three elements are vital:

1. community organization skills that can be applied to mobilize the elderly and to organize the resources that are valuable to them
2. clinical skills that enable practitioners to be competent in working in both an intergenerational and multigenerational family counseling context
3. methodologies and techniques for assessment, for if problems are not understood, then they cannot be resolved effectively.

Little has been said about prevention. Few cases identified programs or practitioners who were concerned about preventing isolation. Most of the time programs were offered to persons who already had serious problems. Maintaining social supports when they were operating satisfactorily usually was not a goal. This is a serious problem in both the intervention orientations of practitioners and in the goals of program developers.

In case after case across the subgroups were examples of caregivers so near burnout that arrangements were likely to collapse. In many cases, informal caregivers had only themselves as supportive resources. If assistance was available in the community, professionals did not seem aware of self-help sources or consider it legitimate to refer the elderly or the caregivers to them. The conceptualized rearrangement of services proposed in some of the analysis of subgroups attempted to build self-help sources into the helping system.

Many of the practitioners interviewed seemed to deemphasize the importance of the relationship between themselves and their isolated elderly clients. This was surprising considering how frequently they were one of the most important, if not the only, social contacts that the elderly had on a regular basis. In case after case it seemed as though the aged persons valued the expressions of caring from a worker as much as a concrete service. Warmth and humor also were anchor points in relationships with the very isolated.

Some of the practitioners said their most seemingly nontraditional ideas had proved most effective in gaining access to an isolated older person or in performing an important advocacy activity. Examples of unconventional means of obtaining access include working with groups of Mexican-American youths, who knew their neighbors better than police and social service workers did, and being aided by neighborhood bartenders, who were at the hub of the social network of older alcoholics. This was mentioned frequently enough to suggest that creativity in formulating helping strategies can be much more effective than the suggestions in a practitioner handbook.

Few documents seem to exist to deal with providing services to any of the groups that were of concern here. Clients' rejection of sincere offers of help was one of the most difficult attitudes for practitioners to accept. To work with these types of clients, it may be very important for the practitioner to have good colleague and supervisory support. Sometimes practitioners were distressed at the lack of the sophistication of their interventions. These almost apologetic responses suggested that clinicians believed high technology therapy would provide greater benefits. The authors' assessment was somewhat different: it seemed that much of the best intervention did not involve highly professional therapeutic activities.

The isolation among the Hispanic and black elderly is a most important, however neglected, area of intervention knowledge. It seemed that so much of what had been written about the minority elderly gave nonminority practitioners little guidance. Minority communities often were resource rich in the midst of the poverty and invisibility of their residents. Minority practitioners should be encouraged and supported to provide their knowledge and experiences in written form and in educational arenas. Their perspectives are vital for knowing how to assess community resources from the standpoint of what they can and cannot contribute to the welfare of the isolated minority aged. Minority elderly and their nonminority counterparts are living lives like other people and are attempting to maintain a continuity from the past to the present and into the future. Mythologies about the minority aged grossly distort that important reality.

In conclusion, it is important to state that the authors' intention was not to write a tragic book about the elderly. However, there is a great deal of human misery and suffering associated with many of the problems and conditions that produce isolation and keep older persons locked into isolation. The sad parts do not necessarily make a tragic totality. In retrospect, few of the elderly highlighted were without someone who cared about them and who attempted to be helpful.

While it would be difficult to find many desirable features in the existence of many of these elders, few of them would say that it was awful to be old. While those who attempt to intervene in their lives may ask why they bother to survive, the answer is clear to them: My life has a precious quality that only I may understand.

Index

Note: Page numbers in *italic* indicate entry will be found in a figure.

About the Authors

ELOISE RATHBONE-McCUAN, Ph.D., is an assistant professor of social work at the George Warren Brown School of Social Work, Washington University in St. Louis. She is director of a graduate training program on the mental health of older women funded by the National Institute on Mental Health. She has published extensively in the areas of geriatric day health care, alcoholism and aging, geriatric abuse, and older women. Rathbone-McCuan is a fellow in the Gerontological Society of America, a board member of the Mid-American Congress on Aging, and a member of the Gerontological Health Section of the American Public Health Association.

JOAN HASHIMI, Ph.D., is an assistant professor in the Department of Social Work at the University of Missouri-St. Louis. She has had considerable experience working directly with elders and supervising social work students in gerontological settings. She has participated broadly in university and community activities directed toward improving intervention with elders in need of assistance and in training persons who are or will be delivering services.